EXPERIMENTAL STUDIES IN

EQUINE INFECTIOUS ANEMIA

MIKLÓS N. DREGUSS, M.D.

ASSOCIATE PROFESSOR OF VIROLOGY
UNIVERSITY OF PENNSYLVANIA

and

LOUISE S. LOMBARD, D.V.M., Ph.D.

RESEARCH ASSOCIATE IN PATHOLOGY
UNIVERSITY OF PENNSYLVANIA

With 28 Illustrations
and 16 Tables

UNIVERSITY OF PENNSYLVANIA PRESS
PHILADELPHIA 1954

UNIVERSITY OF PENNSYLVANIA PRESS

Manufactured in the United States of America

Library of Congress Catalog Card Number: 54-11539

Published in Great Britain, India, and Pakistan
by Geoffrey Cumberlege: Oxford University Press
London, Bombay, and Karachi

This monograph is dedicated
in gratitude to the memory of

RAYMOND ALEXANDER KELSER
(1892-1952)

DEAN OF THE SCHOOL OF VETERINARY MEDICINE
UNIVERSITY OF PENNSYLVANIA

who was responsible for initiating the experimental study of equine infectious anemia at the University of Pennsylvania and who skillfully guided and supervised that work

NOTE BY THE PUBLISHER

Dr. Miklós N. Dreguss received the degree of Doctor of Medicine from the University of Debrecen, Hungary, in 1928. After doing postgraduate research work at the University of Vienna in Austria, he became Assistant Professor of Medical Chemistry at the University of Debrecen. Following this, he did research work in the Children's Hospital of the same University. In 1934 he joined the staff of the National Institute of Health in Budapest, Hungary, and worked there, with interruptions, until 1947. In 1936-1937 he was engaged—under the tenure of a Rockefeller Foundation fellowship—in experimental work on influenza at the Rockefeller Institute, New York City, and at the National Institute for Medical Research in London, England. From 1939 on he was Head of the Virus Research Division of his home institute. After the war he continued his studies on virus diseases at the State Serum Institute in Copenhagen, Denmark. In 1948 he was called to the University of Pennsylvania to participate—under Dean Kelser's guidance—in experimental work on infectious anemia.

Dr. Dreguss has published over forty papers in American, Hungarian, German, and Swiss scientific journals, first in the field of biochemistry, and later in the field of various virus diseases (influenza, measles, poliomyelitis, typhus fever, primary atypical pneumonia, and equine anemia). Three times he received fellowships to do research work abroad, and he was given the Balassa Award and the Högyes Prize by Medical Societies of his native country.

Dr. Louise S. Lombard received her degree of Doctor of Veterinary Medicine at Kansas State Veterinary College in 1944, and the degree of Doctor of Philosophy at the University of Wisconsin in 1950. She taught at Woman's Medical College in Philadelphia, before she became associated in 1951 with the group studying equine infectious anemia at the University of Pennsylvania. Dr. Lombard has published papers in the fields of sterility in cattle and cancer research.

FOREWORD

An intensive study of equine infectious anemia has been conducted at the School of Veterinary Medicine, University of Pennsylvania, under the sponsorship of the Grayson Foundation during the six-year period 1948-1953. This work was initiated by the late Dr. Raymond A. Kelser and had his direct guidance during most of the period. Active direction and execution of the laboratory aspects of the investigation were largely the responsibility of Dr. Miklós N. Dreguss, assisted for varying periods of time while the work was in progress by Dr. Werner Leemann, Dr. Arnold R. Gilman, Dr. Louise S. Lombard, and Miss Jane F. Shirer.

The group applied in their experimental investigations the newer techniques of virology in attempts of adapting the virus to growth in culture and experimental animals, and in developing a more adequate method of accurate laboratory diagnosis. In addition, the research work included the study of the pathology of the disease and its blood picture for clarifying the mechanism of the infectious process. Part of the results of these researches have already been published in various scientific journals.

In carrying out such a diverse attack on equine infectious anemia, an extensive amount of the large literature on the subject had to be reviewed, and Dr. Dreguss became impressed by how scattered and far-flung and frequently poorly accessible this literature was. It seemed to Dean Kelser and Dr. Dreguss that a monograph on the subject, drawing together all of the pertinent information within one publication, would serve a very useful purpose for those interested in either the laboratory or clinical aspects of the disease. The Grayson Foundation heartily concurred in this view and asked Dr. Dreguss to prepare, in cooperation with Dr. Lombard, such a monograph. The arduous task of reading and critically reviewing the hundreds of papers on the subject was carried out while the actual experimental work with equine infectious anemia was in progress at the University of Pennsylvania. The even more arduous task of converting this mass of literature into readable chapters of a monograph has been conducted since the actual experimental work was completed at the University's old Bolton Farm near Bristol, Pennsylvania. The monograph includes not only the work of investigators of equine infectious anemia from all parts of the world, but both the published and unpublished original work of Dr. Dreguss and his group. It outlines in a very complete and concise manner our current understanding of the disease.

The Grayson Foundation is grateful to Dr. Dreguss and Dr. Lombard for their willingness to undertake a task of the magnitude of this monograph and presents it in the hope that it will prove useful and valuable, not only to those interested in diseases of the horse and in animal husbandry but also to those seeking a clearer understanding of pathologic processes in virus diseases.

The Rockefeller Institute for Medical Research
New York, January 1954

RICHARD E. SHOPE, M.D.
Chairman, Scientific Advisory
Committee of the Grayson Foundation

CONTENTS

TABLES

CHARTS

PLATES
(Microphotographs)

CHAPTER 1

HISTORY AND GEOGRAPHIC DISTRIBUTION

Nomenclature.—Since infectious anemia of horses was recognized and described as a clinical entity, many names have been used to designate the condition. At present the generally accepted term is *Equine infectious anemia* in English, or its equivalent in other languages. The following is a list of the more common synonyms used in various descriptions dealing with the disease:

(*English*) Equine infectious anemia, Infectious anemia of horses, Swamp fever, Equine pernicious anemia, Pernicious anemia of horses, Equine relapsing fever (Watson), Equine malaria, American surra (Rutherford), Malarial fever of horses (Torrance), Manitoba disease, Mountain fever, No-name disease, Loin distemper, River bottom disease, Wyoming disease.

(*French*) Anémie infectieuse du cheval, Typho-anémie infectieuse (Carré et Vallée), Hydrohémie du cheval (Lignée), Cachexie aqueuse du cheval (Lignée), Anhémie idiopathique du cheval (Anginiard), Anémie contagieuse du cheval, Anémie eqizootique des équidés, Anémie pernicieuse du cheval, Anémie pernicieuse progressive, Fièvre des malais, Maladie de Carré et Vallée, Maladie de Vallée, Malaria des chevaux.

(*German*) Infektiöse Anämie der Pferde, Ansteckende Blutarmut der Pferde, Ansteckende Anämie der Pferde, Infektiöse Blutarmut der Pferde, Infektiöse Pferdeanämie, Perniziöse Anämie der Pferde, Progressive perniciöse Anämie der Pferde (Zschokke), Malaria des Pferdes, Rekurrierendes Fieber der Pferde (Lührs), Wechselfieber des Pferdes, Sumpffieber, Augsburger Krankheit (Schotte), Augsburger Anämie (Ziegler), Virusanämie der Pferde (Krupski), Vallée-sche Krankheit.

(*Italian*) Anemia infettiva del cavallo. (*Spanish*) Anemia infecciosa de los caballos, Anemia infecciosa de los equinos.

(*Dutch*) Infectieuse Anaemia der Paarden. (*Finnish*) Näivetystautia. (*Hungarian*) Lovak fertözö kevésvérüsége, Fertözö vérszegénység. (*Scandinavian languages*) Infektiös anaemi hos hesten, Perniciös anämi hos hästar, Smittsom blodbrist hos hästar. (*Slavonic languages*) Infekciozna anemija, Infekcni anaemie koni, Virosni anaemie, Niedokrwitosc zakazna koni.

Latin terms suggested for international use: *Anaemia infectiosa equorum* (Fröhner), Anaemia infectiosa equi, Septicaemia intermittens seu recidiva equi.

The disease was first described in France by Lignée (256)* in 1843 under the name of *anhémie du cheval.* He believed that it was of nutritional origin connected in some manner with the artificial diet of horses. Charlier (68) and Dénoc (78) discussed the problem in the same year, while Anginiard (8) concluded in 1859 that the disease was contagious, but Sanson (378) strongly opposed this concept. Bouley (44) and Ledru (241) agreed with Anginiard. In 1883 Zschokke (498) reported a clinically similar condition occurring in Switzerland; he tried, though unsuccessfully, to transmit the disease. In the same decade Fröhner (126) and Ostertag (337) reported from Germany cases of "pernicious anemia" of horses that were apparently infectious in nature. In the New World the first description of infectious anemia in the United States by Watson (480) appeared in 1896 under the name of "equine relapsing fever," and in Canada by Torrance (457) in 1902 as "swamp fever." The identity of these diseases in Europe, the United States, and Canada, respectively, was later established.

The experiments of Vallée and Carré (467,468) at the *École Veterinaire d'Alfort* in France marked the first important contribution to the systematic study of infectious anemia. In their publications in 1904 it was announced that they demonstrated experimentally the infectious nature of the disease and have shown that a filterable virus was the causative agent. Carré and Vallée submitted in a series of articles additional research data of their work in an attempt to clarify the basic problems of the infection (56,57,58). Their findings were confirmed and the clinical, diagnostic, and pathological features of the disease were related in detail during the next decade by Marek (274,275) in Hungary; Ostertag (338), Hempel (160), Lührs (264), and Fröhner (127) in Germany; Francis and Marsteller (123), Mack (271), Van Es, Harris and Schalk (470), and Scott (395) in the United States; Todd and Wolbach (451) in Canada; the Japanese Commission (191) in Japan; Theiler and Kehoe (446) in South Africa; Stadler (414) in Sweden; Wirth (487), Gerlach (132), and Jaffé (188) in Austria; and by many others.

On the following pages a brief review will be presented of reports coming from all parts of the globe about the geographic distribution of infectious anemia and its prevalence all over the world.

---

* Numbers in parentheses are references to the corresponding publications as listed in the bibliography at the end of the monograph.

Europe

In 1843 infectious anemia was reported among horses in the Marne Valley of France (68,78,256). In 1906 it was enzootic (58) in Alsace-Lorraine, in the entire Meuse Valley, in the departments of Aube, Ardennes, Côte d'Or, Haute Marne, Meurthe et Moselle, Meuse, and Seine et Marne. In Lorraine it was considered one of the most formidable of equine diseases attacking about half of the total cart-horse population (181). Lamarre (234) analyzed the regional distribution of the disease in France in 1933 when a serious outbreak occurred at Belfort. In 1935 a good review of the situation was published by Carré and Verge (61).

In Belgium the disease was first reported in 1906 by Béghin (34), and Ries (372) believed that it was introduced into Luxembourg from France.

As early as 1901 Köpcke (213) described an anemia of horses often ending fatally and occurring in epizootic form during the late summer and autumn months in the neighborhood of Metz, Germany. According to Hutyra, Marek and Manninger (181) infectious anemia first occurred in Germany in districts adjoining Lotharingia and later became known in the neighborhood of Augsburg in South Bavaria as "Augsburg disease." It was prevalent also in Hessen, East Prussia, and Schleswig. During and after the first World War the disease was conveyed to most of the remaining parts of Germany by infected cavalry horses (371). This prompted a thorough scientific exploration of the problem by many investigators in several centers. In later years the severity of the disease decreased and it assumed a less acute and fatal form (181). A review of its distribution in Germany from 1918 to 1937 is given by Fortner (116).

Marek recognized the disease in Hungary in 1907 (180,274) and noted its spread during and after World War I when it assumed a more virulent type (181). Later, Mócsy (293-300) published a series of reports. Its occurrence was recorded also in Austria (132,487). Král and his co-workers gave a comprehensive account of the disease in Czechoslovakia (222). In Slovakia it was widespread after 1938 (482); in ten years between 1939 and 1948, 533 cases were officially reported (321). Zwick (500) gave, in 1935, an account of its prevalence in Yugoslavia, while Zenkner and co-workers (495) reported it from Poland.

In Italy the disease was observed in Lombardy (72). Recently, Abbondanza (1) discussed the possibility of mistaking leptospirosis for infectious anemia in the Po Valley. In the opinion of Krupski and co-workers (224,226) true equine infectious anemia is comparatively rare in Switzerland, while an anemia of streptococcus origin is more common. Steck (415,418), however, maintains on the basis of clinical observations that the virus anemia is quite prevalent and that he had seen hundreds of cases during the period of 1932 to 1936. Notification and isolation of diagnosed cases were made compulsory by the federal government in 1942.

In northern Sweden the disease was first observed in 1895 by Ekvall (106), and it was prevalent in central and northern parts of Sweden in 1932. Regulations by the state for its control were in effect in 1934. The morbidity in northern Sweden was listed at about 300 to 400 horses annually as related by Hjärre. In 1942 the State Veterinary Service officially diagnosed 128 cases in Sweden which number decreased to 31 in 1943. From the districts bordering on Sweden, the disease spread to Norway around 1909, but in 1934 only a few cases were observed in the latter country after a period of ten years during which strict control measures were employed (172,448). Infectious anemia was noted about 1909 in Finland (181); Hällfors (148), while checking thousands of horses close to the Swedish border, saw a number of chronic anemic cases.

As recorded by Bartels (31) equine infectious anemia was unknown in Denmark until Niendahl diagnosed some cases in the district near Schleswig-Holstein. Since a law for the control of the disease was established in 1923, no case has been reported. Great Britain and the Iberian Peninsula are reportedly free of the malady (75,28).

America

In western Canada the disease was first referred to near Winnipeg in the Province of Manitoba. Veterinarians settling in Manitoba were confronted, in 1881 and 1882, with equine anemia called "swamp fever" as related by Torrance (456). It was demonstrated to be infectious by inoculation of blood from sick horses into a healthy animal (457). The disease was, in 1902, prevalent among horses in a large area of the Province and in some parts of Northwest Territories; it was first identified in Saskatchewan in 1906. Todd and Wolbach (451) studied the problem of swamp fever experimentally and compared it with infectious anemia as reported from Europe and with equine anemia as described by several investigators in the United States. By 1942, the disease had spread west from Manitoba to the Rocky Mountains and east to Ontario and Quebec. In 1941, 121 cases were officially reported for Quebec while in 1942 the number increased to 218. Mitchell and associates (290) reported in 1944 an outbreak in the Ottawa Valley.

Watson (480) in 1896 described a malady of horses in the United States under the name of "equine relapsing fever" that had first appeared about eight years previously in northern Wisconsin and which apparently was infectious anemia. According to Scott (396) infectious anemia made its appearance in Wyoming during the last decade of the 19th century and, in 1901, caused an extensive outbreak in that state. Brimhall and associates (46) reported the condition in 1903 as observed in Minnesota. Mohler stated in the Bureau of Animal Industry's report for 1908 that the disease was prevalent in seven states (302). According to Mack (271), who made a careful inquiry into the problem of a fatal anemic disease of horses in Nevada, swamp fever was said in 1909 to exist in addition to Nevada, in Minnesota, Wyoming, Montana, North Dakota, Kansas, Nebraska, Colorado, and Texas. In several of these states investigative work was carried out in order to study the condition locally (123,271,395,444,470). The early history of infectious anemia in the United States and Canada is reviewed by Van Es, Harris and Schalk (470) in their monograph on swamp fever, and by Stein (425).

From 1916 to 1928 the prevalence of the disease in the States appeared to have decreased as judged on the basis of reports from veterinarians. Kelser (195) has recognized the nature of a severe outbreak in 1921 in brood mares at Fort Robinson, Nebraska, the infection having apparently been introduced by mares purchased in the vicinity. He also recorded the first occurrence of the disease in the New England states in 1935 (197).

According to a report published by the Bureau of Animal Industry in 1935, inquiries that were made after 1928 showed the disease to be existent in 17 states of the U. S. In 1941, Stein stated that it was apparently more prevalent than originally assumed: authentic accounts of the disease were received from 29 states and in 15 of these the diagnosis was confirmed by horse inoculation test (425). Stein and Mott (435) further discussed the prevalence of equine infectious anemia in the United States on the occasion of a serious outbreak among thoroughbred horses at Rockingham Park, New Hampshire, in 1947, in which 80 horses were lost; this outbreak was reportedly traced to a race horse brought from Florida. They stated that during the past five decades the disease has been authentically reported from 34 of the 48 states, chiefly in the form of sporadic outbreaks. Small local outbreaks, showing little tendency to spread, occurred from time to time in certain areas in Idaho, Louisiana, Montana, Nevada, Oregon, Texas, and Wyoming, while the disease is enzootic in the Mississippi Delta where it exists in mules principally in chronic form. The Bureau of Animal Industry (462) stated that sporadic but unconfirmed equine infectious anemia cases were reported in ten states in 1951.

Information concerning the prevalence of the disease in Mexico, Central and South America is meager, partly because of the difficulties in differentiating it from tropical diseases of the horse. Darling, writing from the Panama Canal Zone in 1910, made mention of a malady clinically corresponding to swamp fever (470). In a description of equine anemia as seen in Venezuela, Kubes (227) states that the disease was first observed in Brazil around 1905. He believed that of two clinical entities, "peste boba" and "derrengadera," the one named "peste boba" is in reality infectious anemia, and the other is an infection with *Trypanosoma venezuelense*. In Uruguay infectious anemia has been also reported and was studied experimentally in horses (62).

Asia

There is no doubt that the disease is prevalent throughout the entire Eurasian continent. As early as 1909 many cases were recorded as occurring in low-lying swampy regions of Russia, particularly around the Rokitno and Pripet marshes (181). Judging from the number of reports in Russian dealing briefly with problems and studies of the malady, without presenting details, it must be widespread in present-day U.S.S.R.

There are early reports of the high incidence of the disease in Japan. In 1909 a special Commission was set up for the study and control of infectious anemia, and in 1914 it submitted a detailed account (191) of large numbers of field and experimental cases and also presented a draft of control measures for adoption. During the last three decades many papers have been published, most of them in Japanese, on experimental work performed in Japan by a number of investigators (Nagao, Nakamura, Ishii, Hirato, Kutii, and their co-workers). As reported by the Japanese Commission (191), the first outbreaks of the disease had occurred in 1895 in the province of Hidaka on Hokkaido Island, in the prefecture of Aomori, and in Yokohama. The Japanese Livestock Bureau (190) listed the disease as known to exist in Java, French Indo-China, Formosa, the islands of Japan, Sakhalin, Korea and Manchuria. In Japan 2,302 cases were officially reported for 1949.

In India equine surra (trypanosomiasis) and equine infectious anemia probably co-exist (582), but apparently no serious effort has been made thus far toward a clear differentiation of the two diseases.

Africa and Australia

In North Africa the disease was intensively studied by Balozet who used the African donkey for experimental transmission (13). Accounts were given concerning the presence of infectious anemia in French Morocco (474,11), Tunisia (29), and Eritrea (598). The disease was first identified in South Africa by Theiler and Kehoe in 1913 (446). De Kock (212) concluded, from a study of records, that it existed in South Africa even before 1904. He stated that there were isolated cases up to 1923, but that an extensive outbreak never occurred in horses; it was enzootic among donkeys of Natal, South Africa.

Infectious anemia has been recognized in Australia whence it spread, according to reports, to the Dutch East Indies (181). Whittem relates that the disease was introduced to the island of New Britain in the Bismarck Archipelago by the Japanese invasion during World War II. However, it was soon eradicated and did not spread to continental Australia.

*

In conclusion, it may be said that infectious anemia has been recognized and reported as being present on all continents and all geographic latitudes from the subpolar regions of Finland and Norway to the tropical climate such as that in Venezuela or Eritrea, with the exception only of Great Britain and the Iberian Peninsula (Balozet (28)).

In a conference, held recently at the *Office International des Épizooties* in Paris (325), prominent workers in this field from all over the world reported the situation in their respective countries about infectious anemia, the incidence of which is rising in some well defined regions of several countries. We may add in this connection that the mere absence of reports from a certain area does not necessarily exclude the presence of the malady among the equine population of that region, but may be attributed to lack of interest in the problem or, in the case of colonial territories and under-developed regions, the lack of competent investigators. Naturally, in countries in which the disease has been quite prevalent at one time or another, thus presenting an economic problem as well as a scientific challenge, more attention was paid to its surveillance and study than in places where its importance seemed negligible.

CHAPTER 2

NATURAL TRANSMISSION OF THE INFECTION

Ever since it was demonstrated experimentally that the disease is infectious, investigators have been seeking to learn how infectious anemia is transmitted from one animal to another under natural conditions. Before discussing the modes of natural transmission, it is well to consider the susceptibility of horses to the virus, and to summarize briefly the views about the regional distribution of the disease.

Observations as well as experiments revealed that the various equine species, including horses, mules, and donkeys, are susceptible to the infection in all age groups. In regions where the disease is enzootic, one may find some immune animals, an obvious explanation for this being that such animals have had a manifest or subclinical infection some time in the past and have gradually grown resistant to re-infection with the virus. In most instances, however, infection with the virus of infectious anemia does not confer immunity, a surprising fact that constantly baffled investigators studying the malady. Horses seemingly recovered from an infection would usually produce a spontaneous flare-up of symptoms from time to time (*chronic cases*); some others would exhibit no symptoms for a long time, but their blood would retain infectiousness, as a rule, for the rest of their lives (*symptomless virus carriers*). In the latter group of seemingly normal horses, symptoms may recur after long quiescent periods without any apparent reason, or may be provoked by various methods, including re-infection with a virulent virus strain; on the other hand, they may reach a stage, after several attacks, when they will exhibit solid resistance to attempts of re-infection. With the sole exception of the latter relatively small group, all horses are more or less susceptible to infection and re-infection with the anemia virus.

The peculiar distribution of cases noted within a given area has often been discussed and the problem analyzed by several authors. Beside noting the seasonal occurrence of the outbreaks during the late summer months and in the autumn, search for a common regional factor was long in progress, since the disease was known to persist in certain well-defined areas in many countries. Lamarre (234) considered the geologic formation of the terrain an important factor in the epizootology of the disease.

Dobberstein and Hemmert-Halswick (85,86) concluded, after an extensive search into the problem and a detailed discussion, that neither the geological structure, nor the watercourses of a given region appeared to have outstanding significance in influencing the dissemination of the infection and the incidence of the disease. In America outbreaks occurred chiefly in undrained, low-lying, swampy areas (hence the name swamp fever) such as, for example, along the valley of the Red River in Minnesota and North Dakota, in the valleys of Wyoming, in the Mississippi Delta, and along the wet coastal plains of the Gulf of Mexico in Texas; outbreaks may occur, however, in any locality regardless of altitude and drainage, provided that infected animals are present or brought into such territories and circumstances are favorable for transmission to susceptible horses (425). The influence of geology and the seasonal incidence in France were recently carefully analyzed by Lucas (262). Steck (419) believes that the local climate has some bearing on the regional distribution and the occurrence of outbreaks.

The first record about the successful experimental transmission of infectious anemia is in the report, for 1902, of the Ministry of Agriculture in Canada (457); according to this report, blood from two horses sick with the disease (swamp fever) was inoculated into a healthy horse that reacted with a rise of temperature on the 12th day and exhibited two subsequent rises 10 to 12 days apart. In Europe, Vallée and Carré (467) were similarly successful in reproducing the disease by inoculation of infectious blood, and also by bacterium free filtrates of the blood serum. While these experiments established the infectious nature of the malady, they did not clarify the question concerning the manner in which the disease spreads under natural conditions. Since observations on naturally infected horses merely suggest possible ways of infection, experiments were devised by a number of authors in order to produce experimental evidence for or against the various concepts advanced with regard to the mode of natural transmission.

Infection by Way of the Alimentary Canal

Carré and Vallée (56,58), analyzing the possibilities of the spread of the disease as it occurred in France, came to the conclusion that sanitary conditions in the stables are mainly responsible, and that the alimentary tract might serve as the portal of entry for the virus, by means of the drinking water and food of the animals. They were able to reproduce the disease in normal horses by feeding them infectious blood, large amounts of urine, or diarrhoeic (bloody) fecal material collected from infected animals. Their concept was accepted and, in the main, their findings were soon confirmed in Europe (388,160), America (124,470), and Asia (191). Nevertheless, attempts by others to transmit the disease by feeding feces from infected horses met with no success (470,191).

Van Es, Harris and Schalk (470) transmitted the infection by intravenous and by subcutaneous injection of blood, of urine, and of filtered serum coming from infected horses, and also by giving the urine *per os,* and by feeding the horses capsules containing virulent blood. However, they were unable to incite the disease in normal horses by giving them subcutaneously 100 cc. of an extract of feces from infected animals, or larger amounts of the same by a stomach tube. Manninger (273) infected horses by feeding them large amounts of blood, or urine. The infectiousness of urine given *per os* was found to be inconsistent or weak (191,273) and was related to albuminuria (58,220). All attempts at oral transmission with urine by the U. S. Bureau of Animal Industry failed, as reported by Stein and co-workers (438). It seems doubtful whether the large oral doses of urine (up to 2500 cc.) used for experimental transmission are frequently duplicated under natural conditions, even in crowded stables kept in very poor sanitary condition; and it is extremely unlikely among horses at pasture.

The fact that the disease does not spread readily by contact casts doubt upon the assumption that the alimentary canal is the main route of entry for the virus. Chances of the contact infection were checked by Francis and Marsteller (123,124) who kept a pony continually exposed to infection for more than two years by intimate association with infected horses; no sign of infection was noted in the pony and its blood was non-infectious when tested by horse inoculation. A number of general observations are on record in the literature with a similar conclusion (160, 444,127,264,399,222,438). Instances are cited that normal horses that were in daily contact with infected animals, or were quartered in stalls adjacent to those occupied by infected horses, did not contract the disease in spite of long exposure, especially if the animals were kept in clean stables, free of bloodsucking insects. This suggests that there must be modes of transmission other, and possibly more important, than by way of the alimentary tract.

The Role of Vectors in Transmission

There is no doubt that infectious anemia can be experimentally transmitted by minute amounts of virulent blood, which is in keeping with the behavior of blood-borne virus diseases. A logical inference would be then the possibility of natural transmission by the intermediate action of bloodsucking insects. Indeed, the seasonal incidence of the disease strongly points to the possible role of some insect vector most abundant in stables and on pastures during the summer and autumn months.

Brimhall, Wesbrook and Bracken (46) in America suggested, previous to the publication of Vallée and Carré's work, the role of insects, when considering the mode of natural transmission from the standpoint of pasture conditions in Minnesota and the seasonal incidence of the disease; they took account of reports that fresh outbreaks of the disease occurred only in the summer or early autumn, and were more frequent during rainy summers. Mack (271) also considered the role of biting flies and mosquitoes as a possibility, and Mohler (302) regarded transmission of the disease by insects as a definite likelihood, according to the report of the Bureau of Animal Industry for 1908. Francis and Marsteller (124) attempted unsuccessfully to transmit the infection through ticks (*Boophilus annulatus*). The observations of the Japanese Commission (191), while investigating the problem of transmission, did not establish the role of a particular species; nevertheless, they seemed to implicate insects, and their conclusion was that, in Japan, horseflies are "the real transmitters."

The first well-controlled experimental transmission by insects was published in 1914 by Scott (395), who demonstrated at the Agricultural Experimental Station in Wyoming on horses kept in screened cages that the stable fly (*Stomoxys calcitrans*) can readily transmit the virus from infected to normal horses. Later he reported, at a meeting in 1917, experimental proof that the infection may also be transmitted by horseflies (*Tabanidae*). Howard (175) published experiments in the same year, the results of which suggested that infection has been transmitted from one horse to another by stable flies, while his experiments with horseflies gave negative result. The possible role of both, stomoxys and tabanus flies, has been experimentally confirmed, among others, by Lührs (264) and Fortner (116) in Germany, by Lehnert (245) in Sweden, by Zenkner and co-workers (495) in Poland, and by Laktionov and co-workers (231) in Russia. Lührs successfully transmitted the infection by using the stomach and intestinal contents of stable flies, and of some tabanids as well, which were collected in stables of infected horses; however, results were negative when he let such stable flies bite susceptible horses. Fortner achieved transmission of the infection by allowing infected tabanid flies to bite the horses repeatedly, while Zenkner transmitted the disease by use of the mouth parts of stomoxys flies that were collected while feeding on an infected horse. Lehnert ascertained the role of insects in transmission by showing that horses in well-screened stables did not contract the disease.

Lührs (264) reported significant results noted in experiments with mosquitoes; positive results were recorded by injecting normal horses with stomach contents of mosquitoes (*Anopheles maculipennis*) collected in stables of horses suffering from infectious anemia, and also by allowing the mosquitoes to bite a susceptible horse; the larvae of mosquitoes did not contain virus. Scott (398) tried to confirm these findings in America, but his attempts of transmission by *Aedes* mosquitoes were unsuccessful. Panisset (340) reviewed in 1922 the evidence related to insect transmission.

Most of the above findings have been later confirmed and extended by the U. S. Bureau of Animal Industry. Stein and co-workers (428,429) have shown in a series of carefully planned experiments that the horseflies (*Tabanidae*) and the stable fly (*Stomoxys calcitrans*) can communicate the infection to normal horses. They also demonstrated that mosquitoes (*Psorophora columbiae*) can transmit infectious anemia in an inapparent, subclinical form. A similar subclinical infection was produced in a susceptible horse by the injection with 1 cc. of a 1:100,000 dilution of infectious serum. Their papers contain a good review of the literature dealing with the problem of insect transmission.

Leeches have also been considered as potential transmitters in low-lying, swampy regions. Indeed, Miégeville (289) collected leeches (*Limnatis nilotica*) from the legs of anemic horses and reproduced the disease in a susceptible animal by the use of the "press-fluid" of the insects. Glättli (140) regarded leeches as possible vectors in spreading the infection. Another ectoparasite of the horse similarly blamed is the louse, *Trichodectes equi* (*Bovicola equi*) (401).

The role of the insects in the transmission is apparently a mechanical one (396). It seems that any type of insect that first feeds upon a diseased horse and then upon a normal animal is a potential carrier and transmitter of the virus. It is immaterial whether the insect belongs to the ectoparasites or the endoparasites. It has been shown experimentally that the parasitic worm, *Filaria equina* (*Setaria equina*), and its eggs and embryos contained virulent, infectious virus (264), and so did adult strongyles (430); these have been collected from horses affected with infectious anemia. On the other hand, extract of third-stage larvae of strongyles originating from the feces of infected horses, and similarly an extract of washed larvae of the so-called botfly (*Gasterophilus intestinalis*), collected from the stomach of a horse that died of acute infectious anemia, failed to produce symptoms when injected into normal horses (430).

Products of insects and their larvae have been thought to be directly responsible for infectious anemia. Ries (372) first suggested this possibility, and Seyderhelm and Seyderhelm (403,404) later presented experimental studies which they believed would indicate that a toxic product (Oestrin) of the larvae of botflies (*Gastrophilus haemorrhoidalis* and *G. equi*)* can produce genuine infectious anemia. Extracts of such larvae, collected from the stomach of slaughtered horses, provoked fever reaction and other symptoms including anemia when injected into normal horses. No experimental proof was presented, however, that they excluded the presence of virus carriers among the horses from which the larvae were collected. In some of their experiments, heated extracts also produced suggestive symptoms.

---

* Recently adopted scientific terms: *Gasterophilus haemorrhoidalis* and *Gasterophilus intestinalis.*

The conclusion of the Seyderhelms was soon rejected by Carré and Vallée (59,60). Theiler reported in 1916 that he was unable to confirm their findings. Similar was the experience of other re-investigators, like Van Es and Schalk (471,472), Klempin (206), de Kock (209), and du Toit (452). They reproduced infectious anemia by use of extracts of larvae from infectious anemia cases, but they failed to reproduce the typical disease with extracts of bots from normal horses. Van Es and Schalk's work indicated that parasitic allergy can produce transient symptoms somewhat resembling those of equine infectious anemia (472). R. Seyderhelm (406) emphasized in 1917 that the Oestrin "as a genuine blood poison" is responsible for pernicious anemia cases of parasitic origin only. Marxer (282) believed that the toxic effect of gasterophilus larvae is anaphylactic in nature as shown by experiments in rabbits.

Various Other Routes of Transmission

The possibility of many other routes and means of transmission has been explored by several investigators experimentally. The disease was successfully transmitted by nasal secretions (399,546), by application of the virus to wounds and to the conjunctiva (359), and by injecting infectious serum into the anterior chamber of the eye (319). Manninger (273) infected horses by the application on their legs of bandages soaked with infectious blood, or urine; on the skin where the bandages were applied, there were no wounds or erosions detectable by the naked eye. Beller and Traub (546) were unable to demonstrate transmission through the intact skin.

Scott (396) demonstrated in a simple model experiment, how easily accidental infection can occur through abrasions of the skin or through surgical manipulations. He reproduced the disease in a susceptible horse with a single prick by a hypodermic needle that was contaminated through first pricking an infected animal. It is apparent from this, that careless use of unsterilized surgical instruments, syringes, and hypodermic needles may well play a role in disseminating the infection among horses. Infection through the skin by the intermediary of harness has been described; and the use of common equipment such as bridles, currycombs, and brushes has also been incriminated in the spread of the disease (438). Many of the accidental infections can be readily explained in face of Scott's experiment just mentioned, or if we recall the experiments with extremely diluted infectious serum (429).

As mentioned above, nasal secretions may contain the virus. Thus, it is conceivable that infected horses or virus carriers can transmit the disease through the respiratory system under suitable conditions, such as at times of catarrhal symptoms in the upper respiratory tract whether the catarrh is caused by the virus of infectious anemia or by other infectious agents. That the nasal mucous membrane may be attacked by the virus is suggested by the observation that two of our experimental horses suffered from severe capillary nose bleeding lasting for over a week during febrile attacks. It is felt, however, that involvement of the nasal mucosa or its capillary system is not a regular feature in infectious anemia; but it may develop in consequence of the petechial hemorrhages observed on different mucous membranes in toxic cases.

Congenital Transmission of the Infection to Foals

The transmission of the virus by infected mares to their offspring is a complex problem. Observations have been reported suggesting the passage of the virus to the fetus through the placenta (431,440,460). The milk of infected mares contains the virus as shown by parenteral injection to susceptible horses (191,399,431), but whether the virus ingested by the milk remains viable in the stomach before it comes to resorption is another question. No conclusive evidence was furnished by investigations of Stein and Mott (431,433) as to whether some foals acquired the infection from being nursed by their infected dams, as part of their experiments suggested, or by close contact with their dams. The semen of infected stallions may contain the virus; subcutaneous inoculation of such semen into a normal mare resulted in a subacute form of infection (431). Trautwein and Schmidt (460) observed a severe outbreak among foals, ten days to nine weeks of age, born of infected mares. They stated that colts are more susceptible to the virus than adult horses. Krauss (223) described an epizootic believed to have originated from five imported stallions that were virus carriers.

The problem of congenital transmission of the infection is probably closely connected with the fact that immune bodies and other blood proteins of the pregnant mare are, as a rule, not transferred to the fetus during the intrauterine life (389), at least not to the same extent as in some other animal species. However, by means of the colostrum, such proteins are readily available to the foal (389); the same was shown by experimental work performed by Wallenstein, Brueckner and Poelma (479) in connection with the Rh-like isoagglutinins of newborn foals. If similar conditions prevail in infectious anemia, as we believe they do, foals may be infected, probably subclinically, during the intrauterine period, or during the first days of their life after birth, when colostrum may pass undigested (and the virus contained in it unaffected) through the mucous membranes of their intestinal canal. It is known that, at this developmental stage, the permeability of these membranes is different from that during the rest of the life.

Oppermann (326) called attention to the fact that infectious anemia is responsible for many abortions in diseased mares. Stein and Mott (433), on the other hand, stated that mares, when experimentally exposed to infection while pregnant, may or may not abort their fetuses during fever attacks.

*

It is now generally accepted that infectious anemia spreads mainly through the agency of insects, in particular of bloodsucking flies (147,201). This conclusion has been reached through experimental research and by logical inference from the seasonal appearance of fresh outbreaks, coincident with the seasonal activity of biting flies and mosquitoes (397). It may be added that there are several virus diseases known to be transmitted by bloodsucking insects; for example, yellow fever is spread in tropical regions through mosquitoes, and Kelser (196,198) demonstrated experimentally that mosquitoes (*Aedes aegypti*) can transmit equine encephalomyelitis, a neurotropic virus disease of horses, that has been shown to be transmissible also to man (Meyer (287)).

The source of virus in the spread of infectious anemia is the sick horse or the virus carrier. It is known that once a horse is infected, it remains a life-long carrier of the virus. Several authors tested the blood of such carriers systematically for 12 to 16 years, and noted positive results (116,119,221,380,462). An unsuspected virus carrier among horses, naturally, constitutes a dangerous reservoir of the virus and continues to spread the disease until eliminated from the group.

There is no indication that an intermediate reservoir of the virus exists. The role of insects is considered plainly as a mechanical transfer of the infectious material, usually blood, and no evolutionary cycle is postulated in the development of the virus within the insects. Whether some insects or parasitic worms may harbor the virus in a masked form for a long time is not known. Shope (410), in a series of interesting experiments, has demonstrated that swine influenza virus can survive in lungworm larvae of the swine, or in earthworms in masked form for at least two years. The possibility of such latent, masked persistence of infectious anemia virus in an intermediate host has not been explored so far; it could explain the repeated outbreaks on pastures where the disease notoriously flares up every year, and yet the infection cannot be traced to virus carriers.

Although the most important, insect transmission is not the only mode responsible for the spread of the disease. Many authors believe that the disease has little or no tendency to spread among horses by contact under good hygienic conditions. On the other hand, infection can readily occur through abrasions of the skin, or via the mucous membranes of the animal, and by accidents capable of bringing the virus to resorption.

If the infectious material does not reach the blood stream quickly, either directly, or by resorption, it is probably retained in the regional lymph glands and is apt to produce a mild, latent type of infection, or to bring about the usual clinical symptoms after a prolonged incubation period. It appears, as if merely a sensitization had been achieved first, with no manifest symptoms, to be followed by clinical symptoms later on. Steck (420,421) states that, in certain localities where infectious anemia is enzootic, many latent infections occur among horses that have frequent contact with one another. Such cases are usually not recognized until some provocating factor activates the disease and brings about manifest symptoms in the horse. According to the above concept, the latent, subclinical infection may exist for a long time before it is recognized on the basis of clinical symptoms, and then it is regarded as a relatively "rare" instance of contact infection.

It may be said in conclusion then that natural transmission of infectious anemia can take place in many different ways, the most common of which seems to be insect transmission; but there is sufficient evidence that the disease may spread by contact and by a number of other ways of accidental infection.

CHAPTER 3

SYMPTOMATOLOGY

As a study of the symptoms of infectious anemia was not one of our prime objectives, we shall report only a few pertinent observations made on horses that had been injected with material known to contain virulent virus.

The *acute* cases comprise those animals suffering severe symptoms that either terminated fatally or the horses were destroyed in the early phase of the disease. In this stage the febrile attacks either occurred at short intervals (one to four days) or the fever continued unabated until death. The incubation period varied from 8 to 17 days. The peak of the temperature at the time of the febrile reaction ranged from 104° to 108° F. (40° to 42.2° C.). The pulse was 46 to 56 per minute when taken on the resting animal.

Symptoms usually accompanying the exacerbations were thirst, often perspiration, debility, and depression. Epistaxis, sublingual and nasal hemorrhages, were occasionally observed. Pallor of the mucous membranes was noted only when the anemia was severe. A papular eruption was observed on the neck of one horse at the time of the second attack; the rash, which lasted four days, spread over the entire body.

In fatal cases a marked debility was indicated by the animal's inability to rise from a lying position. The acute phase of the disease was usually less than a month in duration; it either terminated in death or, evidencing gradually less severe attacks, changed its character to become a subacute or chronic case.

Subacute cases consisted of those horses repeatedly manifesting fever paroxysms at afebrile intervals of 6 to 24 days for a longer period of time, usually for several months. The attacks were milder; the temperature ranged from 102° to 105° F. (38.9° to 40.6° C.)* during attacks and the accompanying symptoms were similar to those observed during the acute phase. Many of our horses were remarkably free of severe symptoms during the first and second febrile attacks; symptoms became more notice-

* For converting temperature readings given in Fahrenheit degrees into centigrades (C°), see Table 1.

able and increased in severity during subsequent attacks in spite of the usually milder fever response. Loss of weight, depression, marked debility, edema of the dependent parts, and unsteady gait were most apparent after the second month. In this stage, pallor of the mucous membranes was usually quite apparent.

TABLE 1

COMPARATIVE TEMPERATURE FIGURES IN DIFFERENT SCALES

Fahrenheit (F°)	*Centigrade (C°)*	*Fahrenheit (F°)*	*Centigrade (C°)*
97.0	36.1	103.0	39.5
97.5	36.4	103.5	39.7
98.0	36.7	104.0	40.0
98.5	36.9	104.5	40.3
99.0	37.2	105.0	40.6
99.5	37.5	105.5	40.8
100.0	37.8	106.0	41.1
100.5	38.0	106.5	41.4
101.0	38.3	107.0	41.7
101.5	38.6	107.5	42.0
102.0	38.9	108.0	42.2
102.5	39.2	108.5	42.5

In the *chronic* form, the febrile periods occurred at intervals of one month or more and were less severe. Chronic cases may be divided into two groups: those animals whose condition gradually grew worse, and those maintaining a relatively favorable state of health. In the former group, emaciation, edema of dependent parts, incoordination, depression, and debility were prominent characteristics. In the latter, the animals appeared healthy and produced no manifest symptoms, but their temperatures, taken twice daily, revealed mild elevations at about monthly or longer intervals.

Mortality.—Accurate figures on mortality are lacking because animals afflicted with inapparent or mild forms of the malady would escape diagnosis; consequently no dependable figures are available to serve as a basis for calculation. Nevertheless, some estimates have been made in various countries and a few of the figures reported in such estimates should stand here.

Watson (480) emphasized the high mortality, when reporting in 1896 about the disease as seen in Wisconsin. Francis and Marsteller (123) stated in 1908 that the mortality was 80 per cent in Texas. The U. S. Bureau of Animal Industry (462), reporting on the outbreak of infectious anemia in a group of several hundreds of valuable thoroughbred horses during 1947, made the statement that "this outbreak in New England took a toll of 80 horses." In the Province of Quebec, Canada, the mortality was set at 31 per cent in 1941, and 21 per cent in 1942.

In Switzerland, Wyssmann, in 1915, estimated the mortality 57 per cent from a series of cases studied. In the enzootic areas of France, the mortality was considerable (181). In 1933, 30 horses died of infectious anemia at one single establishment of the army in Belfort, France. In Württemberg, Germany, 65 animals died of the disease in 1931, and 218 in 1932.

The Japanese Commission (191) reported a mortality of 30 to 70 per cent depending upon the form of the disease, the climate, and the care of the animals. They stated that, during a summer month in 1911, of 107 horses present in one village a total of 52 were lost, of which 24 died, and 38 were destroyed.

*

The symptoms exhibited by our experimental horses were essentially the same, although not as severe as those reported by other investigators. The reason for this difference in severity is not quite clear but it may partly be attributed to the feed and care that our animals received. While under experiment, our horses were housed in screened isolation stables and were not subjected to work or any physical strain.

Division of the disease into acute, subacute, and chronic forms was made by Carré and Vallée (58) on the basis of the fever attacks. In the acute stage, there were usually no remissions, the attacks were severe, and the duration of the phase was from five to fifteen days. In the subacute phase the symptoms were attenuated, remissions were clear-cut and the duration was a few weeks to several months; whereas in the chronic form, fever attacks were infrequent and the symptoms were those of extreme progressive anemia.

Hutyra, Marek and Manninger (181) characterized the three divisions on the same basis but in greater detail. They reported the duration of the acute phase in adult animals as three to four weeks with no remissions or only a few at very short intervals; in the subacute phase, attacks occurred two or three times a month and the duration of the stage was a few weeks to several months. Febrile attacks in the chronic form were milder and recurred at intervals of one to three months or more over periods lasting from months to years. These authors emphasized that one animal may pass through all three stages of the disease, moreover that the disease, after becoming quiescent, may resume an acute, fulminating course. Other classifications found in the literature do not vary essentially from the above (28,191,264,426,470).

There are reports that the incubation period as observed in artificially induced infections may vary from one day to three months or more (28,181,191,426,470) depending upon what is taken as the first sign of infection. The most frequently observed incubation usually extends from one to three weeks (181,426,470). Martin (278) concluded from his observations on experimentally inoculated animals that the actual period of incubation is two to five days, at which time the first reaction is observed in the form of a mild temperature rise; the first marked fever reaction occurred in ten to nineteen days. Gerlach (132) noted incubation periods lasting as long as three months. His experimental animals were hyperimmune serum horses; this may account for his findings, as such animals have high immune globulin level. On the basis of our experiments, we believe that the fever reaction to the virus is delayed in such cases because of the high unspecific immune globulin, as discussed later in the chapter dealing with the pathogenesis.

Factors which are believed to influence the length of the period between inoculation and the appearance of symptoms are the serial passage of the virus (58,217), the route of injection (271,398,470), and the material containing the virus, i.e., whole blood, serum, urine, milk (191,219,398, 470). Variations in the virulence of the virus and differences in the susceptibility of the experimental horse are factors as yet not sufficiently understood (28,470). According to Stein, Lotze and Mott the incubation period was lengthened by dilution of the virus as the dilutions became greater. A latent form of the disease was produced by inoculation of a 1:100,000 dilution or through transmission by mosquitoes (429). These authors also provided evidence that the incubation period was lengthened when transmission was through stable flies (428).

With the exception of the rapidly fatal acute and the latent chronic phases, the disease has as its main characteristics: intermittent fever attacks, progressive debility, marked depression, emaciation, and edema of dependent parts (28,181,191,470).

Other symptoms reported as occurring in the course of the disease include lack of appetite (181,191,426), nocturnal polyuria (46,123,181, 426), diarrhea (58,181,426), increased irritability (28,181), incoordination (28), weakness or paralysis of the hind quarters (123,181,337,426), pallor of mucous membranes (28,181,470), yellowish discoloration of the conjunctiva (28,123,271,426), urticaria (152), sublingual and nasal petechial hemorrhages (257,417,3), abnormal cardiac activity (191,424), accelerated pulse (181,191,426), increased respiratory rate (191,426), and also splenomegaly as detected by rectal palpation (191), just to mention a few references from the voluminous literature on symptomatology of equine infectious anemia.

Symptoms in the chronic and latent cases have been studied by Zeller (494) and by several other investigators; it has been concluded that symptoms in this stage are not distinctive for the disease. However, when combined with the history of the case and hematology, they should arouse suspicion. Apparently recovered and symptomless cases have been known to undergo relapses when exposed to strenuous labor (181), inclement weather (191), and surgical manipulation (426), or by profuse bloodletting ("provocation").

CHAPTER 4

CLINICAL DIAGNOSIS

The only definite means of diagnosis of equine infectious anemia which is now available is the horse inoculation test. On account of the expense involved, this is utilized only if the sick horse is valuable or there are other reasons for which it is essential to arrive at a definite and final diagnosis in a horse suspected to suffer from infectious anemia. The test consists of inoculating blood from the suspect case into a normal horse, and its result is considered positive, if characteristic symptoms develop after an incubation period.

In many cases, however, the diagnosis can be made with a reasonable degree of accuracy by considering collectively the history of the case, clinical symptoms and the results of blood examination, particularly in the acute and subacute stage of the disease. Diagnosis may be difficult in an early severe case or in a chronic carrier. It may be relatively easy when a new case with typical symptoms appears in an endemic area. A tentative diagnosis is often made when signs of anemia are present and fever is observed, but it hardly is necessary to point out that more data than these are requisite before arriving at this conclusion.

When the disease takes a rapidly fatal course, it may closely resemble acute septicemia (181). The first attack may persist as a high continuous fever with death occurring before the usual sequence of symptoms develops. Anemia may be absent or mild. Other symptoms that may appear are marked weakness, prostration, mental depression, and slight icterus. The disease in the acute form may be confused with anthrax, influenza, purpura hemorrhagica, acute equine encephalomyelitis, and other acute febrile conditions (191,399).

According to Hutyra, Marek and Manninger (181) it may be impossible to distinguish between anthrax and infectious anemia without bacterial examination of the blood or inoculation tests. These authors noted that equine influenza spreads more quickly among a group of horses, taking a rapid and usually more favorable course than that of infectious anemia. The former is characterized chiefly by catarrhal manifestations.

Other conditions which have been confused with equine infectious anemia in its early stages are piroplasmosis, pneumonia (181), acute helminthiasis, leukemia, and neoplasms (416). In tropical countries piroplasmosis, trypanosomiasis, as well as other protozoon diseases present a definite problem in differential diagnosis (227). Such conditions have been reported to co-exist with infectious anemia (350). In piroplasmosis there is usually icterus and often hemoglobinuria. In piroplasmosis there are petechial hemorrhages on the conjunctiva, whereas in infectious anemia they are sublingual. In piroplasmosis large numbers of parasites are found in the blood at the time of the fever peaks. Hematologic examination of the blood in early stages of infectious anemia should be done during or right after the fever attacks, as the lowered values tend to return to normal during remissions in this phase of the disease.

Sublingual hemorrhages have been claimed as a diagnostic criterion in distinguishing equine infectious anemia from other diseases (257,416, 417,420). In equine infectious anemia the petechiae are minute and often occur in numbers ranging from hundreds to thousands. In septicemic diseases the hemorrhages are larger, and in petechial fever they vary in number and distribution, most often being found on the nasal mucosa.

When the course of infectious anemia is less severe and of longer duration, the usual chain of symptoms is: intermittent attacks of fever, rapid loss of weight, debility, pale mucous membranes or some degree of jaundice, and dropsical swellings of the dependent parts, the anemia as well as other symptoms being usually most pronounced in the febrile attacks.

In the subacute form, the disease may be mistaken for trypanosomiasis or strongyloidosis (181). Other diseases from which the subacute form must be differentiated are nutritional and other types of anemia (53,179, 224,310,418), filariasis (181), chronic articular rheumatism (146,158), and tumors (416).

Nutritional anemia almost always runs an afebrile course (181). Chronic articular rheumatism has been described as showing signs of anemia and producing from time to time an irregular remittent type of fever (146). Symptoms of joint pain may aid in differentiating the condition from infectious anemia; however, Habersang (146) reported lameness due to tendosynovitis, and Sokolowski (413) observed lumbago in infectious anemia.

Differentiation from anemia due to neoplasms is illustrated by the following cases: Two horses suspected of having infectious anemia were brought to our attention. Both revealed malignant tumors at autopsy. Clinically they had displayed irregular temperature elevations, marked anemia, progressive debility, and mental depression. The lack of any regularity in the occurrence of the fever attacks, especially in the early stages, as well as the past history of the case are factors which might assist in making a differentiation. In the cases just mentioned, our laboratory tests (hemagglutination and blood protein determination) were helpful in ruling out infectious anemia.

In chronic cases in which the characteristic symptoms of progressive emaciation, debility, anemia, and intermittent fever attacks from time to time are apparent, diagnosis is not difficult. However, in the symptomless, balanced virus carrier the disease easily escapes detection; during this stage, the animal may look as healthy as any other horse. Though it has been claimed that a constant lymphocytosis is present in such horses, this is apparently not always true, and even so is not sufficient to establish a criterion of carriership.

There have been numerous reports of mixed infections of infectious anemia and tuberculosis, such as those by Eilmann (105), Ghier (133), Lamarre (234), Panisset and co-workers (341,342), and others. Behrens (35) reported that seven out of eight horses, suspected of having infectious anemia on clinical examination, were shown at autopsy to have tuberculosis. One must be careful in making or rejecting the diagnosis of infectious anemia on the basis of the presence or absence of a positive tuberculin test. Several investigators reported positive tuberculin skin tests in a large percentage of their infectious anemia cases (105,341). However, in most of them the two diseases might have been co-existent in the same animal. Panisset and Pflieger (342) came to the conclusion that the tuberculin test is of no value in the differential diagnosis of infectious anemia.

Stein (426) stressed the fact that, although chronic parasitism can present similar symptoms, it is also possible that intestinal parasitism and infectious anemia may be present in the same horse. An aid in their differential diagnosis is the microscopic examination of the feces for eggs of intestinal parasites and examination of blood films for eosinophilia. One should bear in mind, however, that changes occur in the number of eosinophils also in infectious anemia.

*

Beside analyzing the aggregate of clinical symptoms, various tests can be used as additional tools of the diagnosis. The problem of differential diagnosis on the basis of histopathologic findings has been investigated by many workers, among them Ziegler (496), Nöller and Dobberstein (322), Oppermann (328), Hjärre (168), Moszczenski and Krupski (310), and Steck and Hauser (423).

Liver biopsy has also been advocated to decide diagnosis in the living animal. Richters (369), Wall (478), Hjärre (168), and many others reported the results of this method for histological diagnosis. Wall (478) made suggestions for modifying the trocar to be used for this purpose. Akerström (3) believed that liver biopsies are a valuable aid in making a diagnosis and implied that the procedure was relatively safe and easy to perform. He noted that sublingual hemorrhages and liver biopsy were of some value in detecting carriers.

Histological examination of the tissues of slaughtered horses has been practiced for some time to determine the incidence of infectious anemia in a certain area, and several reports have been published on the subject. However, as many investigators rightfully pointed out, it is quite false to make a diagnosis of infectious anemia in the abattoir without the knowledge of the clinical history of cases, as many other conditions may cause similar pathologic changes, particularly hemosiderosis in the liver (375).

Tests other than histological investigation that might be helpful in supporting the clinical diagnosis will be considered in the chapters on Hematology, Hemagglutination, and other Laboratory methods of diagnosis.

Taken separately the clinical, laboratory, and pathological findings can serve merely as suggestions for tentative diagnosis. Combined with one another, however, they often can be of definite value in deciding the differential diagnosis. Nevertheless, the horse inoculation test remains the only means of assuring, beyond any doubt, a final diagnosis of infectious anemia.

CHAPTER 5

PROPERTIES OF THE VIRUS

While some of the main characteristics of the virus of infectious anemia are known, many of its properties have not been sufficiently explored as yet. The reason for this is the lack of simple and inexpensive methods of demonstrating the presence of the virus in a material under study. The horse inoculation test is the one dependable way of indicating the presence of an active virus strong enough to provoke clearly recognizable symptoms; but, for obvious reasons, the test cannot be utilized to any great extent. In order to determine the ultimate strength of a virus, inoculation of graded dilutions into a considerable number of experimental animals is required. Such titration is, in most cases, not feasible in infectious anemia; neither is the application of indirect methods, which are readily available for the study of many other virus diseases.

A brief summary will be given below on what is known at present with regard to filterability, size, and biological identification of the virus; its distribution within the body fluids and tissues; its resistance to physical and chemical agents; and finally, current views concerning its nature.

Filterability and Size

The virus etiology of the disease has been established by the experiments of Vallée and Carré (468). They transmitted the infection to normal horses with infectious blood and were equally successful in reproducing the disease by giving a susceptible horse 100 cc. of a bacterium free filtrate of horse serum obtained from a case of infectious anemia. They determined the efficiency of the filter in a collateral experiment; it removed all organisms from a highly infectious broth culture of Pasteurella, one of the smallest among pathogenic bacteria, as verified by a test in guinea-pigs. The filterability was soon confirmed by several authors, among them Ostertag (338), Hempel (160), and Theiler and Kehoe (446).

Balozet (27) determined the approximate size of the virus by horse inoculation experiments following filtration through Elford's collodion membranes of known porosity. He estimated the size of the virus to be between 18 and 50 mμ, since it passed through membranes having a pore size of

100 mμ, but was retained by those of 52 mμ. Reagan and collaborators (364) attempted to determine the size and shape of the virus by means of the electron microscope; in the sediment of an infectious horse serum filtered and then centrifuged at 52,000 rpm for 3 hours, they noted spheric formations ranging from 11 to 59 mμ (average 30 mμ), which they considered the virus of infectious anemia, since no particles of similar size were noted in normal horse serum. The size thus determined seems to be in fairly close agreement with that found by Balozet.

On account of its very small particle size, the virus cannot be detected through the use of the ordinary light-microscope, as the diameter of the virus remains much below the resolving power of such microscopes. Inclusion bodies have not been demonstrated in infectious anemia. The small, ringlike formations to which first Mack called attention were regarded as artefacts by Swingle (444).

No bacterial organism was ever cultivated with any regularity, or found to be present in the blood or various organs in horses suffering from infectious anemia. Miyagawa and co-workers (292) reported the cultivation of spirochetes on Noguchi's medium from the blood of infectious anemia horses, but Hoskins (174), Mócsy (294), and others were not able to confirm their findings. If we consider that Atoxyl and various Salvarsan preparations have been found ineffective in the therapy of the disease, this fact itself would indicate that infectious anemia is not caused by spirochetes or protozoa. Such infections, however, may very well co-exist with infectious anemia, or may be mistaken for it, as Abbondanza (1) suggested. Such may be the explanation of the unusual findings reported by Pigoury and collaborators (350), who studied equine surra (trypanosomiasis) and infectious anemia in laboratory animals. The close similarity, particularly in the clinical manifestations, between streptococcus anemia and virus anemia as observed on horses in Switzerland was discussed by Krupski, Grumbach and Leemann (226). The question of alleged etiologic significance of parasitic toxins was mentioned in Chapter 2.

Identification of the Virus and Its Distribution in the Body

The virus can be identified by its pathogenic effect in susceptible animals. The typical symptoms and the differentiation of the disease from clinically similar conditions have been briefly reviewed in the preceding chapters. Additional means of studying the pathologic condition in horses experimentally infected with the virus or in animals naturally ill with the disease will be discussed in subsequent chapters.

Attempts at neutralization of the virus by immune serum did not lead to any appreciable success (427). Although differences in virulence have been noted by several authors, it is uncertain whether this is a permanent property of any virus strain. As a rule, it is influenced by the rapidity and the type of passages which it undergoes in horses (56), but it is immaterial whether 1 cc. or 750 cc. of blood is injected. Strain differences of serologic type have been suspected by some research workers (290,546), but it is difficult to produce evidence for this because of the lack of proper serologic methods. The findings on which the assumption of strain differences is based can, in our opinion, be explained in several different ways.

For identifying the virus, susceptible individual animals are needed; equines (horses, mules, donkeys) are regarded as equally susceptible, although a strain adapted to one of these species within the equine family is usually more virulent to that particular species. Susceptibility of other animals than equines will be discussed in connection with the transmission experiments on laboratory animals (in Chapter 10).

Although there are a few reports (265,347,221) suggesting that the infection has been accidentally transmitted to man, it is believed that such infection in humans is exceptionally rare, or else it runs an unrecognized subclinical form. Otherwise more cases would occur among persons having frequent contact with horses ill with the disease. We may quote here an observation in our laboratory. During a *post mortem* examination of an experimental horse killed in the subacute stage of the disease, a laboratory worker cut his finger while cleaning a sharp surgical knife stained with blood of the horse. The person in question did not develop any symptom and has remained in perfect health ever since. Stein and Mott (434) noted negative results when they tested in horses the blood of two human patients suffering from aplastic and hypoplastic anemia, which conditions have been suggested by Peters (347) to be possibly related to equine infectious anemia.

Because of its constant persistence in the blood, the virus may be regarded as *ubiquiter* in the body of the infected animal. Its presence has been demonstrated in the milk (191,264,399,431,433) and in nasal secretions (399,546); it is present in urine exhibiting albuminuria, as is known from the work of Vallée and Carré. Experiments would tend to show that it is not contained in saliva (338,160,253), or in tear and sweat (28,253,399). Evidence is conflicting about the virus content of feces; most workers believe, however, that it is not eliminated through the bowels (470). Nakamura and co-workers (319) tried to estimate the relative concentration of the virus in various organs of infected horses. Specific affinity of the virus to certain tissues or to a particular organ system has been assumed, to erythrocytes and the hematopoietic system, although it has not been demonstrated; but it was repeatedly stated as an inference from histologic findings that the virus has a tendency to attack the capillary walls and shows a definite affinity to the reticulo-endothelial system. Holz (171), who noted in some infectious anemia cases histologic alterations of the central nervous system reminiscent of those seen in acute encephalomyelitis has assigned a neurotropic tendency to the virus. In one of our experimental horses, which we injected with virulent virus intracerebrally, no recognizable disturbance was noted in the nervous system; the horse reacted with a typical fever response and other symptoms after an incubation of 16 days.

Resistance of the Virus to Physical and Chemical Agents

In general, the virus of infectious anemia is relatively resistant as compared with other viruses and may survive outside of the animal's body for a comparatively long time. Early reports indicated (470) that the virus is well preserved when exposed to freezing. Later work confirmed that the virus remains viable in serum or plasma for at least 6 months, if preserved at or below freezing temperature. Under bacterially sterile conditions, infectious serum may remain virulent for several months at room temperature. In our laboratory, infectious serum and plasma samples were kept frozen in rubber stoppered vials at –15° to –20°C., and also at about –70°C. on carbon dioxide-ice, without the slightest reduction of virulence in 4 years. The virus is fairly resistant to desiccation. According to Avramenko (520) it remained viable on hay as long as 180 days. Investigators at the U. S. Bureau of Animal Industry found the virus fully active after 6 years storage in lyophilized form (462). Balozet (26) tested the effect of ultraviolet light by irradiating virus samples in Petri-dishes with a mercury vapor lamp for 5 minutes to 7 hours; all irradiated samples remained viable as tested in donkeys. It has been known from early experiments that heating at 58° to 60°C. for one hour renders the virus noninfectious (58,191).

Inactivation of the virus for the purpose of disinfection or its attenuation for immunization was studied by many investigators. The effect of phenol (191,267,128,20), formalin (246,475,299,300), and a number of other chemical substances (199,222,16,17,279,439) has been investigated and the products so treated were tested in horses for infectiousness. Phenol seems to possess less inactivating capacity unless it is used in somewhat higher concentration, while formalin inactivates the virus in a relatively short time. Balozet (20) reported that 0.1 per cent phenol inactivated the virus in 4 months, or at room temperature in 16 days (22). By using 0.5 per cent phenol, serum samples kept at refrigerator temperature lost their virulence in 3 months (222). Mócsy (299) found that 0.3 to 0.5 per cent formalin destroyed the virulence of the virus in 38 days. Glycerine first attenuated the virus, in about 4 months; while 7 months contact with glycerine inactivated it (17,20). Saponin (16) and bile (18,19) were very effective in inactivating or attenuating the virus. It is thought to be alcohol resistant (459), and according to Richters (371) strongly alkaline disinfectants are favored by Waldmann.

The problem was reviewed and a series of experimental studies related to the resistance of the virus were reported in 1944 by Stein and co-workers (439). In serum samples kept at 5°C. the virus was inactivated in a month by the addition of 0.5 per cent phenol, or 0.1 to 0.2 per cent formalin, and also by a combination of crystal violet and phenol. It is often difficult to decide on the basis of the test inoculation in horses whether an attenuation or a final inactivation occurred, because of the mild subclinical infection that may result from such experiments.

Nature of the Virus

On the basis of the histology and his studies related to the infectiousness of the protein fractions as present in virulent horse serum, Mócsy (297, 300) assumed that the inciting factor of infectious anemia is merely a "stimulating substance" (*Reizstoff*) formed within the body of infected animals and that it is a nonliving protein acting as a virus, being present in the albumin fraction. He came to these conclusions partly because the virus survived repeated precipitation of protein fractions without a decrease in its virulence and because it was not inactivated by irradiation with X-rays. Balozet (25) opposed this concept on grounds that the supporting evidence was not satisfactory; he believed that the virus was simply adsorbed to the protein fractions tested by Mócsy, and that the dosage of X-ray used by him was too small. Martin (279) demonstrated that the virus is present in both the albumin and the globulin fractions of infectious serum. At present the prevailing view is that the virus of equine infectious anemia is a filter passing, living microorganism.

CHAPTER 6

METHODS OF LABORATORY DIAGNOSIS

Infectious anemia, in any of its stages, can by proper means be transmitted to normal horses for the purpose of confirming the diagnosis. Because of the expense involved, however, this method cannot be utilized as frequently as may be necessary. Therefore, efforts have been made to develop laboratory procedures, such as specific serologic tests or other methods, that could be used in making a decision in the practical diagnosis. The peculiar nature of the disease and the fact that the virus has not been cultivated so far are mainly responsible for the present limited success in developing diagnostic procedures that will meet all the requirements of a practical test, since it is not yet possible to overcome many of the difficulties involved. Nevertheless, there are a number of laboratory methods that can be used in combination either to support or disprove the clinical diagnosis of equine infectious anemia.

The Problem of Specific Serologic Diagnosis

Complement-fixation Test.—Many infectious diseases of bacterial or virus origin give rise to the occurrence of specific complement-fixing antibodies in the blood serum of the affected host. Such antibodies can, as a rule, be detected after the symptoms have been present for some time and usually last for a considerable time following the clinical recovery of the animal. In the case of equine infectious anemia, the latter observation should be of great value in identifying clinically recovered, symptomless virus carriers.

As long ago as 1909 Hempel (160) reported that the complement-fixation test is of no value in the diagnosis of equine anemia. Wirth (487), using boiled extracts of clotted blood as antigen, also recorded negative results. Lührs (267), on the other hand, found that in a few cases of infectious anemia an extract of kidney, spleen, and liver furnished a suitable antigen that reacted with sera taken during the fever reaction; cases in the afebrile stage gave negative results. Zeller (494) came to a similar conclusion, but noted that not all febrile cases react positively with good antigenic extracts. He also tried with inconclusive results the conglutination technique similar to the one reported by Schoening and first utilized by Pfeiler and Weber in the diagnosis of glanders. Mohler (303) prepared water extracts from the spleen of infectious anemia horses to be used as antigen, and published a preliminary note in 1936 reporting positive results in some cases. However, there seemed to be no regularity in his findings; the same animal that produced a suggestive positive result on serum from one bleeding, gave a completely negative reading at the next bleeding, and some of the proven cases of experimental infectious anemia never produced a positive reaction in the test, thus making the test useless for practical diagnosis. Traub and co-workers (458) hyperimmunized horses with 10 to 16 injections of infectious material and obtained positive results when testing their sera against suitable antigenic preparations (spleen extracts). They concluded, however, that the method cannot be used for practical diagnosis, since only one out of 25 field cases of infectious anemia gave positive result in the test.

As part of the present studies here to be described, much time was spent in working out a suitable complement-fixation test by the use of modified and improved techniques. Some of the findings of earlier investigators were duplicated, but consistent and reproducible results were not obtained.

At first, attention was mainly concentrated on preparing a suitable antigen from various organs and from the blood of infected horses.* The technique of the test proper was a somewhat modified complement-fixation test as described by Kelser and Schoening (201) for the serological diagnosis of glanders. Spleen and liver extracts often gave positive fixation with lower dilutions of sera from some of our experimental horses, but in general the experience was similar to the one recorded by Mohler: the results were inconsistent and transitory even in the same horse, and some animals failed to present a positive reading in the test during the whole course of their illness. An attempt was made to adsorb an eventual reacting antigenic component of infectious anemia blood to normal red blood cells of horses and also to chicken red blood cells at refrigerator temperature. This was then eluted at incubator temperature from the cells, centrifuged, and the clear supernatant used as an antigen against serum samples of normal, diseased, and seemingly recovered horses. Experimental antigenic preparations, kindly furnished by Doctors C. D. Stein and W. M. Mohler of the U. S. Bureau of Animal Industry and prepared by various methods of extracting red blood cells and plasma of infectious anemia horses, were also utilized. The results obtained in both groups, i.e., with eluted antigens and with the rest of the antigen preparations, were largely negative; some slightly positive readings noted in serum dilutions of 1:4 to 1:16 were not readily reproducible.

* The first group of complement-fixation experiments were carried out by Dr. Werner Leemann of the University of Zürich, Switzerland, working in our laboratory.

Since a laboratory test for checking the results in other types of experiments, such as cultivation of the virus and its adaptation to laboratory animals, seemed to be essential for us, renewed efforts were made later in order to work out a procedure sufficiently sensitive at least for experimental purposes. For working with small amounts of serum and antigen, the technique described by Dreguss and Farkas (98) for serologic studies in typhus fever was adopted. In this method 0.2 cc. of each constituent is used (diluted serum, complement, antigen, and physiologic salt solution), giving a total volume of 0.8 cc. in the first phase of the test, before adding the hemolytic system. The sensitivity of the method was checked by an immune rabbit serum prepared by repeated injections of horse serum. The rabbit serum gave a definite four-plus fixation up to a dilution of 1:160 when tested against antigens of normal or infectious horse serum diluted 1:1200, or against suspensions (clear supernatants) made from organs of horses in dilutions of 1:200, while proper controls included in these tests were completely negative.

Using this refined technique, a number of antigen preparations were tested against serum samples collected in all phases of the illness and also following recovery. Graded dilutions, rather than an empirically selected amount of the serum, were tested against antigens of various strength.

Antigens were prepared from tissues of infected horses collected aseptically at the time of autopsy, with physiologic salt solution as the suspending material; the clear supernatant obtained after centrifugation was used in dilutions ranging from 1:5 to 1:200 to the original wet weight of organs (liver, spleen, kidney, lungs). Hemolysed red blood cells of normal and sick horses were tried as antigens; hemolysis was achieved by sterile distilled water, and the hemolysate was made isotonic by adding the proper amount of sodium chloride before use.

Lung suspensions were included, as they often render good service as complement-fixing antigens in virus diseases. One of us (Dreguss (97)) used saline suspensions of the lungs of mice infected with human and swine influenza virus for thousands of complement-fixation tests in studies related to influenza. Recently, Randall, McVickar and Doll (361) published a procedure of complement-fixation test for infectious abortion of mares, utilizing lung tissue of the affected horses as antigen. The advantage of lung tissue is that unspecific organ-fixation is less common with this type of antigen.

Since none of these antigens proved to be satisfactory so far as a practical complement-fixation test is concerned, no detailed account will be given here. Although fixation to a lesser degree occurred with many of them, it is uncertain whether it was specific. The difference between normal and pathologic sera was mostly too slight to be sufficient for differentiation. A somewhat higher degree of fixation might have a theoretical significance, even though nonspecific. For instance, positive fixation with liver antigens could be regarded as a sign of liver damage, although this might occur in many diseases other than infectious anemia. Such finding would indicate that the liver tissue became antigenic during the disease process and provoked the production of auto-antibodies.

In this connection, following a technique similar to that of Björneboe and Krag (39) in their report of positive complement-fixation with liver

TABLE 2

COMPLEMENT-FIXATION TEST WITH VARIOUS ANTIGENS AND SERA

Antigen Made of	*Serum Tested*	*Positive in Dilution*
Lungs (Horse 21)	Rabbit 392	1:80
Lungs (Horse 21)	Rabbit 390	1:20
Lungs (Horse 21)	Rabbit (20th transfer)	1:10
Red blood cells (normal horse)	Rabbit 392	1:40
Lungs (passage mice)	Rabbit 22	1:50
Lungs (passage mice)	Rabbit 22 (normal)	1:10
Lungs (normal mice)	Rabbit 22	1:20
Lungs (normal mice)	Rabbit 21	(neg.)
Cultured virus (4th passage)	Horse 10 (16th day)	1:40
Cultured virus (4th passage)	Horse 10 (24th day)	1:20
Cultured virus (13th passage)	Horse 17 (20th day)	1:20
Cultured virus (13th passage)	Horse 17 (before inoc.)	1:10
Serum, Horse 20 (4th day)	Horse 2 (26th day)	1:160
Serum, Horse 20 (4th day)	Horse 17 (before inoc.)	1:40

extract antigen in cases of human hepatitis, we attempted to use liver suspensions of normal and infected horses as the antigen. However, these usually exhibited such a high degree of anticomplementary effect that they had to be greatly diluted, and this in turn made positive fixation unlikely. For example, a normal liver suspension in saline used as the antigen in a final dilution of 1:3200 produced all negative results with a number of infectious anemia serum samples taken during fever attacks or remissions; on the other hand, stronger liver suspensions could not be utilized as they were anticomplementary. Liver extracts were not tried.

Some of the results in the complement-fixation tests are summarized in Table 2. Tests that gave negative readings, and antigens or sera exhibiting anticomplementary effect, are not listed in the summary of results.

As already mentioned, the positive findings in these tests were irregular and often inconsistent, and the titers were too low to be of practical value for diagnostic use.

We made an attempt to bring about a reaction between acute phase sera, and sera collected in the later stages of the illness or during convalescence. Davis (76) and Hudson (177) have described a complement-fixation test for yellow fever in which they used with satisfactory result acute phase serum of experimentally infected monkeys as the antigen against sera of humans and monkeys recovered from yellow fever infection. In our tests, using a similar technique, a slight suggestion of a positive reaction was noted. The serum of an infected horse taken on the 4th day after infection, and used as an antigen in a dilution of 1:5 and 1:10, evidenced positive fixation when tested against the serum of horses taken on the 26th to 42nd day of infection. The positive titers of the latter sera were as high as 1:80 to 1:160, and the results were reproducible. However, normal horse sera in lower dilutions also produced positive readings.

It is known that some mammalian and avian sera, among them certain immune horse sera, do not fix complement in spite of the presence of the corresponding specific antigen. This applies, for example, to the reaction between pneumococcus antigens of carbohydrate nature and their antisera prepared in horses (365). In such instances the so-called indirect complement-fixation can be used to disclose the presence of specific antibodies. Therefore, in addition to the tests performed with the usual (direct) technique, the indirect complement-fixation was utilized in our work in a few instances; however, there was no appreciable result. The technique followed was largely the one suggested by Rice (365), and a simplified version as described by Wolfe and co-workers (491) for testing avian sera for Newcastle disease antibodies. In the application of these indirect methods for the test in infectious anemia, immune sera prepared by injection of materials containing horse protein cannot be used in the direct phase of the reaction, unless the antibody to horse protein is first removed.

Immune sera obtained from our laboratory animals in attempts at transmission of the virus to them, produced surprising results in complement-fixation tests. Many serum samples of rabbits gave positive readings against antigens prepared from the lungs of infected horses. But the same sera also fixed complement with normal and infectious horse blood. These results were not attributable to antibodies to foreign protein (horse blood), since they were noted in tests with sera of rabbits that were injected with rabbit passage material during serial transfers of the virus in them. Similar positive results were recorded when organs, usually lungs, of presumably infected mice were set up as antigens against sera of infectious anemia horses. However, organs of normal mice also fixed complement to lower titers with the same sera. At the time when the experiments on complement-fixation were performed, we regarded these findings as indicating unspecific fixation. But after reviewing all the evidence at present on hand, we are inclined to believe now that the results as outlined above may have more significance than we at first suspected. We shall return to this question in the discussion below.

The unsatisfactory results of complement-fixation tests recorded by other research workers as well as by ourselves may be explained in various ways. One explanation may well be that antigenic materials that were used in the experiments contained too low a concentration of the specific antigen, thus the latter did not reach the threshold value required for good results in any *in vitro* test. In general, viruses comparable in size to the virus of infectious anemia (e.g., poliomyelitis virus) do not readily supply antigens strong enough for complement-fixation tests.

The inconsistency of slight fixation noted in blood samples of the same horse taken at different times can be best explained by assuming that the relative concentration of the antigen, and possibly also that of the specific antibody to the virus, varies from time to time. Therefore, the amounts are not always sufficient to be detected by complement-fixation. In certain phases of the illness, the antigen may be coupled and thus partly neutralized by the antibody, while at other times there may be more free antigen within the blood stream or in some of the organs of the infected animal.

The behavior of the small laboratory animals' sera (particularly the sera of rabbits exhibiting a rather constant serologic response) and the results noted when testing, in combination, acute phase sera of horses and those collected during a later stage of the disease, require special consideration. It is conceivable that in the early phase of the disease an antigenic product is present in the blood of sick horses, probably derived from the erythrocytes attacked by the virus, to which antibodies are produced during the further course of the illness, and that this component has a common counterpart in the blood of other animal species. If so, any blood (or organs containing blood) might have the role of one reactive component in the chain of the serologic reaction. There are in our work indications, to be discussed later, that the course of events may be close to or at least compatible with this description. The working of the serologic test would be then somewhat analogous to the situation as seen in connection with human syphilis. As it is known, the "Wassermann antigen" used in the serologic diagnosis of that disease may be obtained from normal beef heart. If the seemingly conflicting results that we noted in some of the tests are based on a "tissue" antigen, the reaction may not be expected to be strictly specific.

It is possible that more concentrated and, in particular, purified antigens may lead to a complement-fixation test at least for immunologic studies in the laboratory, even though its practical application for diagnosis of the disease or for identifying virus carriers might be limited. Cultivation of the virus offers the possibility of eventually preparing better antigens.

Moreover, it might be profitable to investigate further the use of lungs and lymph nodes of infected animals collected in the early, acute phase of the disease.

Precipitin Test.—Hughes (178) reported that sera taken from monkeys or humans recently recovered from a severe yellow fever infection contain a precipitin capable of reacting with a precipitinogen present in the blood of monkeys during the acute phase of the illness. The concentration of the latter reflected the severity of the illness, although it was not considered identical with the virus of yellow fever.

Adopting the technique of Hughes, we made some precipitin tests with sera of our experimental horses. Into a narrow serologic test tube, 0.2 cc. of the serum to be tested for the presence of precipitins was pipetted; then graded twofold dilutions of the acute phase serum (antigen) were prepared in saline, and 0.5 cc. of each dilution was carefully layered on the top of the test serum. Readings were taken after the tubes had stood in the incubator for 120 minutes. Formation of a ring-like precipitate at the contacting surface of the two layers was regarded as a positive reaction. Results were expressed in the highest dilution of antigen that would bring about the formation of a precipitate.

Many combinations were tried. Some early serum samples gave good reactions, while others did not. Considerable difference was noted also in the behavior of sera from later bleedings tested against the same antigen. Many tests were performed in which a serum sample (Horse 4) taken at the peak of the first marked fever attack served as antigen.

No definite conclusions could be drawn from the positives in the tests. However, the impression gained was that a positive precipitin test would first occur about the time of the second fever attack. Titers ran as high as 1:1280 or higher. In later stages of the disease the positivity declined. No direct correlation was noted with the albumin-globulin ratio or the gamma globulin content of the sera tested.

A number of false positive tests were seen. In some instances a precipitate would form at the juncture of the liquids upon the addition of saline instead of diluted antigen. Naturally, such sera gave a false positive reaction at any dilution of the antigen used for testing. This phenomenon was probably connected with the altered colloid stability of the sera in question. The sera of some horses (often the normal sample also) would give positive reactions from the very beginning of the experimental infection, when tested against an early phase serum. We were not able to discover the reason for these unspecific positive results.

No explanation of the precipitin test will be attempted here, as the data collected are not sufficient for an analysis. The preliminary work was discontinued because of the questionable value of the conflicting results.

Sedimentation Rate of Erythrocytes

The sedimentation rate of the red blood corpuscles was suggested for diagnostic purposes in infectious anemia by Noltze (323). He adapted the technique used in connection with human diseases to larger amounts of horse blood (25 cc.) and concluded that an evenly accelerated settling out of red cells is diagnostic, or at least highly suggestive of infectious anemia. Kuhn (228) and Lührs (268) disputed Nolze's conclusions on the grounds that several other diseases may produce the same phenomenon, while some infectious anemia cases, particularly during remissions, would not show an accelerated sedimentation. Schermer and co-workers (387), on the other hand, considered the test as a useful aid, if used in combination with hematologic tests and protein determinations. Later, many authors contributed to a proper evaluation of the test (149,234,251,293, 321,330,343).

In this country, Hammersland and co-workers (150) and also Griffin and Brose reported on increased sedimentation rates in infectious anemia. The former investigators utilized Cutler's technique and noted on citrated blood an average sedimentation of 18 mm. in normal horses, while infectious anemia cases showed an average of 26 mm. On account of the different technique they used, their values cannot be compared with ours. Since many factors including the anticoagulant, the instruments used, and the timing of reading the results, etc., exert a definite influence on the numerical values recorded in the sedimentation test, only such results as were obtained with identical techniques can be compared (Nichols).

Gilman (135), who investigated the sedimentation rate in this laboratory on our experimental horses, used oxalated blood samples and tested them within two hours of collection under strictly uniform conditions by a somewhat modified Westergren technique, which is widely employed for studying the sedimentation in human diseases. Readings were made at 10, 15, 20, 30, 45, and 60 minutes, recording the fall of erythrocytes in millimeters. The sedimentation rate was compared with the hematocrit values and it was found that in acute cases there is a fairly good correlation between the two. Increase of the sedimentation rate largely paralleled the drop in the red cell volume. When the mean sedimentation rate per ten minutes (SR/10) was calculated according to van Zijl from the readings at 30 and 60 minutes and the values were corrected for an average red cell volume of 42 per cent, no significant changes were found in these calculated figures during the course of the acute stage of the disease. From this Gilman concluded (135) that the changes in sedimentation rate in this particular phase of the disease were largely due to changes in red cell volume. According to the present concept of the nature of increased sedimentation rate, alterations in the plasma proteins are the main factors responsible for the phenomenon, particularly the increase in the fibrinogen and globulin components. These changes seem to run parallel with the decrease of the red cell volume (hematocrit) in acute infectious anemia.

In general, our findings in connection with the changes in the sedimentation rate during the course of infectious anemia suggest that the readings can be used (without correction), in conjunction with the clinical diagnosis, for judging the activity of the infection prognostically. But the behavior of the sedimentation rate can neither prove, nor rule out a diagnosis. We shall here summarize the observations on general trend as seen in our experimental horses.

TABLE 3

SEDIMENTATION RATE OF ERYTHROCYTES IN INFECTED HORSES

Days foll. infection	*Horse 29 (acute case)*						*Horse 22 (subacute case)*					
	Temp. F°	*R.B.C. mill.*	*Sedimentation in* 10	20	30	60	*Temp F°*	*R.B.C. mill.*	*Sedimentation in* 10	20	30	60
			minutes						*minutes*			
(before)		7.8	2	11	33	88	99.4	8.6	3	9	19	55
4	100.0	7.1	5	31	64	105	99.6	9.0	3	47	73	86
6	102.2	7.4	3	29	65	108	99.2	9.1	4	33	76	96
11	99.8	5.6	13	55	96	125	103.4	7.1	26	92	103	111
16	104.8	5.8	21	95	118	125	99.0	6.3	26	65	83	104
20							101.2	7.6	13	38	60	89
24							101.4	7.4	30	57	72	89
30							103.4	6.6	14	43	61	90
36							104.4	6.5	6	22	42	74
42							104.0	6.8	14	35	54	85
50							103.0	4.5	28	97	113	127

Individual variation of the sedimentation rate in normal horses covers a fairly wide range; therefore, no strictly valid figures can be given for all horses. The sedimentation is much more rapid in horse blood than in that of most domestic animals or of humans. In 10 minutes, values are reached with horse blood equaling those noted at about 60 minutes with human blood. By using the above-mentioned method, the large majority of normal horses presented a sedimentation rate of 2 to 12 mm. in readings at the end of 10 minutes, while in 20 minutes the range was from 10 to 60 mm., and at 60 minutes between 15 and 90 mm. If extreme values are noted temporarily in a seemingly normal horse, the animal must be considered as not in normal condition.

The sedimentation rate in our infected horses varied considerably. Generally, during or even before the first marked fever attack, the sedimentation rate would increase and readings from about 20 to 50 would be noted in 10 minutes, while after 30 minutes the range was between 50 and 130 mm. These were the readings most often observed, but deviations were not infrequent. Table 3 illustrates some of the readings obtained in an acute (Horse 29) and a subacute case (Horse 22) during a typical course of experimental infectious anemia. Horse 29 was observed for a total of 18 days following infection. The figures as shown in the table represent direct readings expressed in millimeters.

The extensive investigations carried out on our horses indicate that in cases of longer duration no strict rules seem to exist. In some of the chronic cases the sedimentation rate would remain in about the normal range even during fever attacks. The same applied also to the horses that failed to exhibit anemia following challenge inoculation. Others would show a definite increase in the sedimentation rate early in the course of the disease and, in spite of an apparent recovery, the sedimentation rate would remain at a relatively high level suggesting that the pathologic condition of the animal did not sufficiently balance in spite of seemingly improved clinical health. Such animals would, sooner or later, experience an unexpected flare up of symptoms. Taking our results as a whole, it may be said that an increased sedimentation rate is a regular feature in acute and subacute cases; not so, however, in the chronic stage of the disease, when the sedimentation rate either would run largely parallel to the activity of the infection or would remain within or close to the normal range in spite of clinical symptoms, as mentioned already.

We were not able to determine in our experimental animals whether the sedimentation rate would increase under strenuous labor in chronic cases or virus carriers, because our horses were not worked or exercised. Attempts have been made in the past to use the sedimentation test for screening herds in order to eliminate latent infectious anemia cases. However, it must be remembered that there have been reports (149,234,385), confirmed by our investigations, that the sedimentation test often fails, particularly during remissions and in asymptomatic virus carriers.

In view of the fact that also other disease conditions may show an increased sedimentation rate of the erythrocytes, the test is not well suited to decide alone the differential diagnosis in infectious anemia (228,268). According to Lamarre (234), Panisset (343), and Oppermann (330), the sedimentation can be used for differentiating infectious and parasitic anemia. This is apparently not always the case. Schermer and co-workers (385,387) stated that accelerated sedimentation may be observed in parasitic anemia as well, but in the latter condition no relative lymphocytosis is present, while it is often noted in subacute or chronic infectious anemia.

Lemétayer (251) pointed out that serum horses exhibited a definite increase of sedimentation rates following injections of antigenic material to them during the process of hyperimmunization. This observation fits well into the present concept about the mechanism of accelerated sedimentation of corpuscular elements, which is generally believed to be the result of alterations in the relative concentration of plasma proteins, causing the erythrocytes to clump and settle faster than under normal conditions.

The findings of Knisely and his collaborators (810) tend to show that an increased sedimentation *in vitro* is not equivalent to agglutination *in vivo*. Intravascular agglutination of the latter type (sludged blood) was demonstrated by them experimentally in certain pathologic conditions (33,207). It is conceivable, that a similar *in vivo* hemagglutination takes place temporarily in certain phases of infectious anemia. (See Chapter 8.)

In our opinion, an increased sedimentation of the erythrocytes cannot be considered a diagnostic test for infectious anemia, but it might add pertinent information in diagnosed cases as to the status of the infection. It may be used for supporting the clinical diagnosis in early cases, provided other conditions, which may produce a similar increase, can be ruled out.

Colloid Stability Tests

The pathologic condition of a horse suffering from infectious anemia is reflected in qualitative and quantitative alterations of the colloids present in the liquid portion of its blood. The changes which occur in the relative amount of the protein fractions, lipids, etc., exert an influence on the stability of the various colloids suspended in the blood fluid. Several authors have attempted to use these pathologic changes of the blood serum or plasma as an aid in the diagnosis of infectious anemia. It is to be assumed that none of them would be specific; nevertheless they may serve as supporting evidence for confirming the diagnosis. A great number of colloid stability tests were suggested for use, among them the so-called sublimate test, the dependability of which was widely discussed.

Tests based on the lipid content of infectious horse serum were suggested by several workers. However, Richters (368) stated that a Meinicke-type lipid binding test gave positive reaction in some cases of infectious anemia, but it was not considered specific. Mócsy (296) compared as many as eight stability tests and noted that none of them gave results reliable for practical diagnosis. Wittfogel (489) and also Member and coworkers (285) found elevated cholesterol values during fever attacks in infectious anemia. As a contrast to this, the cholesterol content was found to decrease during the hyperimmunization of serum production horses (Lemétayer (251)).

Boshyan (42) concluded that while the protein level decreased, the nucleic acid and polypeptid content of the plasma increased during fever attacks. On this ground he devised a colorimetric test that was supposedly 90 per cent accurate in detecting infectious anemia cases. His findings were not confirmed and the results were not duplicated by others. Further tests which were suggested for use in infectious anemia are the inhibition test of saponin-hemolysis (Abderhalden and Frei (2)), and the formol-gelatine test. Lührs (264), Lehnert (244), and Slagsvold (412) stated that the saponin test is of little value for diagnostic purposes, while Wittfogel

(490) concluded that the formol-gelatine test can be used as an aid in diagnosis, but it is not specific. Although based on the serum colloids, the colorimetric test and the saponin-hemolysis test are not devised to probe the stability.

Recently, Leemann (242) described a simple test in which cadmium sulfate solution is used for studying the colloid stability of horse serum. Based upon a similar test used in human medicine, it was considered by Leemann as a supplementary aid in the diagnosis of suspected infectious anemia cases.

Another method often used to investigate the colloid stability is the Fulton test. Originally devised by Bennett and Kenny for the diagnosis of trypanosomiasis in camels, Fulton (129) adapted it for use in infectious anemia. According to him the serum of healthy horses gives a precipitation with solutions of mercuric chloride (sublimate) in dilutions of 1:20,000, but not with weaker solutions. On the other hand, the serum of horses afflicted with equine infectious anemia gave a positive reaction with dilutions of mercuric chloride up to 1:100,000. The mechanism of the reaction is based on alterations in the serum proteins. The value of the test as a diagnostic aid has since been considered by a number of authors, as Urbain et al. (464), Lemétayer (249), Oppermann (329), Hecke (156), Hillmer (162), Hamerski (149), Derrick (80), and others. Many considered the reaction nonspecific, or misleading (80,156,162); some infectious anemia horses have been shown to give a negative reaction (149,156, 329), usually the symptomless carriers. On the other hand, positive reactions have been observed in clinically healthy horses (464), in horses hyperimmunized to produce therapeutic sera (249), and in horses with equine encephalomyelitis (80) and strangles (464). In cases of parasitic anemia the test was found negative (464).

As expected, none of the serum colloid stability tests can be considered specific for equine infectious anemia. Nevertheless, they may furnish information of value for proper critical evaluation of other data.

Albumin-Globulin Ratio of Blood Serum

Since it is known from the histopathologic findings that the liver is seriously affected in infectious anemia, we conducted a detailed study of the blood proteins because of the role the liver plays in the protein metabolism. The relative amounts of the two main groups of proteins present in the serum were determined in the experimental horses. It was expected that the determination of the albumin-globulin ratio would be helpful in the diagnosis, as it is in some human diseases, and might furnish useful information concerning the disease process, particularly with regard to the development of debility, emaciation, and edema.

It has been known for some time that blood proteins undergo changes and globulins increase during the disease (244,381). Schermer (384) suggested that the hyperglobulinemia can be used, along with the hematologic findings, as a criterion in the differential diagnosis. In two carefully studied cases of infectious anemia he noted globulin values of over 80 per cent of the total protein, as against the normal figure of approximately 50 per cent. He probably used Howe's method for determination of the globulins, which gives a higher albumin-globulin ratio than is obtained with more recent methods.

Howe's technique applied 23 per cent sodium sulfate concentration for salting out the globulins and it was in general use until recently. Careful comparison of the chemical and physico-chemical methods has shown that a practically complete precipitation of the globulins can be achieved only at a 26 per cent saturation with sodium sulfate; this will furnish results that are in fairly close agreement with those obtained by electrophoresis analysis (203). Using such recently developed methods, we obtained values of serum protein fractions comparable to those given by electrophoresis (81); these deviate significantly from the figures recorded by the use of older techniques (73,381,384), working with 23 per cent sodium sulfate.

Part of the findings, mainly the ones noted in acute cases of infectious anemia, have been published from this laboratory by Gilman (136) with a detailed description of the methods. In the studies on which our present report is based, the total protein was determined by a slightly modified Greenberg procedure (690) through the addition of a 10 per cent sodium hydroxide solution and Folin's phenol reagent to the properly diluted horse serum; the blue color thus developed was read in a Klett-Summerson photoelectric colorimeter standardized by the use of known tyrosine solutions. For determination of the serum albumin, the globulins were precipitated at 26 per cent sodium sulfate saturation and filtered, both at incubator temperature. The amount of albumin in the clear filtrate was then determined in the colorimeter after the addition of Folin's phenol reagent and sodium hydroxide as above. The globulin was calculated by subtracting the value of albumin from that of the total protein. The proportion of albumin to globulin was calculated and expressed as A/G, that is, albumin-globulin ratio (136).

Recent data taken from the literature (81,82), as well as our own results, indicate that the globulin fraction constitutes the greater part of serum proteins in normal horse blood. In normal horses with a total serum protein of 6.0 to 8.5 grams per 100 cc. the globulin fraction amounts to about 4 to 5 grams per 100 cc. that is approximately twice the figure given for albumin. The normal A/G ratio in our horses before experimental infection as well as in a group of other healthy horses generally ranged between 0.5 and 0.8. In a few instances values of 0.8 to 1.0 were noted.

A detailed analysis of the results from more than 400 serum samples of experimentally infected horses is not warranted; instead, a brief summary of the pertinent findings will be presented. Gilman (136) published an account of several acute cases in our series. It may be said generally that a significant decrease of the albumin-globulin ratio was observed in the serum of infected horses during the acute and subacute stage. This was brought about by a primary drop of the albumin level, closely followed by a marked rise in the globulin fraction. A slight decline in the ratio may be noted as early as the 9th or 10th day following infection, then, as a rule, a very marked decrease occurs between the 14th and 23rd day of infection. The lowered ratio is maintained through the active phase of the disease. As the illness progresses, the *A/G* ratio progressively declines.

In the majority of our horses infected for passage of the virus, a decreased ratio of 0.45 to 0.20 was found within the first three weeks of infection, and values as low as 0.12 or 0.10 were seen in some cases. Such horses manifested debility and considerable loss of weight. In chronic cases the ratio either fluctuated at a somewhat decreased level or returned to the lower normal range, with only slight drops from time to time coincident with the relapses. A well-balanced, symptomless carrier produced *A/G* values which did not differ from those obtained in normal horses.

During the experimental immunization with organ suspensions, an early decline of the *A/G* ratio was noted in one animal (Horse 25); when challenge inoculation was attempted, this horse first exhibited a transient increase in the ratio followed later by a marked drop. Another animal similarly treated (Horse 30) did not show a decreased *A/G* ratio when receiving the first few doses of vaccine; but when the horse received the second group of immunizing injections and following challenge inoculation the ratio dropped. It is not certain whether the early reactions were due to eventual subclinical infection by the vaccine used, or to the vaccine as such having provoked the production of antibody globulins.

It may be added that egg culture materials, presumably containing infectious anemia virus (Chapter 11), only slightly influenced the *A/G* ratio in the serum of recipient horses. On the other hand, virus that was carried in serial mouse passages, when injected to horses, brought about a marked drop of the ratio from 0.61 to 0.35 in 22 days (Horse 10), and from 0.47 to 0.29 in 39 days (Horse 15), respectively.

As already mentioned, the numerical values of albumin-globulin ratio recorded in the literature were obtained with a different technique, therefore they are not directly comparable with our results; but they indicate the same general trend. Schermer (381) noted a physiologic increase in the relative amount of globulins in hard working horses; other horses on a starvation diet also showed a relative globulin increase in their sera, while the total protein remained within normal limits (meaning a decrease in the *A/G* ratio), but the alteration was not as marked as in infectious anemia. Furthermore, he found that in chronic infectious anemia cases the relative percentage of the globulin fraction was, in average, one and one-half times higher than the average in 30 normal horses. It is conceivable that infection, hard work, and poor diet may act together in some field cases to produce an extremely low value of A/G ratio.

The diagnostic value of the albumin-globulin ratio is, naturally, limited because of the close to normal values often recorded in chronic cases. On the other hand, a marked decrease of the ratio during the acute and subacute stage is quite regularly observed, and seems to be an integral part of infectious anemia. It must be kept in mind, however, that similar changes occur also in other conditions associated with liver damage.

Liver Function Tests

Serious impairment of the liver function can be detected by liver function tests performed on the serum of patients. A great selection of such tests are used in human medicine (48), but they cannot be applied to horse serum without adaptation because of the differences in the composition of human and horse blood.

The various liver function tests that yield information concerning certain types of hepatic lesion do not, as a rule, disclose early and mild pathologic changes, since the liver can maintain its function with only a small part of relatively intact liver tissue and also because of the great regenerative capacity of the liver. Thus, some of the liver function tests, if definitely positive, usually indicate an extensive liver damage.

Within the scope of the present studies, an attempt was made to use two types of liver function tests. 1) Among the precipitation tests, the thymol turbidity test was selected. When positive, this was found to indicate very severe liver damage (136). 2) One of the flocculation tests, Hanger's cephalin-cholesterol test (151), was studied in some detail; it gave satisfactory results, after adaptation for testing horse sera, considerably more diluted than in the case of human serum, and if a suitable pH was maintained (137).

By testing a large number of normal and infectious anemia sera in this laboratory, Gilman (137) observed that the modified cephalin-cholesterol test became positive between the first and second marked fever attacks and usually remained so during the acute, subacute, and chronic phase of the experimentally induced disease, indicating that an impairment of the liver function is a regular part of the infectious process. The delicate test, the reading of which requires some experience, was regarded positive when three- or four-plus flocculation occurred in a dilution of 1:85 or higher. The dilution is expressed in a relationship of the amount of serum to the cephalin-cholesterol emulsion present in each test tube.

Both, the thymol turbidity test and the cephalin-cholesterol flocculation test, are known to indicate parenchymal liver damage in humans (48,204). The latter seems to be the more sensitive of the two when used as suggested for horse serum (136,137). It is noteworthy that it gave consistently positive results in one of our experimentally infected horses (Horse 10, a chronic case) that, although suffering a few relapses, was in good health for long periods of time. The liver was apparently so much damaged that its function remained impaired. It remains to be seen by future studies whether balanced, symptomless carriers (with no relapses) would behave in the same way. If so, the test may help in picking out suspect virus carriers from a group of horses, provided that other chronic conditions associated with liver damage can be ruled out.

Obviously, neither of these liver function tests can be considered as specific for infectious anemia. Nevertheless, they can contribute to following the course of the disease and understanding the mechanism of the infection.

Various Chemical Components of the Blood

Chemical constituents of the blood other than proteins were also studied by several investigators, but none of them revealed changes of diagnostic significance. Wright (493) found the iron content of blood and spleen decreased. Hammersland and co-workers (150) determined the urea nitrogen, dextrose, chloride, calcium, phosphorus, and iron content of the blood serum in infectious anemia and compared the values with those of normal horses. The average values showed a significant difference only in the iron and calcium content. In the infected group, iron was lowered while the calcium was elevated. The former probably has some relationship to hemosiderosis in various organs, while the latter can be explained by changes in the blood proteins and their inter-relationship to calcium and phosphorus content as described by Craige and Gadd (73). The average values for blood sugar were somewhat diminished in the anemia group (150). An apparently detailed study on chemistry and physico-chemistry of the serum in infectious anemia was published by Lay (240), but it was not accessible to us either in original, or in abstract form.

In our work, calcium determinations did not reveal any unusual changes. The same was true for attempts to follow non-protein nitrogen and blood sugar values. The sodium content of serum and plasma was extensively studied by means of a volumetric method described by Dreguss (91), but aside from some decrease at the final stage of the disease, no alterations beyond the limit of physiological fluctuation were noted in the sodium level.

*

Although there is as yet no specific test for the laboratory diagnosis of infectious anemia, a combination of several tests may render a good service in the diagnosis, if considered in conjunction with a careful clinical observation and repeated hematologic investigations. Histopathologic findings, *post mortem,* can add further data of diagnostic significance, although they are not specific, and liver biopsy may serve to follow the evolution of characteristic pathologic alterations in the liver, while the animal is alive. Methods of laboratory diagnosis, which were not dealt with here (Hematology, Hemagglutination, and Histopathology) are discussed later in subsequent chapters.

Chapter 7

HEMATOLOGY

Descriptions of equine infectious anemia contain many contradictory statements on hematologic findings noted in the condition. This is partly due to the fact that various authors studied the changes of the blood in different stages of the disease and did not take into consideration that the blood picture is constantly changing during the course of the infectious process reflecting, to a certain extent, the systemic response of the organism to the infection. Another possible source of the controversy may well be that the unusual hematologic findings were noted either in anemic horses suffering from mixed infections, or in sick animals with no satisfactory evidence that the anemia observed was in fact caused by the virus of infectious anemia. With the hope of clarifying some of the controversy, and also of collecting basic information about the nature of anemia in this disease, we regularly followed the hematologic changes in most of our experimental horses. Altogether over 600 bleedings were done. In one group, bleedings were performed when required by the particular experiment in progress. In a second group, devoted to a closer study of the hematology, blood samples were taken every second to fourth day or at about weekly intervals.

We shall briefly summarize our findings here, then relate them to those described by other workers, and finally analyze the relative value and eventual practical use of the conclusions derived from these studies. Gilman (134) has published from this laboratory hematologic observations in the acute phase of the disease. In the present analysis based on the total of our data, part of which was collected by Dr. Gilman while he participated in the experimental work, we shall discuss, in addition to findings in the acute stage, those noted in subacute and chronic cases of longer duration.

Methods.—The horses were inoculated with the New Hampshire strain of equine infectious anemia virus. Of the total number of horses used by us for experimentation, complete hematologic studies were performed in twenty animals. Three of these will not be considered here because an interpretation of their values is difficult at this time owing to the type of experiments performed upon them. The rest of the horses received virulent virus, infectious plasma or serum, taken at various stages from our passage animals.

The technique for collecting blood and for making the differential blood smears, total red and white cell counts, hemoglobin and hematocrit determinations, and also the methods of calculating the mean corpuscular hemoglobin, and mean corpuscular volume were identical or similar to those which Gilman (134) referred to and which are in general use in such studies. Total serum protein was determined by a modified Greenberg procedure (690) as mentioned in the previous chapter on Laboratory Diagnosis (p.43). Determinations performed on the blood of individual

TABLE 4

HEMATOLOGIC RESPONSE OF AN ACUTE CASE (HORSE 29)

Days foll. inoc.	*Temp. F°*	*Total Serum Protein*	*R.B.C. million*	*W.B.C. thous.*	*Neutr.*	*Lymph.*	*Mono.*	*Eos.*
					per cent			
(before)	100.2	6.81	7.78	8.55	59	30	2	4
4	100.0	6.58	7.05	6.50	49	35	4	4
5	101.6							
6	102.2	6.90	7.35	6.95	48	35	7	5
9	100.0							
11	99.8	6.84	5.58	7.40	73	19	2	1
15	103.2							
16	104.8	7.86	5.79	5.95	59	20	1	3
18	105.4	7.98	4.51	7.60	47	39	3	0

animals prior to infection were used as controls, in addition to a number of other normal horses tested.

The results of the hematologic investigations will be presented in two groups, those collected on changes in the red blood corpuscles, and the ones related to alterations in the number and relative percentage of the various types of white blood cells. The findings will be grouped according to changes noted in the acute, subacute, and chronic phases of the disease.

Red Blood Corpuscles

Acute Phase.—There is a primary fall in the number of erythrocytes between the second and fifth day after inoculation (Tables 4 and 7). Recovery of approximately one-half of this loss occurs within the next few days. Between the tenth and sixteenth days there is a further fall in the number of red blood corpuscles that usually is accompanied by a marked temperature rise, which in most cases ranges from 102 to 106°F. (Tables 4 and 7). At the time of the first fever attack the average decrease of erythrocytes per cubic millimeter is about 2 to 2 and one-half million. In the interim between the first and second fever attacks, a gradual increase in red cells ensues and the greater part of the original normal value is often attained (Table 7). During the first and second attacks, there is no apparent change in staining qualities, size, or shape of the erythrocytes. After

TABLE 5

HEMATOLOGIC RESPONSE OF A SUBACUTE CASE (HORSE 22)

Days foll. inoc.	*Temp. F°*	*Total Serum Protein*	*R.B.C. million*	*W.B.C. thous.*	*Neutr.*	*Lymph.*	*Mono.*	*Eos.*
					per cent			
(before)	99.4	7.64	8.00	10.02	64	27	3	3
3	99.6	8.16	8.88	5.80	58	30	6	3
5	99.4	9.46	9.04	7.50	59	36	3	2
6	99.2	7.60	9.09	10.50	55	38	4	2
8	99.8	7.52	8.04	8.75	56	36	7	0
9	99.6	6.96	8.64	7.85	57	28	7	5
10	104.2	7.26	7.14	6.70	64	28	3	3
12	103.6	7.12	8.61	8.95	73	20	6	0
13	102.4	7.36	7.51	7.80	80	13	4	0
15	104.0	7.36	7.50	8.15	67	22	3	0
16	99.0	7.44	6.27	7.50	60	24	4	1
17	100.6	7.04	6.95	8.60	62	25	2	0
19	101.2	8.16	7.58	7.40	53	30	8	0
24	101.4	7.92	7.41	14.50	68	21	2	0
29	103.4	7.52	6.59	9.05	76	19	3	0
33	102.0	7.84	6.56	11.40	39	45	9	1
36	104.4	7.84	6.53	10.90	70	15	12	0
42	104.0	6.64	7.20	9.00	69	25	4	0
44	103.6	7.04	6.75	5.60	67	19	8	0
50	103.4	7.68	4.53	7.85	62	28	5	0
60	103.0	8.64	4.54	8.20	71	22	3	1

three or more severe exacerbations, as the case tends to become subacute in nature, a few immature forms, usually normoblasts, are seen.

Table 4 illustrates the findings in a typical acute case during the first 18 days following infection. The temperature was taken twice daily, but only the higher daily reading is given. Horse 29 was injected intravenously with 1 cc. of infectious serum from Horse 25 on April 28, 1950. On the fifth day following infection a mild temperature rise occurred, and a marked fever reaction began on the 13th day; the temperature reached 105.4°F. on the 18th day. At this time the animal was destroyed for another experimental purpose. As may be seen from the table, at the time of the mild temperature rise a slight decrease occurred and by the 11th day the erythrocytes decreased by two million as compared with the normal value. A week later the loss of red blood corpuscles exceeded three million.

Subacute Phase.—When fever attacks occur at longer intervals and are less severe in nature, the loss of red cells proportionately diminishes (Table 7. The total serum protein, although varying little at the fever peaks, exhibits an increase between attacks (Table 6). In the instances in which the fever attacks are marked, a further diminution of the total red cell count occurs at each ensuing fever attack, with less and less reparation (Tables 5 and 6).

TABLE 6

HEMATOLOGIC RESPONSE OF HORSE 33 (SUBACUTE CASE)

Days foll. inoc.	*Temp. F°*	*Total Serum Protein*	*R.B.C. million*	*W.B.C. thous.*	*Hemogl. (gram)*	*Hema-tocrit*	*Neutr.*	*Lymph.*	*Mono.*	*Eos.*
							per cent			
(before)	99.6	7.66	6.71	8.60	13.8	40	59	35	1	5
14	105.6	7.84	4.62	4.95	9.2	24	61	34	1	1
24	99.2	8.05	5.82	9.65	11.6	33	60	32	5	3
27	106.0	7.79	4.46	7.85	10.2	28	67	20	4	1
34	100.9	8.16	3.71	5.90	7.7	22	41	50	5	1
41	101.4	7.34	3.20	8.70	6.3	18	41	49	8	2
65	105.0	7.84	1.41	3.80	3.0	8	60	31	6	0
72	99.8	8.30	2.60	10.85	5.2	15	45	40	11	0

Table 5 demonstrates the values in an experimental horse that was under observation for 60 days after it had received a single inoculation of 1 cc. of virulent virus (infectious serum). It produced three typical fever attacks; the third started on the 36th day following infection and the temperature did not drop below 103°F. until the horse was destroyed on the 60th day. Although the animal exhibited an initial rise and a definite decrease of red blood cells by the 16th day, it did not develop a marked anemia until the 50th day.

The values presented in Table 6 are those recorded after another animal (Horse 33) received a challenge inoculation with a known virulent virus (5 cc. serum). This animal was previously injected twice for experimental purposes with serum pools, but did not show a clinical reaction. After the challenge inoculation the horse had several marked fever attacks usually exceeding 105°F., as may be observed from Table 6. On the 64th day following infection, epistaxis occurred and continued until the horse was destroyed.

Chronic Phase.—As the febrile periods are less frequent and as they diminish in severity, the erythrocyte count often falls only slightly below the normal and the counts between attacks are in most instances within the normal range (Table 7).

Running largely parallel with the changes in the number of erythrocytes, alterations can be noted in the total volume of red blood corpuscles (hematocrit) as determined by strong centrifugation of fresh whole blood after addition of anticoagulants. The hemoglobin content of the blood likewise exhibits marked fluctuations. Some early investigators of infectious anemia laid particular emphasis onto the proportionate or disproportionate diminution of hemoglobin content as compared with the decrease of the number of erythrocytes; some of these authors ascribed diagnostic value to the behavior of the relative amount of hemoglobin. However, we were unable to confirm this in our experimental horses. We shall summarize below our findings related to hematocrit and hemoglobin values as noted in infected horses.

Hematocrit.—Concurrent with the first fall in the number of erythrocytes and hemoglobin, taking place during the first week of the infection, the average hematocrit value drops 6 to 8 per cent and improves in the following days, only to diminish markedly at the onset of the first marked fever attack. In subsequent attacks, a similar pattern is discerned. The hematocrit value at the time of the first attack averaged 29 per cent, whereas the normal average before inoculation was 41 per cent in 15 of our horses (Table 7). During remissions the hematocrit value increases.

Studies dealing with sedimentation rate of the red blood corpuscles, as determined under controlled laboratory conditions on spontaneously sedimenting blood of infected horses, are discussed under methods of laboratory diagnosis (Chapter 6).

Hemoglobin.—In acute phase there is a primary decrease in hemoglobin content between the second and fifth day after inoculation, with an average loss of 1 to 2 grams in 100 cc. of blood. In the next few days there is an average gain of approximately 1 gram. Between the tenth and the sixteenth day of the experimental infection, there is an additional loss of hemoglobin (average 3 grams). In the period between temperature rises, the hemoglobin value increases until it reaches the lower normal range (Table 7). In the majority of our cases, a decrease in hemoglobin content, a fall in the erythrocyte count, and a temperature rise occurred simultaneously.

Mean Corpuscular Hemoglobin, Mean Corpuscular Volume.—When these values were calculated, no significant changes were noted in our experimental horses during the acute phase of the disease, as stated by Gilman (134). With the disease progressing, the rate of corpuscular hemoglobin may increase, evidently to compensate somewhat for the loss of erythrocytes and to promote oxygen transport needed for respiration and metabolism of the tissues. Such a need particularly exists in animals working or being exercised.

White Blood Cells

During the first few fever reactions, the total number of white blood cells decreases, exhibiting values in the lower normal range or a definite leukopenia. The decrease is manifested early during the course of infection, making its initial appearance in most cases during the first week, usually on the third to fifth day following an experimental infection. As a rule a decrease is clearly indicated before or during the first marked fever attack (Tables 4, 5, and 6). At the onset of the fever response, or before, there is a shift in the relative proportion of the lymphocytes and the polymorphonuclear neutrophils: the number of the former diminishes considerably, thus producing a relative increase in the number of the neutrophil leukocytes (Tables 4 and 5). During remissions between the first two or three fever attacks, the total number of white blood cells shows a tendency to return to the normal values; this is often accompanied by a transient relative lymphocytosis.

TABLE 7

AVERAGE OF HEMATOLOGIC VALUES IN 15 EXPERIMENTAL HORSES

	Phase of Infection	*Temp. F°*	*R.B.C. million*	*W.B.C. thous.*	*Hemogl. (gram)*	*Hematocrit*	*Neutr.* per cent	*Lymph.* per cent	*Mono.* per cent	*Eos.* per cent
	(Normal)	99.6	7.5	8.6	13.6	41	57	35	2	3
Acute cases	2 - 5 Days Foll. Inf.	100.7	6.8	6.9	12.8	35	51	40	2	2
Acute cases	1st Fever Attack	105.8	5.8	6.0	9.8	29	67	24	2	0
Acute cases	Remissions	99.7	7.2	9.1	13.3	38	63	28	4	2
Subacute	At Fever Attacks	104.3	3.9	8.2	10.5	32	60	32	3	1
Subacute	Remissions	99.9	5.8	8.9	11.8	34	52	38	5	1
Chronic cases	At Fever Attacks	102.6	5.1	9.8	11.3	34	58	30	3	2
Chronic cases	Remissions	100.6	6.9	9.0	12.6	36	45	41	8	2

In more advanced stages of the disease, the relative lymphocytosis remains a fairly constant feature of the blood picture. During relapses in subacute or chronic cases a reduction may be observed in their relative number, but this is not as pronounced as in the early, acute phase of the infection.

Some symptomless and well-balanced virus carriers show practically normal values in their differential white cell counts. On the other hand, some chronic cases which, following very much prolonged remissions, produce relapses from time to time may exhibit a fairly constant relative lymphocytosis. It is probably for this reason that, in the past, lymphocytosis was considered by some observers pathognomic of infectious anemia. There are descriptions in the literature, in which the correctness of infectious anemia diagnosis was criticized because of the low percentage of lymphocytes recorded in the condition. Careful observers, however, expressed the view that, simultaneously with the decrease of the red blood corpuscles, lymphopenia occurs during fever attacks (11,116,252,89).

Our experience indicates that this is true for the first few fever attacks, but later the decrease of the lymphocytes during relapses is, in most instances, insignificant, especially following prolonged afebrile remissions.

Long-standing chronic cases, manifesting clinical symptoms time and again, generally exhibit a relative lymphocytosis with little tendency to a decrease in spite of fever relapses. This may be illustrated by the hematologic findings in one of our experimental horses. In this animal (Horse 10), while it exhibited no clinical symptoms whatever for about six months, the average red cell count was 8.1 million, and the average of total white blood cell counts 9,700 in 18 bleedings performed in the afebrile period. During the same time in the same bleedings, an average of 39 per cent lymphocyte was counted in the differential blood smears. This horse has had several fever relapses afterwards, for about five months; in this period the lowest erythrocyte and white blood cell counts recorded were 6.6 million, and 6.300, respectively. However, the lymphocytosis remained unaffected during this time, as 12 differential counts gave an average of 36 per cent lymphocytes.

The lymphocytosis, as seen in most chronic cases, is not quite stable, there is a fluctuation of the values up and down. In our experimental animals the highest lymphocyte count was 60 per cent in the records; in general, values over 40 per cent were often noted in chronic cases. It must be added—as already mentioned—that symptomless virus carriers may show normal hematologic values, indicating that an equilibrium of the infectious process is reached in such carriers.

A definite decrease in the number of eosinophils was regularly observed during fever reactions particularly in the acute stage, but in most cases also during relapses of the subacute and chronic cases. After fever attacks their number reached the normal level again. In Horse 10 a normal eosinophil count was revealed averaging 3 per cent during the six-month symptomless period mentioned above. When fever relapses occurred later, the eosinophils disappeared or decreased to 1 per cent several times.

The number of monocytes often increases during remissions following a few fever attacks (Tables 6 and 7).

Immature, young forms of the neutrophil granulocyte series are not recorded in the tables; usually neutrophilic metamyelocytes and staff cells, rarely myelocytes are sometimes seen in cases of prolonged duration and frequent exacerbations. In our cases, as in most findings recorded in the literature, very little tendency was noted in the differential counts toward a shift to the left.

Occasionally, leucocytosis was noted in the horses in a range of 11,500 to 15,800. No correlation could be detected between these relatively rare values, making about 5 per cent of all total white blood cell counts, and the symptoms of the disease. It is our impression that such higher values were more common in horses with a tendency to become chronic cases, and also in the ones receiving several injections in attempted immunization. Whether they indicate an increased reactivity of the hematopoietic system, or an easier mobilization of the white blood cells, is an undecided question.

In brief, our findings indicate that, beside the fluctuating decrease and increase in the number of the erythrocytes, a tendency to leukopenia and, later, a general trend to relative or absolute lymphocytosis can be noted during the disease process. However, it is difficult to set solid rules, as the blood picture is constantly changing. The findings in our horses concur, in general, with those obtained by most investigators reporting about the blood changes. There are, however, some differences between our findings and those recorded in the literature, especially with respect to the severity of the alterations, which we shall discuss later.

*

It was early recognized that anemia is a regular symptom of the typical disease (256), as may be seen from the names used in various countries to designate the condition; it was considered characteristic of the disease by all of the early investigators. Lignée (256), who first described infectious anemia as a clinical entity, referred to the condition as *anhémie du cheval.* Zschokke (498) and Ostertag (337) used the name "pernicious anemia of horses," indicating that they assumed some analogy between the human disease and that of the horse. Torrance (456) observed marked anemia in cases of swamp fever in Canada, but he emphasized that poikilocytosis was never seen in those horses.

Carré and Vallée (58) reported that, in their experimental horses, the drop in the number of the red blood cells preceded the fever reaction as the first sign of the disease. On the 10th to 16th day following infection, they noted a decrease by one and one-half to two million against the normal number of red blood cells, setting the latter at 7 million. In acute cases there was a further decrease until death of the animal ensued, while cases of longer duration showed values as low as about one million per cubic millimeter. During remissions an increase was observed; this, however, did not reach the level of the original normal values. They also recorded a slight decrease in the number of white blood cells and remarked that the lymph glands were always involved in the process, showing hyperemia and slight hemorrhages in acute cases and a marked swelling in the chronic phase; enlargement of the spleen was also present in most of their cases.

Other investigators soon confirmed and extended the findings reported by Carré and Vallée. Studying equine anemia in the United States, Mack (271) stated that the decrease in the number of red blood cells occurred gradually and reached low values similar to those recorded by the French investigators; the total number of the white blood cells remained in the normal range or decreased slightly. Kinsley (205) has presented a good description of the changes in the blood. He studied not only the behavior of the red cells, but also the alterations in the differential count of the white blood cells. Van Es and associates (470) were struck by the regular presence of a marked anemia in field cases and its rather uncommon occurrence in cases in which the disease was experimentally produced.

Seyderhelm (405) recorded observations similar to those of Van Es and co-workers and expressed the view that the equine disease is closely related to pernicious anemia in man. Wirth (487) did not concur with this opinion, as he had not observed anisocytosis in equine infectious anemia; therefore, he considered it a severe type of anemia with no relation to human pernicious anemia. Jaffé (188) concluded from his careful histologic studies that the bone marrow is not primarily involved in the equine disease, but may show signs of reaction in very severe, prolonged cases; he found the main cause of anemia in an injury to the red blood cells and in their massive destruction during fever attacks. Seyderhelm (405) described the hematologic picture both in the circulating blood and in the organs. He found in the blood stream no indication of an increased hematopoiesis but observed, at the same time, markedly reddened bone marrow along with myeloid changes in the secondary blood-forming organs; he noted all stages of erythropoiesis and leukopoiesis in the liver and the spleen of infected horses. His conclusion that the condition is related to human pernicious anemia was not accepted by others. Most authors agree now that there is no direct relationship between the two diseases, a view expressed by Hutyra and Marek (180) as early as 1910. Dobberstein (84) related that in the equine disease no alterations can be noted in the shape of the red blood cells; he concluded from this that the anemia is not caused by the primary action of the virus exerted on the hematopoiesis.

For the unusual findings of some investigators (poikilocytosis, elevated color index, etc.), two explanations may be offered. One of them is that the changes noted in a very much prolonged stage of the disease may differ considerably from the typical blood picture, most likely on account of the exhaustion of the blood-forming organs. The other possibility is that the controversial hematologic findings were noted in horses with mixed infection (page 24); this is frequently found in the temperate zone and is probably quite common in tropical regions.

Normoblasts and other immature forms of the erythrocyte series are seldom found in the blood even in prolonged cases. Lührs (264) stated that in hundreds of differential counts made on blood of infectious anemia horses, normoblasts were noted in a single instance only. We saw nucleated red blood cells in two of our experimental horses; one of them (Horse 4) had a red cell count of 2.5 million when this was recorded during the 9th prolonged fever attack. In earlier blood smears of the same horse no normoblasts were noted.

Marek (275) stated in 1921 that the volume of the packed cells (hematocrit), which amounts to from 40 to 50 per cent in normal horses, drops considerably in the early stage of infectious anemia.

Although statements have been made to the contrary, it would seem that the hemoglobin decrease largely follows the decline in the number of the red blood cells (493, 134). The resistance of the erythrocytes, as measured in solutions of different osmotic strength, was found to be generally increased (560, 317, 261). On the other hand, there is also observation on record that it decreases during the fever paroxysm (11).

Leukopenia and a decrease or disappearence of eosinophils during fever attacks was mentioned in the early reports (456, 58, 205). There was a divergence of opinion for a considerable time as to the relative participation in the decrease, or increase, by the lymphocytes and the polymorphonuclear neutrophils, but the dispute may at present be considered settled (11, 250, 149, 116). The findings vary according to the phase of infection, as briefly discussed on page 54. Variations are noted also in the reaction exhibited by individual animals.

Similarly, the degree of anemia as noted in individual horses varies considerably. From the normal figures the red cell count may progressively go below one million (58, 11, 317, 250). There are some differences according to countries and authors in what is considered normal value. Scarborough collected the data published by 23 authors on normal horses; the average found in 318 counts was 7.8 million RBC (red blood corpuscles). It is known that the values in thoroughbred horses are considerably higher: according to a study recently published by Hansen and co-workers (153) in America, the average red cell count in 65 thoroughbred mares was found to be 10.5 million.

In our horses the average normal count noted was 7.5 million RBC (Table 7). The lowest figure that we recorded in our investigations was 1.4 million, and the average of the *lowest* values in 20 infected horses sufficiently well studied was 4,150,000 RBC. This indicates that the cases on which we are reporting may be considered less severe than the average field cases, probably because our experimental horses were not worked and were kept under optimum conditions.

Concerning the *nature of anemia,* it may be said that the disease cannot be classified as one of the more common anemias. According to a widely used classification (216), the anemias form two large classes: 1) the anemias due to blood loss and destruction, characterized by hyperactivity of the bone marrow, and 2) anemias due to decreased blood production with hypoactivity of the bone marrow. A further classification is based on size and hemoglobin content of the red blood corpuscles: the common deficiency anemias are usually microcytic and hypochromic, while pernicious anemia is characterized by macrocytic, hyperchromic cells.

In our infected experimental horses the erythrocytes appeared normal in size, shape, and staining qualities; accordingly, the anemia is normocytic, and normochromic in its general character. This is in line with the experience of the large majority of other investigators in this field. The anemia is chiefly due to an excessive destruction of the red blood cells (188) indicated by the marked hemosiderosis in the liver (*see* Fig. 9 on page 128). Still it does not completely fit into the first class as mentioned above. It cannot be listed among the so-called secondary anemias, neither can it be grouped with the hemolytic anemias, and it is not related in its pathogenesis to human pernicious anemia. With this negative characterization, equine infectious anemia must be placed in a separate subgroup of its own. There is a possibility that anemias of somewhat similar behavior reported to occur in sheep and goats (90, 662) and in cattle (87) might have a relationship to the equine disease.

It is often difficult to differentiate infectious anemia from other types of anemia that are fairly common in some countries. In Sweden, Finland, and Switzerland nutritional anemia seems to occur side by side with genuine infectious anemia in certain regions. Huguenin (179) considered many of the anemia cases in Switzerland as a deficiency disease due to undernourishment. Krupski and associates (224, 226) believed that most of the equine anemias noted in Switzerland are of streptococcus origin; Keller (194) has shown by experiments that transmissible and nontransmissible anemias exist, while Steck (415, 418) maintains that equine infectious anemia is widespread in Switzerland. Svanberg (443) considers the soil and vegetation responsible for the noncontagious anemias in Sweden. Laurell (239) and Carlström and Hjärre (53) also stated that two types of anemia exist in that country, one of them being of nutritional origin. In the latter type the reticulo-endothelial system is not involved (53).

The use of the hematologic findings for the diagnosis has been reviewed by several authors (122, 169, 170, 235, 252, 385). According to Schermer and his co-workers (385, 387) the diagnosis may be ascertained in 70 per cent of the cases by following the changes in the blood regularly.

A systematic study of the blood changes on repeated occasions may be a valuable aid in making a diagnosis, if combined with other laboratory tests and careful clinical observations.

CHAPTER 8

HEMAGGLUTINATION

Hirst (164) discovered in 1941 that cultured influenza virus would cause agglutination of the erythrocytes of the chicken embryo in which the virus was cultivated. When the test was performed with cells of normal chicks, the same phenomenon occurred. The hemagglutination was considered a result of the specific action of the virus. This concept was supported by the fact that a specific influenza immune serum would inhibit the agglutination (165). Since 1941, a number of human and animal viruses have been shown to produce hemagglutination as seen in the Hirst test, e.g., the viruses of variola and vaccinia (52), Newcastle disease (51), mumps, etc.

An attempt was made to develop a similar hemagglutination test in equine infectious anemia. For this purpose one of us began a systematic study of the problem at the early phase of the present investigations during the summer of 1948, and reported the preliminary findings in a note published in 1949 (Dreguss (94)). Before discussing the results of the hemagglutination test and their significance in infectious anemia, an outline of the method will be given and the preliminary findings will be summarized.

Methods and Preliminary Results.—To obtain the chicken red blood cells, normal chickens were bled aseptically by heart puncture or from the wing vein; about an equal volume of 3.8 per cent sodium citrate solution was used as anticoagulant. The red blood cells were washed three times with sterile physiologic salt solution in the centrifuge and a 10 per cent suspension of packed cells was prepared. This stock cell suspension, well stoppered, should be "aged" at room temperature for a few days before use; it will then remain usable for several weeks, if kept at refrigerator temperature under aseptic conditions to prevent contamination.

Small test tubes, 10 mm. wide and 75 mm. long, with round-shaped bottoms are suitable for setting up the test. First, two-fold dilutions of the serum are made (1:10, 1:20, etc.); then to each 0.5 cc. of diluted serum is added an equal volume of 0.3 per cent suspension of the chicken red blood cells freshly prepared in physiologic salt solution from the stock suspension. Proper controls should be included, such as normal serum, a known positive serum, and a red blood cell suspension with no serum added.

In general, the technique similar to that used in hemagglutination tests with the viruses of influenza (165), or Newcastle disease (32), was followed. Reading is done after 60 to 75 minutes standing of the tubes undisturbed at room temperature. If the test is negative, the sedimented cells form a compact, sharply demarcated disc at the bottom of the tubes. Positive hemagglutination is indicated by small clumps of cells finely dispersed throughout the bottom of the tube in an unevenedged wide layer. Results are expressed in terms of the highest dilution of serum or other test material which produces a definite hemagglutination.

As described in the preliminary report (94), all 16 horses that were inoculated with the virus of infectious anemia until the time of the report developed agglutinating substances in their blood for normal chicken red blood cells. Titers were recorded up to serum dilutions of 1:320 during the early stage of the illness, while they decreased somewhat during the subacute stage; a symptomless carrier elicited low titers. For the purpose of control, a number of normal horses were tested. Their sera either did not produce hemagglutination or did so in dilutions of 1:10 to 1:20 only. There were indications that positive results may be obtained in conditions other than infectious anemia. It was assumed at the time of the report that the hemagglutination is caused either (a) by the infectious agent, (b) by antibodies, or (c) by some pathologic compound produced during the course of the disease and present in the blood of infected animals.

From these preliminary findings it seemed worthwhile to pursue further the investigations in two main directions: first to find out whether the hemagglutination can be utilized as a means of diagnosis if a specific inhibition test can be developed; secondly, to clarify the mechanism of the reaction for better understanding and for gaining insight into the infectious process. The results of these efforts will be briefly presented below.

Diagnostic Application of the Hemagglutination Test

First it was assumed that the hemagglutination is analogous to that seen with influenza and other viruses. This assumption had some support in that the severity of the disease appeared to be correlated with the agglutination titer of the serum or plasma of the infected horses. In a few experimental horses that exhibited less pronounced symptoms than the average, the agglutination titer not only developed slowly but never reached as high a level as in the majority of animals. Horse 2, which at first showed marked clinical symptoms and, at the same time, evidenced a high agglutinating titer in its blood serum (up to a dilution of 1:320), became a symptomless virus carrier after a few attacks, and from then on was in robust health, resisting re-infection with large doses of highly virulent virus; coincident with this the original high titer dropped sharply, and soon reached the level considered to be in the normal range.

In order to demonstrate the specific nature of the hemagglutinin, inhibition tests were set up with serum of horses considered as being in the convalescent stage. In general, no specific inhibition was demonstrated by the use of such serum samples, or of any other type of serum or plasma collected in various stages of the disease. The results were contradictory and failed to show any regularity. If inhibition was noted in certain setups, normal serum seemed to produce a similar effect.

It was realized after much unsuccessful effort that the system being tested was too complex. Although acute-stage serum samples were utilized as the source of hemagglutinin (virus?), and later-stage serum samples as inhibitors, theoretically both could contain virus as well as antibody, since horses once infected usually remain lifelong carriers of the virus. Moreover, a specific reaction, if it did occur, would probably be influenced by such side reactions as were seen in the precipitin and colloid stability tests when diluting or mixing normal and pathologic serum samples.

We were confronted with a situation different from the known inhibition tests in which immune sera are tested against cultured virus or, in some instances, clarified supernatants of organ suspensions containing the virus. Most of the inhibition tests in our experiments were performed according to the technique used in influenza work (165) or in Newcastle disease (32). Many modifications of these methods were tried in an effort to overcome the difficulties and eliminate nonspecific reactions; because of the inconclusive results, the details are not given here.

During our experimental studies the hemagglutination test itself was routinely applied to our horses and the changes were closely followed in all of them. There was not a single experimental horse in our series that did not show a rise of hemagglutination titer following infection by an active virus, whether it was a primary infection or a challenge inoculation. Therefore, the conclusion seems to be justified that hemagglutination, using serum or plasma of infected horses and suitable chicken red blood cells, is a regular feature in typical infectious anemia. Thus, a characteristic, even if not quite specific, alteration in the blood of infected horses is strongly suggested. In Table 8 we have summarized the highest titers observed in individual horses receiving primary inoculation of a virulent virus; the day when this titer was noted and the gamma-globulin level, determined simultaneously, are also recorded.

Horses with marked fever attacks during the acute and subacute stage, usually soon developed a high hemagglutination titer that persisted for a longer time, lasting even during remissions of fever, although with a tendency slowly to decrease. In cases of a more chronic nature, the severity of repeated fever attacks was not as closely correlated with the hemagglutination titer of serum: some horses showed a definite rise, while others exhibited only minor changes in the titer during relapses.

If we analyze the titers in horses subjected to experimental immunization, or utilized for testing cultured virus material and virus strains carried through mouse passages, the results are not as uniform as in inoculations with the typical active virus. Three horses (H.24, H.27, and H.28) used in testing chick embryo material in attempted cultivation of the virus elicited an early mild elevation of the titer on the 5th to 8th day following inoculation; about a two- to three-fold rise was noted. A similar slight, early increase was noticed in a few instances following infection with horse passage strains, if frequent bleedings were done. Such titers would decrease before a sharp rise occurs later about at the time of the first marked fever attack.

Such early mild reactions were also noted in horses that received material which had been subjected to mouse passages previously. Even in the third serial passage (Horse 38), made for the purpose of regaining the virulence of the virus to horses, only a very slight increase was recorded in the hemagglutination titer of the serum accompanied by a marked, although delayed, fever attack. The impression was that the cultured virus and the mouse passage strains had lost the ability to provoke a marked hemagglutinin production.

TABLE 8

HEMAGGLUTINATION TEST IN EXPERIMENTALLY INFECTED HORSES
(Primary Inoculation with Virulent Virus)

Horse No.	*Highest titer*	*Day foll. infection*	*Gamma-globulin*	*Note*
Horse 3	1:160	29th	2.43g	
Horse 4	1:240	28th	2.06	
Horse 7	1:160	32nd	*	*Not done
Horse 8	1:80	63rd	1.96	
Horse 16	1:320	17th	2.32	
Horse 17	1:160	20th	2.27	
Horse 20	1:240	27th	2.98	
Horse 22	1:320	29th	2.52	
Horse 26	1:1280	10th	2.21	
Horse 29	1:320	18th	2.35	

Horses inoculated with formalinized organ suspensions for immunization, exhibited fairly high titers in their serum (1:80 to 1:160) during the process of immunization, one of the horses in the early phase (H. 25), another at the later stage of immunization (H. 30). A possible explanation is that the virus was attenuated but not completely inactivated in the vaccine used, thus causing a mild subclinical infection indicated by the positive hemagglutination test.

Following challenge inoculation, the hemagglutination titers showed further increase in all immunized horses, as well as in those injected for testing the egg culture virus. The same was true for horses injected with mouse passage material, if and when they were subjected to challenge inoculation with horse passage virus. As may be seen from Table 9, the peaks of the hemagglutination titers reached after the challenge inoculation are comparable with those noted following primary inoculations. (For more details on these experimental horses, see Chapters 10, 11, and 12.)

To obtain comparative values in horses other than the ones used in our experiments, a considerable number of normal blood samples were tested, in addition to those coming from field cases suspect for infectious anemia, or horses suffering from other diseases.

Normal Blood.—Over 100 normal horse serum samples were tested, including those taken from the experimental horses before inoculation.

TABLE 9

HEMAGGLUTINATION TEST FOLLOWING CHALLENGE INOCULATION

Horse No.	*Highest titer*	*Day following inoculation*	*Gamma-globulin*		*Remarks*
H. 5	1:640	20th	2.64g	Primary inoculation(s):	monkey blood
H. 10	1:320	16th	2.28		mouse material
H. 15	1:320	14th	2.20		mouse material
H. 21	1:640	22nd	2.66		immun. (alum)
H. 24	1:160	15th	1.89		egg culture
H. 25	1:240	21st	2.60		immun. (organ susp.)
H. 27	1:320	23rd	1.94		egg culture
H. 28	1:320	22nd	2.00		egg cult. (passage)
H. 30	1:640	22nd	2.37		immun. (organ susp.)
H. 31	1:160	23rd	2.46		immun. (organ susp.)

The overwhelming majority of both groups either did not produce hemagglutination, or elicited a positive test in a 1:10 dilution only; some possessed a titer of 1:20; these groups comprised about 90 per cent of the normal horses. Thus, hemagglutination in a 1:20 dilution or less was considered as the normal range.

The other 10 per cent of the clinically normal horses showed higher titers (1:40 to 1:80). The question naturally arises, whether they were normal in every respect. Their past history was not known to us: they were usually old horses, and it is entirely possible that a recent illness or some chronic condition—not readily recognizable clinically—was responsible for the positive result. The higher titers observed in the blood of the horses were probably not due to a past infection by the anemia virus, since the disease was not prevalent in the environment from which these animals had come; but it is not quite impossible that some of them were infected previously. Owing to the limited facilities at our disposal, no horse inoculation test could be performed using the blood of these horses to rule out such a possibility, except in connection with crucial experiments. Horses with higher than normal titer were utilized for plain passage of the virus.

Blood of Sick Horses.—Many blood samples were received taken from horses suspected of infectious anemia mainly because of unexplained fever attacks, weakness, and anemia. Hemagglutination was often helpful to clarify the diagnosis, although in some of the field cases it was impossible to follow the case history as, often, no further information or additional blood samples were available. From regions where the disease is known to be prevalent (e.g. in the South), serum samples were sent to us, coming from horses diagnosed on the basis of clinical observations as having infectious anemia. They often exhibited positive hemagglutination of similar titer as seen in horses infected experimentally. Unfortunately, these laboratory results could not be verified by horse inoculation tests; nevertheless, part of these investigations is interesting enough to warrant a brief description.

In 1950, we received 41 blood samples from Florida without any preliminary information about the individual horses. The first 25 blood samples came from one farm: in this group 20 were positive, 4 questionable, and 1 negative by the hemagglutination test. Information received from the veterinarian in charge, after he had learned the results of the hemagglutination test, stated that "these animals are all very eligible for swamp fever. The horses are pasture animals and are in poor condition. Many of these tested animals show severe anemia and five of the horses have clinical symptoms of swamp fever." It may be added that all of the five horses, identified by name, exhibited strongly positive hemagglutination. It was also stated that "six or seven horses have died from clinical swamp fever" during the preceding year on the same farm.

The next 16 blood samples came from a thoroughbred horse farm at which two clinical cases of swamp fever had been observed previously. Four of the samples were positive, although the corresponding animals seemed to be in good health at the time of testing. One horse that, at an earlier date, had shown symptoms suggestive of infectious anemia—but was reported healthy at the time of the test—gave a negative result. When the same animal had an atypical temperature flare-up three months later, blood was received again and, because it showed positive hemagglutination this time, 2 cc. of the serum was injected into a test horse. This horse produced mild fever reactions on the 18th and 25th day following inoculation, but without significant anemia; thus, the result was inconclusive. Challenge inoculation with a known virus strain on the 38th day was followed by marked fever attacks accompanied first by an increase of the red blood cell count to 9.1 million, and later by anemia within a month (5.8 million R.B.C.). Thus, in the Florida group, laboratory findings were in a fairly good agreement with the clinical observations indicating that the hemagglutination test was of practical value in supporting the diagnosis.

Value of Negative Evidence.—As already mentioned (p. 23) repeated tests were made on two horses suspected of having infectious anemia but proved finally to have malignant tumors. The clinical manifestations were

TABLE 10

HEMAGGLUTINATION IN VARIOUS CLINICAL CONDITIONS OF HORSES

Identification	*Hemagglutination Titer*	*Clinical Diagnosis and Observations*
Th. Br. 1	1:80	Anemic since one year; not doing well
Texas H.	1:320	Equine infectious anemia
H. 3003	1:160	Intermittent fever, pale mucous membranes
W. N. C.	1:160	Suspect of equine infectious anemia
H. 2086	1:160	Edema of the abdomen. Anemia
Th. Br. 3	1:80	Lost much weight recently
R. W.	1:80	Jaundice
H. 708	1:160	Epizootic lymphangitis
C. 2	1:320	Infectious abortion
Th. Br. 4	1:160	Temperature elevations, edema of legs
Th. Br. 4	1:20	(Same horse as above, one year later)
C. 4	1:80	Mare; aborted
N. J.	negative	Purpura haemorrhagica
L. Md.	negative	Epidermoid cancer of the stomach
F. S.	negative	Does not use hind legs at turning
Phil.	negative	Healthy animal (check up). Was sick earlier
V. Hosp.	1:10	Chronic heart condition
S. H.	negative	Past contact with infectious anemia case
H. 702	negative	Lost much weight recently
H. 702	negative	Weakness, diarrhoea
H. 806	negative	Sick horse. No closer information
A. S. C.	negative	Brucellosis?
H. 448	1:10	Chronic anemia
V. H.	negative	Anemia following accident
C. 1	negative	Streptococcus anemia
C. 3	1:10	Anemic mare. Aborted
H. 644	negative	Anemia following trauma
B. S.	negative	Aborted two weeks ago. *Salmonella* aggl. pos.
Th. Br. 2	1:20	Mild icterus. Not doing well
F. T.	negative	Lost much weight
W. G.	negative	Disseminated tumor of parench. organs

similar to those of infectious anemia, and fever reactions were noted from time to time; the total protein and the albumin-globulin ratio were considerably lowered. The hemagglutination titer, however, was consistently negative in both animals and the immune-globulin level of the serum remained in the normal range. On the basis of the latter two laboratory tests, we considered the diagnosis as negative for infectious anemia, but the horses were kept on the suspect list on account of the clinical symptoms. The laboratory diagnosis was fully verified by post-mortem findings. The autopsy disclosed, in the first case, a large epidermoid cancer of the stomach extending to the abdominal cavity (post-mortem diagnosis by Dr. J. W. Mills of the Veterinary School, University of Pennsylvania); and disseminated tumor of the liver, lungs, and kidneys in the second case (information received from the veterinarian who observed the case clinically and performed the post-mortem investigation).

In some other instances, where bacterial origin of secondary anemia was established by showing the causative organism or high titer of specific antibodies (Streptococcus-infections, *S. abortus equi,* etc.), it is worthy of note that the chicken red blood cell hemagglutination was either completely negative, or produced a titer of low range.

Table 10 summarizes part of the results obtained with serum samples of horses suspected of infectious anemia or some other disease. Many of these samples were received on request, as it was intended to test blood samples of horses in different pathologic conditions in order to compare the results with those obtained in infectious anemia. Other samples were sent in for diagnostic purposes to confirm or exclude infectious anemia in febrile conditions. The clinical diagnosis as listed in the table must be regarded as tentative in most instances.

According to the experimental results as outlined above, it would seem, as observed in the preliminary report (94), that a negative outcome of the hemagglutination test with serum of horses showing febrile reaction and other symptoms is fairly good evidence against infectious anemia; also, virus carriers in the quiescent period would usually exhibit titers close to the normal range. On the other hand, interpretation of a positive test requires more caution. Combined together with other tests, it may be of use in confirmation of the clinical diagnosis, but it might well indicate also a pathologic condition other than infectious anemia possessing a similar infectious mechanism.

The test described in 1949 (Dreguss (94)) has since been utilized by other investigators and the positive results have been confirmed by the use of serum from experimentally infected horses tested against different individual chicken cells. (Personal communication by Dr. C. D. Stein, 1951.) Mention has been made of the fact that the hemagglutination test, like many other laboratory procedures suggested for supporting the diagnosis, is not specific for equine infectious anemia (390), which of course was never claimed.

Mechanism and Significance of the Hemagglutination

Efforts were made to clarify the mechanism of the hemagglutination test as observed with chicken red blood cells and infectious anemia serum of horses, with the hope that understanding of the hemagglutination may eventually throw light on the infectious mechanism of the disease. It would be beyond the scope of the present report to describe in detail the long series

TABLE 11

HEMAGGLUTINATION OF RED BLOOD CORPUSCLES OF THE HORSE

Red Blood Corp. of Horse	*Blood Serum Tested*	*Taken Days Foll. Infection*	*Hemagglut. Titer*
Horse 32 (5th d.)	Horse 17	(before)	1:40
	Horse 10	13	1:640
	Horse 10	70	1:2560
	Horse 32	(before)	1:10
	Horse 32	17	1:1280
	Horse 32	20	1:640
Horse 32 (5th d.)	*H. 856	(carrier)	1:80
	H. 884	(carrier)	1:160
	H. 1042	28	1:320
	H. 1251	13	1:160
	H. 1389	(before)	negative
	H. 1389	13	1:40
	H. 1389	15	1:80
	H. 1389	23	1:320
Horse 33 (5th d.)	Horse 17	(before)	1:10
	Horse 17	20	1:160
	Horse 33	19	1:640
	Horse 33	25	1:1280

* Serum samples H. 856 to H. 1389 were received from the B.A.I., Washington.

of experiments which were performed for this purpose. Instead, a brief summary of the more important investigations will be presented.

Hemagglutination of Horse Blood Cells.—Attempts were made in the early phase of the investigations to produce hemagglutination with red blood cells of normal and infected horses, but no hemagglutination was noted in the range of serum dilutions comparable to that seen with chicken cells. Sometimes, agglutination occurred in lower dilutions (1:2, 1:5) attributable to iso-agglutinins of blood groups. In a few instances spontaneous agglutination was observed after collecting blood from infected horses; the horse blood cells evidenced a definite clumping together in their own plasma while standing at room temperature or in the refrigerator. Such cells, after they had been washed three times in physiologic salt solution, would either tend to agglutinate even when diluted with saline, or would lose their agglutinatinability following washing. The results were not better when the cells were "aged" in the laboratory for a few days, as was done with the chicken cells. By considerably prolonging the period allowed for this, some good results were recorded later.

Three horses were injected for challenge inoculation, each with a few cc. of virulent serum, and five days later blood was drawn from all three animals, with the assumption that the blood cells would have had contact with the virus by this time. The red blood cells were washed and utilized for the test as usual, but they gave completely negative result with infectious horse sera in a series of repeated hemagglutination tests. A 10 per cent stock suspension of the washed cells was preserved at 5° C. and the tests were repeated after two months, this time with positive result. The results were improved after the preserved cell suspension was washed in salt solution and the test was set up with 0.4 per cent cell suspension instead of the usual 0.3 per cent. The blood cells were free of bacterial contamination and gave clear-cut results, particularly those which came from two of the horses exhibiting a mild fever response on the third day following infection, and several marked fever attacks thereafter.

Table 11 illustrates some of the results noted by the use of two horse cell suspensions (those of Horses 32 and 33). As may be noted, the red blood cells of both horses were agglutinated by their own sera collected after infection. Normal sera showed considerably lower agglutination titers. The second group of sera originated from horses experimentally infected with the virus of infectious anemia and kindly furnished by Dr. Stein and Dr. Mohler of the Bureau of Animal Industry in Washington. The results with the samples of H. 1389 illustrate the development of hemagglutinins from the preinoculation time to the 23rd day following infection. The first two of the Washington serum samples came from long-time virus carriers; these evidenced moderate hemagglutinin titers, as seen in the Table. The results were readily reproducible.

Hemagglutination with Various Red Blood Cells.—As reported earlier (94), red blood cells of sheep, guinea-pigs, and hamsters were also tested for their suitability to the hemagglutination test; they occasionally gave a positive result in tests with infectious horse serum, but generally the results were inferior to those noted with chicken cells. Rabbit cells produced conflicting results and often manifested spontaneous agglutination. Red blood cells of preinoculated rabbits, injected with normal or infectious serum of horses, elicited strong hemagglutination with any horse serum as an indication of a serologic reaction to the foreign protein.

Experiments were conducted on a large scale for closer study of the agglutination of chicken red blood cells. Adsorption of the hemagglutinin and its elution was effected at various temperatures. The red cells thus treated were further studied in additional experiments devised mainly for concentrating the agglutinin; a moderate concentration was achieved in these experiments, and some properties of the hemagglutinin were noted. Lack of space precludes a more detailed description of these experiments, most of them of theoretical significance; they were originally designed for concentrating the virus of infectious anemia, in case it were accompanied by, or were identical with, the substance causing agglutination of the erythrocytes.

Serum Protein Fraction Containing the Hemagglutinin.—Chemical determinations, combined with hemagglutination tests, disclosed that the hemagglutinin is contained in the immune-globulin fraction of the serum proteins in infectious horse blood (p. 76). This finding raised the question, whether the substance responsible for the hemagglutination represents the virus itself, or is rather an antibody of peculiar nature. The latter possibility is supported by many analogies found in the modern literature dealing with the problem of hemagglutination in various infectious diseases; beside, it fits into the concept of the pathogenesis of infectious anemia (95) developed on the basis of our experimental studies, as discussed in Chapter 9.

*

In the literature of infectious anemia, there are a few reports related to hemagglutination. Several investigators, among them Balozet (11), observed auto-agglutination (spontaneous agglutination) on some samples of infectious anemia blood. We noted the same phenomenon several times, particularly when bleeding horses in the early phase of a strong fever attack. Oppermann and Lauterbach (333, 334), on the other hand, tried to apply the hemagglutination for diagnostic purpose in utilizing red blood cells of rabbits which had been previously injected with infectious horse serum; they attributed diagnostic value to the positive results recorded in the test. The procedure did not prove useful in the hands of re-investigators (28, 222, 296), apparently because of the serologic reaction to the foreign protein which dominates the test, as mentioned above.

Before attempting to explain the possible mechanism of the hemagglutination test with chicken red blood cells and with those of horses, we shall list several analogies which may contribute to an understanding of the phenomenon:

1) Several *viruses* are known to produce hemagglutination of chicken cells as mentioned in the introduction (p. 59). Hirst (164), who first described such hemagglutination in influenza, has shown that it is specifically inhibited by the corresponding immune serum (165). The same is true for Newcastle disease virus (32, 51), and several other viruses. Moolten and Clark (304, 305, 306) recently attempted to use the hemagglutination test in clarifying the infectious mechanism of hemolytic anemia and other blood-borne human diseases suspected to have virus origin; they attribute an important role to auto-hemagglutination in these diseases. In our case, it could not be proven by inhibition tests that the hemagglutinin is identical with the virus (p. 60).

2) By the very nature of the hemagglutination, the analogy with *blood group iso-agglutinins* is fairly close. There is, however, a difference in the strength of the reaction, which is manifested by the high titers of infectious anemia hemagglutinin during the active stage of the disease, and by its independence from the blood groups of the individual horses.

3) In several human diseases hemagglutinins have been detected which are thought to represent a particular group of *antibodies*. These are the heterophile antibodies in serum sickness (74), in infectious mononucleosis (345, 130), and in leukemia (55); the cold agglutinins in primary atypical pneumonia (348, 173); and the heterogenetic antibodies described in acute hepatitis (102), etc. In the case of the heterophile agglutination with sheep red blood cells, the heterophile antibodies do not indicate an etiologic or other direct relationship to the red cells which they agglutinate. The cold agglutinins belong to the group of auto-hemagglutinins. The division between the agglutinin types in this group is not sharp.

4) There are hemagglutination tests known, in which an *in vitro* reaction of the antibody is brought about with red blood cells previously sensitized by various substances (e.g., with specific polysaccharides), or by adsorption of viruses (usually Newcastle virus) to their surface. The sensitizing substance seems to modify the surface of the erythrocytes used in these tests, and thus prepares them for the hemagglutination reaction with the antibody to be tested. Such tests may be considered relatively specific, as in the case of the Middlebrook-Dubos test (288) for tuberculosis; or unspecific, as in the tests used for experimental studies in infectious mononucleosis (109, 112), and in rheumatoid arthritis (159). The type and behavior of the hemagglutination noted in infectious anemia seems to be nearest to that mentioned in the groups under 3) and 4).

It is probable that the hemagglutinin present in the serum of infectious anemia horses is an antibody of heterogenetic nature. The hemagglutination test with chicken red blood cells may be readily explained by this. The details and the supporting evidence for this assumption will be presented in a separate publication (95). The antigenic material that gives rise to the heterogenetic antibodies is, in all likelihood, derived from the break-down products of horse erythrocytes. Therefore, the hemagglutinin possesses a specific affinity to the red blood cells and is probably responsible for their excessive destruction in the horse. This concept is supported by the results noted in hemagglutination with long-stored horse blood cells (Table 11); it seems very likely that a partial (enzymatic) break-down made these cells suitable for hemagglutination by infectious horse sera. The problem will be further discussed in the next chapter when the pathologic process as a whole is considered.

CHAPTER 9

PATHOGENESIS

Equine infectious anemia is perhaps one of the least understood infectious diseases. It has been known, since the fundamental experiments by Vallée and Carré, that the disease is caused by a filterable virus but the closer mechanism of the infection has not been clarified, in spite of the great interest centered around the malady and the many efforts to reach a better understanding of the disease and to gain a deeper insight into its infectious process. Although some features of the disease have been clarified by careful observations and experimental studies, there remain a number of important questions unanswered which have been summarily called "the problem of infectious anemia."

The disease is unquestionably infectious, but it does not behave as do most infectious diseases. With rare exceptions, no immunity follows a past infection in animals apparently recovered; such horses may experience relapses at any time, and their clinically healthy state can change to an acute fatal disease for no apparent reason.

Jaffé (188) concluded, after a careful analysis of the histologic changes, that the Kupffer cells of the liver take up an extremely large number of crushed red blood cells that have been previously destroyed for an unexplained reason. Schermer (382, 383) stated that the virus is insufficient to produce the disease and to explain the pathologic process. Both he and Dobberstein (84) remarked that the histologic findings in infectious anemia are reminiscent of those produced by break-down products of a foreign protein and that the reticulo-endothelial system and the capillary walls are seriously involved in the process. Many others analyzed the question of pathogenesis (139, 184, 297, 318, 386) to explain part of the changes, but the main problem—that is, the real cause of the alterations and the way they are induced—remained unsolved.

Systematic investigations, as part of our study, disclosed the fact that hypersensitivity plays an important role in the pathologic process of the disease and that the allergic state is responsible for many of the paradoxical findings. Hypersensitivity of shorter or longer duration can be observed in a number of other infectious and non-infectious diseases as shown by von Pirquet (352–356) who coined the word "allergy" in 1906. The monograph on human serum sickness published by von Pirquet and Schick (356) in Vienna is the first systematic study on hypersensitivity, with theoretical deductions still valid five decades later. In a broader sense the term "allergy," or allergic state, means altered reactivity of the organism; the more restricted meaning of allergy is a delayed reaction that follows the action (inoculation) of a sensitizing antigen (infectious or non-infectious in nature), while anaphylaxis (357) is an immediate response to such antigen in a sensitized organism. The term "hypersensitivity" can be applied to both conditions. The allergic sensitivity causes the sensitized organism to react in a more intensified manner, different from the reaction expected from an immune organism. Allergy and immunity, although they are frequently present together, are not considered to be interdependent conditions (276).

In the following, the evidence indicating the role of allergy in the pathogenesis of infectious anemia will be briefly outlined. A more detailed description will be published elsewhere (95).

Early Fever Reaction and Marked Fever Attacks

The incubation period most frequently observed in infectious anemia moves in a range from one to three weeks, the average being about 14 days, based on the occurrence of the first marked fever reaction and other symptoms. In most of our horses we noted that a mild temperature response, between the 2nd and the 6th day, preceded the sharp rise in temperature, which as a rule followed the first elevation 8 to 9 days later. There was a striking regularity in this interim period between the two temperature rises. Chart 1 illustrates the fever response in a young horse (Horse 17) that had been injected with 1 cc. of a virulent infectious anemia serum collected from Horse 10. The disease took an acute course in Horse 17 and the animal died on the 28th day following infection. Further analysis of all temperature charts showed that in the early phase of the disease the temperature peaks often occurred after remissions of 7 to 10 days.

We are convinced that the early fever reaction, that may be termed the "virus peak," is the first sign of the action of the virus within the body of the infected horse. It is safe to assume that a blood-borne virus does not require two to three weeks for multiplication in the original host; rather it would reach within a few days sufficient concentration to cause noticeable symptoms, even if mild in character. Coincident with this, there is a decrease in the number of the red blood cells (p. 49). We were able to show by horse inoculation the presence of virus in the blood at this time.

On account of the regular time interval between the fever reactions, and because of a papular eruption noted on an infected horse at the time of the second fever attack, the allergic nature of these manifestations was considered. It is known that in serum sickness and other allergic conditions the incubation period, as a rule, is from 8 to 10 days, sometimes longer. The fever response in human and experimental measles (92) seems to have a similar pattern; as it is known, von Pirquet (355) considered the skin eruption in measles as an allergic manifestation. The early mild fever reaction, noticed also by others (193, 278, 280), was not noted in some of our horses in spite of other systemic reactions present.

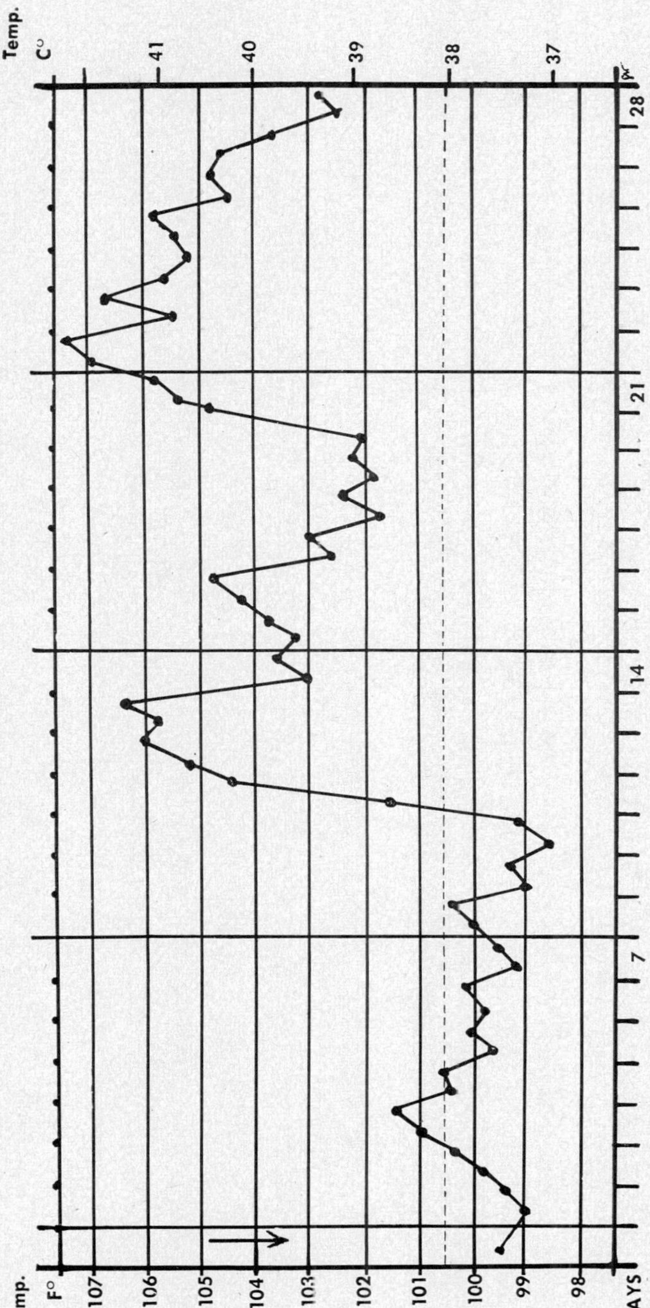

CHART 1. FEVER RESPONSE IN AN ACUTE CASE OF INFECTIOUS ANEMIA (HORSE 17)

It seems that the virus causes in the first days following the infection a slight initial reaction with or without a mild fever response. Then stronger symptoms and marked fever attacks follow, presenting the pattern of typical allergic fever reactions. Small laboratory animals injected with the virus seem to develop only the early mild reaction, if any.

Challenge Inoculation and the Possibility of Re-infection

The existence of an allergic state in infectious anemia is strongly supported by the fact that all of our experimental horses reacted to challenge inoculation with minute amounts of virulent virus, even if there was plenty of evidence that they had passed a milder infection previously; often, the response following the second infection was stronger than that following the primary inoculation. To bring additional proof, Horse 10 was injected with 0.5 cc. of its own blood serum, collected at the first marked fever reaction and preserved frozen in a sterile vial until it was used. This animal had been in a quiescent, afebrile period showing no fever reaction or other clinical symptoms for over five months when it was re-inoculated with its own serum, to which it responded with a somewhat accelerated fever reaction with a peak of 103.5° F. This finding leaves no doubt that horses seemingly recovered from an infection may be re-infected with the virus, the only exception being the resistant virus carriers which are apparently sufficiently desensitized. Observations concerning re-infection, or increased susceptibility are noted also in the literature (p. 123).

Antibody Level in the Blood and Activity of the Disease

According to our present knowledge the allergic symptoms are based on antigen-antibody reactions which are believed to take place on the surface of the cells within the sensitive tissues (463). Therefore, the serum proteins in the blood of our infected horses were subjected to an intensive study. Attention was focused on the gamma-globulin fraction that contains most of the antibodies in infectious diseases (103).

The gamma-globulin has been determined routinely by the chemical method of Kibrick and Blonstein (203), using 15 per cent sodium sulfate concentration for salting out this fraction of the serum proteins. In addition, a few preliminary determinations were performed by electrophoresis (81).

In Table 12 are recorded the highest gamma-globulin values that we noted in the individual horses after infection. The total serum protein values given in grams for 100 cc. serum, and the erythrocyte counts recorded on the same day are also included. Normal values, as determined in the same horses before inoculation and in a number of other healthy horses, moved in a range from 1.17 to 1.68 grams of gamma-globulin per 100 cc. serum. As may be seen from the table, an unusual increase was noted in practically all horses. It is noteworthy that Horse 8 had a low value. This horse never showed marked clinical symptoms during the several months of observation following infection. In a resistant virus carrier (Horse 2), the level of gamma-globulin, which reached very high values during the acute symptoms, returned close to the normal range, when the animal showed a complete clinical recovery. The peak of the gamma-globulin level was reached in all horses while they were in the active stage of the disease.

Generally, an increased antibody level in the serum is considered as an indication of a past infection and—at the same time—as a sign of relative or solid immunity. If the rise of the gamma-globulin level in infectious

TABLE 12

SERUM GAMMA-GLOBULIN LEVEL IN THE BLOOD OF INFECTED HORSES

Horse No.	*Highest γ-globulin*	*Day Foll. Inf.*	*R. B. C. million*	*Total Protein*	*Remarks*
H. 4	2.96 g.	94th	3.8	7.84 g.	
H. 5	3.29	27th	4.8	8.39	
H. 8	1.96	63rd	*	5.90	
H. 11	3.60	80th	4.3	6.56	
H. 15	3.33	36th	5.9	9.0	
H. 21	3.61	78th	6.2	8.45	
H. 22	3.57	59th	4.5	8.64	
H. 27	2.14	30th	6.9	8.61	
H. 28	2.82	24th	7.4	9.36	Several chall. inoc.
H. 30	2.57	33rd	5.7	8.77	
H. 31	3.21	74th	9.8	7.38	
H. 32	2.45	25th	6.5	7.03	
H. 33	3.28	24th	5.8	8.05	
H. 36	1.84	22nd	7.6	7.10	Mouse pass. virus
H. 38	2.75	17th	6.7	9.30	Mouse series, 3rd
H. 40	2.96	35th	10.0	8.91	Cult. series, 2nd
H. 44	2.49	23rd	5.5	8.15	Mouse series, 3rd
H. 46	2.81	17th	8.2	8.25	Shock foll. inoc.

* Not done.

anemia represents an increase in antibodies, as it does in other infectious diseases, one would expect an amelioration or ceasing of symptoms coincident with the rise. But, as the case of Horse 2 clearly shows, recovery and apparent immunity occur rather parallel with the decrease of gamma-globulin approaching the normal level. This strongly suggests that the excess amount of antibody present in the circulating blood of infected horses is an indication of their allergic state, that is, of an increased readiness for antigen-antibody reactions, recognized as characteristic for allergy.

In recent years, marked hyperglobulinemia, similar to the one noted by us, was reported in various human diseases such as lupus erythematosus (71, 473), leukemia (38), rheumatic arthritis (47), lymphogranuloma venereum (477), and liver diseases (125), with extremely high values in hepatic necrosis (497). In all of these, the increase was attributed to elevated gamma-globulin level as determined by chemical methods or by electrophoresis; in two of the reports (38, 125) the subfraction was more closely identified as gamma-one globulin (also called beta-two fraction). Vaughan and co-workers (473) noted correlation between the gamma-globulin content of serum and the duration of the disease in lupus erythematosus. It may be added that Longcope and Rackemann (260) demonstrated the relation of circulating antibodies to manifestations of serum sickness.

Antibodies, considered as modified serum globulins (Mudd (314)), are mostly contained in the regular gamma-globulin (i.e., in the gamma-two globulin). The gamma-one fraction corresponds to a protein which has about six times as high molecular weight as the regular antibodies; its molecular weight (in the horse serum) is 990,000 as against 150,000 of the normal gamma-globulin (461). According to Tiselius and Kabat (449) pneumococcus antibodies, produced in horses by hyperimmunization, migrate with the gamma-one fraction in the electrophoretic field. It seems from our preliminary electrophoresis analyses that the excessive amount of antibody present in infectious anemia serum belongs to the same group of heavy globulins and its mobility is that of the gamma-one globulin. Van der Scheer and co-workers (408) studied the antibody in hyperimmune horse sera prepared against 15 different bacterial antigens; they found that some of these antibodies were contained in the regular γ-globulin fraction (gamma-two), while others migrated with the "T" component.

We made a few analyses by electrophoresis with a Tiselius type of apparatus at the Department of Medical Physics, University of Pennsylvania.* This confirmed the unusual increase in the gamma-globulin fractions of the serum proteins in sick horses. By comparing the electrophoresis pattern of normal horse serum (Chart 2) with that recorded on serum of an infected animal (Chart 3), an enormous increase may be noted in the so-called gamma-one fraction which is located between the beta- and gamma-globulin fraction and is considered by most investigators as a gamma-globulin variety; it is also called "T" component, or beta-two globulin (461). The albumin boundary (*A*) indicates a marked drop in that component. The sera of horses indicating a drop in the gamma-globulin—as determined by the chemical method—presented an electrophoresis pattern of considerably diminished gamma-one globulin fraction.

The Role of Hemagglutinin in the Pathologic Process

As already mentioned in Chapter 8, the component responsible for the hemagglutination was found to be present or to be associated with the gamma-globulin fraction of infectious anemia serum. By salting out this fraction and dissolving it in saline, the hemagglutinin was almost quantitatively separated from the rest of the serum protein fractions.

---

* The electrophoresis analyses were performed with permission of Dr. Britton Chance, head of the Department, in collaboration with Dr. Andreas C. Maehly, and Dr. Gerhard Fromm.

The gamma-globulin fraction of infectious sera probably contains several types of antibodies (to the virus, and to the "secondary" antigens). Among these the hemagglutinin seems to possess considerable significance as to the role it might play in the pathologic process. It causes agglutination *in*

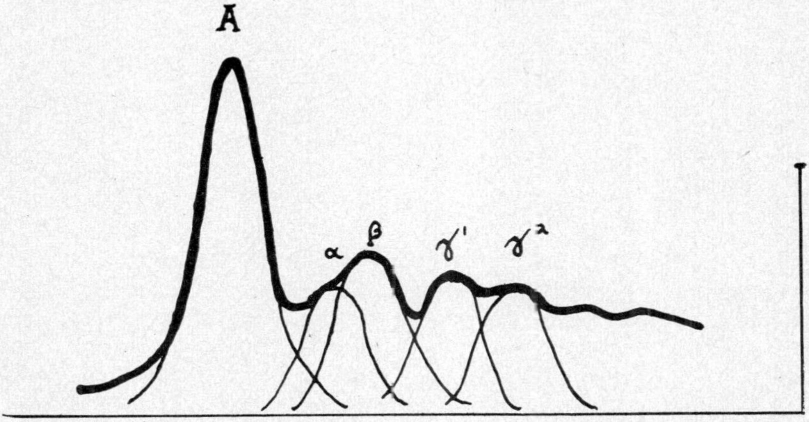

CHART 2. ELECTROPHORESIS PATTERN OF NORMAL HORSE SERUM

vitro with both chicken red blood cells and horse erythrocytes. It is most likely that the same hemagglutinin will produce hemagglutination *in vivo,* that is, in the circulating blood of the infected horse, when present in the serum in sufficient concentration. Bull showed in 1915 the occurrence of

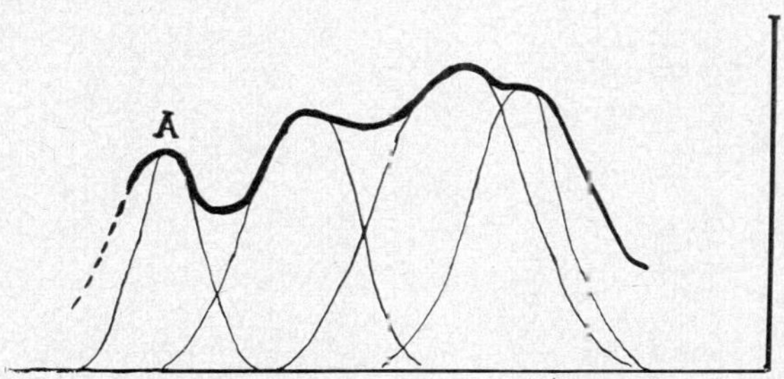

CHART 3. ELECTROPHORESIS PATTERN OF INFECTIOUS ANEMIA SERUM

intravascular hemagglutination by bacterial antibodies, and Knisely and coworkers convincingly demonstrated such agglutination (sludged blood) in several pathologic processes of living animals (207, 33). Blanchard and Vedel (40) reported thrombosis in the hepatic (portal) and splenic veins in infectious anemia. We observed in histologic preparations of the spleen of an infected horse, destroyed after prolonged fever reaction, a marked agglutination of the red blood cells. All this points to the direction that the excessive destruction of the red blood cells is at least partly due to the hemagglutinin present in the serum; the virus probably acts in sensitizing the red cells and breaking down some component of the cell stroma. At high temperatures (fever) the hemagglutinin may be eluted from the red blood cells, which become refractory to repeated hemagglutination.

It is assumed that the antigen which gives rise to the production of hemagglutinins in infectious anemia is a polysaccharide of hapten nature, probably derived from the stroma of the red blood cells of the infected horse. This is based, in part, on analogies of experimental work reported in the literature (50, 393, 394, 453, 454). Tomcsik and his co-worker (454, 393, 394) studying similar problems in connection with serum sickness and the heterophile agglutination in infectious mononucleosis, have shown in their experimental studies the role of haptens.

Microscopic Evidence of Allergic Inflammation

Although no histologic alterations exist which would specifically indicate the presence of an allergic state, there are characteristic changes which regularly occur in allergic inflammations. These have been observed in infectious anemia. Here, a brief reference will be made to a few of them, while the details will be discussed later (Chapter 13).

In our experimental horses infiltration, mostly perivascular, by leukocytes and lymphocytes in various organs, including the heart, has been noted with regularity. In the myocardium the perivascular infiltration (Fig. 1) is followed by proliferation of connective tissue elements, often resulting in lesions strongly resembling Aschoff bodies (9) considered to be specific for rheumatic heart fever (*see* Fig. 15 on p. 131). Eosinophil cells infiltrate in large number the liver (Fig. 2), the lymph nodes (Fig. 3), and the spleen (Fig. 12). The increase of plasma cells (Fig. 4) indicates antibody production, as often seen in hyperimmunized animals as well as in allergic inflammation. The kidney changes, as shown in Figs. 5 and 6, are similar to

---

EXPLANATION OF COLOR PLATE

(opposite page)

FIG. 1. HEART. Perivascular infiltration in the myocardium. Lymphocytes and polymorphonuclear leukocytes are surrounding an arteriole. (Horse 9, Hematoxylin-Eosin, approx.500x)

FIG. 2. LIVER. Marked infiltration by round cells and by numerous eosinophil cells. The liver cells show signs of regression. (Horse 38, Giemsa, approx.565x)

FIG. 3. LYMPH NODE. Moderate infiltration by eosinophil cells. (Horse 9, Methylenblue-Eosin, approx.500x)

FIG. 4. HEPATIC LYMPH NODE. The marginal sinusoids are packed with plasma cells. (Horse 10, Hematoxylin-Eosin, approx.1200x)

FIG. 5. KIDNEY. Perivascular infiltration by round cells in the cortex of the kidney. Signs of fibroblastic activity may be noted. (Horse 9, Methylenblue-Eosin, approx.500x)

FIG. 6. KIDNEY; segment of a glomerulus. Proliferation of the capillary endothelium, obliterating the Bowman space. (Horse 21, Hematoxylin-Eosin, approx.500x)

Microphotographs by Dr. Steven C. Mohos

Plate: Equine Infectious Anemia

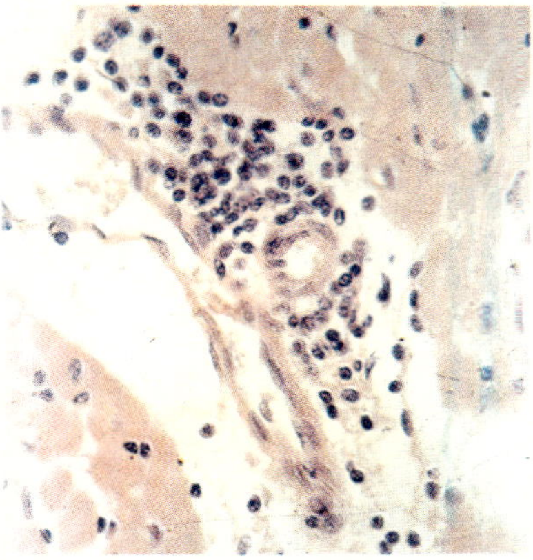

Fig. 1

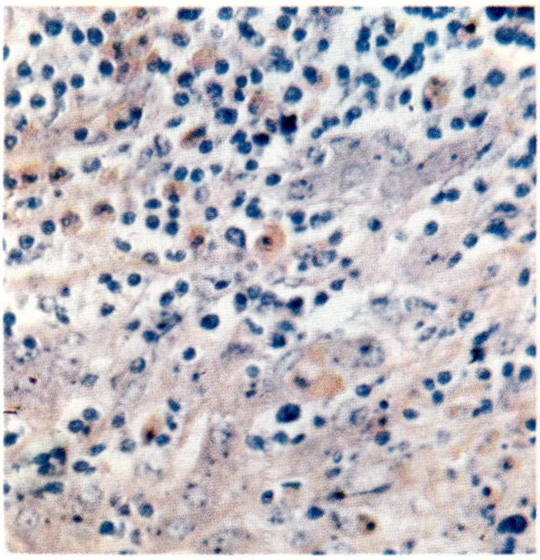

Fig. 2

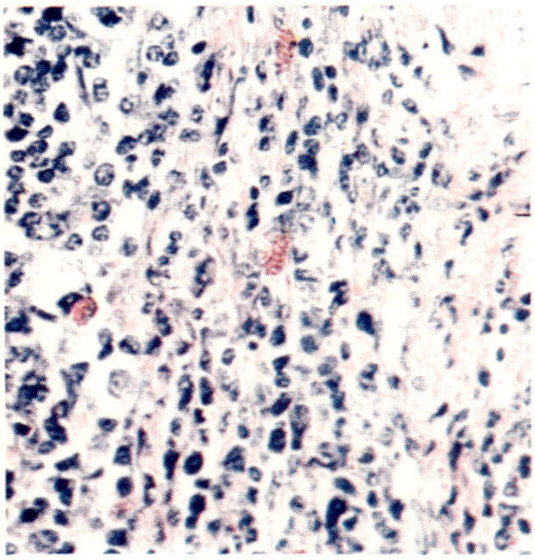

Fig. 3

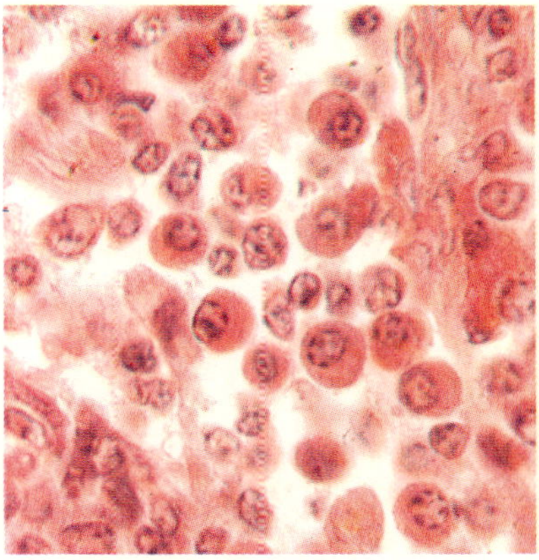

Fig. 4

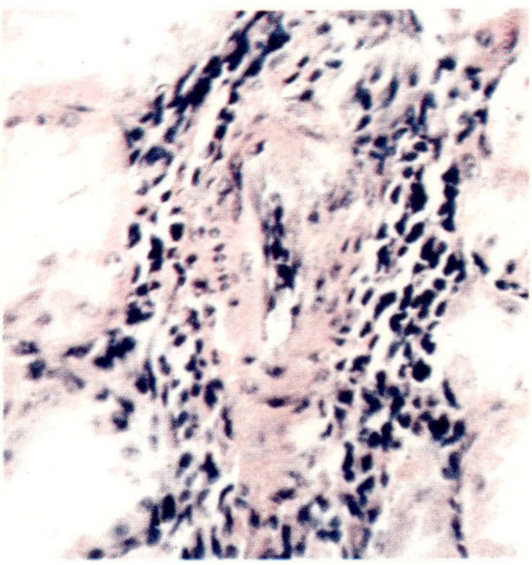

Fig. 5

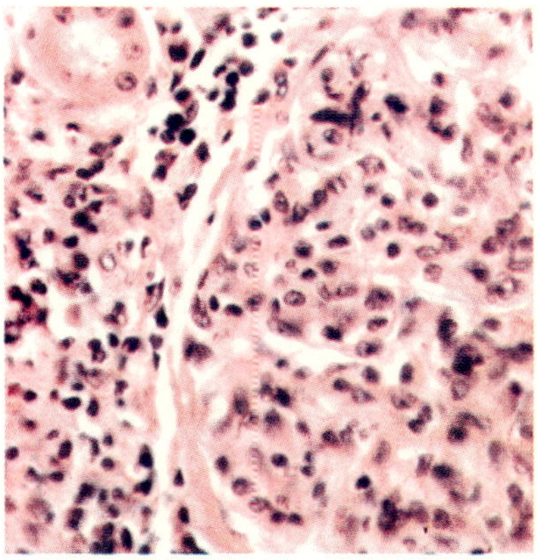

Fig. 6

those noted in acute glomerulonephritis, which is considered as an organ allergic reaction. A very marked involvement of the reticulo-endothelial system in the disease belongs to the typical pathologic picture (*see* p. 137); the same has been observed by several authors (382, 319, 110).

Pathologic alterations in the heart have been noted by many investigators (58, 123, 270, 283, 88, 379) but the Aschoff body-like structures have not been described in infectious anemia so far. The significance of Aschoff bodies, first described in 1904 (9, 484) and of the cardiac histiocytes (Anitschkow cells) (Fig. 16) is variously interpreted (70, 484), but all agree that the Aschoff body is frequently found in rheumatic fever and it is considered pathognomonic for that disease. Similar formations were produced in laboratory animals by the injection of foreign proteins or organ extracts (366, 367, 65, 66, 308), providing experimental proof that they are formed on an allergic basis By a similar experimental technique, other changes have also been provoked, e.g., glomerulonephritis (259, 63, 67, 307) or allergic focal necrosis in the liver (154). All of these changes have been attributed to organ auto-antibodies.

There are striking analogies between the symptoms of infectious anemia and those of the experimentally produced organ allergic conditions; they include fever, anemia, hypoproteinemia, edema, etc. The role of allergy is suggested also by such manifestations, observed in infected horses, as urticaria (152), lumbago-like symptoms (158, 400, 413), and occasional high red cell count (384), probably a sign of hemoconcentration as known from observations in human anaphylactic shock (41). Torrance (455) tried to work out an allergic skin test with promising results, but the investigation could not be carried to a final conclusion.

*

In attempting to reconstruct the pathologic process on the basis of what was said above, in order to find out how the allergic state is brought about in infectious anemia, the following can be said.

The infectious virus acts on the blood within the vessels and, in addition, it provokes a reaction along the vascular system throughout the body, in a particularly accentuated form in the parenchymatous organs, especially the liver. The red cells pass the capillary walls causing petecchial or more extensive hemorrhages in the tissues. Around the vascular system degenerative and necrotic processes appear in the major organs, and the site of these necrotic processes and hemorrhages is invaded, in the early stage, by polymorphonuclear leukocytes, macrophages, and eosinophil cells which are all engaged in removing the break-down products of the injured cells by phagocytosis or by local catalysis. Then the various inflammatory cells partly or completely disappear except for the lymphocytic elements which continue to infiltrate the sites of the primary injury in large number for building up a local barrier of resistance; through this process the organs are equipped for an intensified, though in many respects incomplete and unpractical, local defense reaction (allergy). The lymphatic cells which take part in the excess antibody production (104), react in the infiltrated tissues locally (allergic inflammation) when the infectious process is re-activated.

If the animal does not succumb to the infection during the acute phase, regenerative processes follow to replace the necrotic tissue; this is achieved by regeneration of the tissue cells, and proliferation of the reticulo-endothelium and connective tissue elements, leading eventually to scar formation. As it is known, the virus is not eliminated from the body of the infected horses, rather it seems to co-exist with the antibody indefinitely (79). Thus, the process repeats itself and renewed attacks occur, until the animal reaches a partly or wholly balanced stage of desensitization.

On the basis of the evidence provided by the experimental studies in producing allergic inflammation by parenteral injection of foreign proteins, and the strikingly similar microscopic picture seen in natural equine infectious anemia, it may be assumed that the break-down products of the injured cells (red blood cells and those of the necrotic tissues) act in infectious anemia as if they were foreign proteins, provoking increased antibody production and allergic inflammation in the tissues. These antibodies are directed against the "secondary" antigens (not against the virus) and they distort the pathologic picture of the virus infection by the complex of allergic reactions. The latter closely resemble to the toxic effect caused by repeated injections of foreign proteins ("protein intoxication") as described by Pentimalli (346). In this connection, it may be mentioned that a marked increase in gamma-globulin (antibodies) is frequently found in otherwise unrelated diseases in which an extensive tissue breakdown takes place, causing the formation of antibodies to homologous tissue (144). The influence of the high gamma-globulin level on the activity of the disease process has been discussed above. In our experimental work there was indication that an elevated unspecific gamma-globulin level (of other than infectious anemia origin) may exert a delaying influence on the clinical symptoms (p. 96), but would not prevent the infection. The prolonged incubation period noted in hyperimmunized serum production horses (p. 20) may be explained on a similar basis.

It is beyond the scope of this report to analyze the possibilities of desensitization and how it is achieved. It seems that in some recovered animals such a desensitization occurs spontaneously (resistant virus carriers). In our experiments, we have seen both spontaneous desensitization and some partial desensitization brought about by immunization, combined with repeated injections of less virulent virus.

The results of our experimental work (95) indicate that the pathologic process of equine infectious anemia is initiated by a relatively mild virus infection, followed by an allergic condition in the infected animal. During the course of the disease the allergic reactions, superimposed upon the virus infection, dominate the pathologic process.

Chapter 10

TRANSMISSION TO LABORATORY ANIMALS

The experimental study of infectious anemia has been severely handicapped by the lack of small laboratory animals susceptible to the virus. The initial price of horses and the expense of their upkeep under strict quarantine during the experimental period make it impossible for most laboratories to use them in sufficient numbers, or even at all. Therefore, many attempts have been made by investigators in the past to find some small experimental animals susceptible to the action of the virus that could replace the horse as a test animal in laboratory studies concerning the disease. We conducted a series of experiments, as other experimenters did, in an effort to find a suitable laboratory animal for such purpose.

It has been repeatedly demonstrated that viruses, not originally infectious for a given laboratory animal, may be adapted to the latter by appropriate methods (199). Such adaptation is usually achieved by making serial passages of the virus in the selected laboratory animal. Ordinarily, complete adaptation of a virus to a new host requires a number of repeated passages. Sometimes, in the early passages, no sign of illness is apparent, and animals of the later passages only become noticeably sick. A wide range of viruses has been adapted by this technique to small laboratory animals that originally were believed to be refractory to the particular virus. Well-known examples are the adaptation of the viruses of human and swine influenza, as well as some strains of poliomyelitis virus, to the white laboratory mouse.

The principle of the serial passage technique was utilized by us for the purpose of finding a laboratory animal suitable for the study of infectious anemia. In the great majority of experiments recorded in the literature, the technique of serial transfer was not applied by investigators of the problem. We first tested various laboratory animals in preliminary experiments to determine whether any one species might show indication of a quick adaptation of the virus; then a longer series of experiments was conducted in rabbits and mice. After a brief description of the methods and a summary of the preliminary attempts, some details of the experiments proper will be presented.

Methods.—The virus used was the "New Hampshire" strain of infectious anemia obtained during the New England outbreak in 1947. Dr. C. D. Stein of the Bureau of Animal Industry furnished us with a filtered lyophilized serum sample of their horse No. 1401. This serum was reconstituted with sterile distilled water to the original volume, and 5 cc. was injected into the jugular vein of each of two horses; further passages were made by the same route in normal horses.

Intravenous inoculations were made by way of the jugular vein in monkeys and the ear vein in rabbits by using strictly aseptic technique. Intracerebral injection was performed aseptically by puncture of the skull with a fine hypodermic needle in the case of mice and hamsters, or by first preparing a small hole in the skull with a dental drill in the case of rabbits. Intraperitoneal (intra-abdominal) injections were made through the skin of the lower portion of the abdomen after proper cleaning and disinfecting of the site of injection. The intranasal inoculations were performed by using the technique as employed in work with influenza viruses. The animals were given, under slight ether anesthesia, drops of the fluid to be inoculated, in an amount of 0.03 to 0.05 cc., onto their nostrils, which they aspirated while in ether narcosis. In a few instances, subcutaneous inoculations were also utilized; this was performed as usual. For making dilutions of the inoculum, sterile physiologic salt solution or a phosphate buffer of pH 7.2 was used.

All inocula had been tested for bacterial sterility on solid and liquid media before they were used. Samples of blood and organs collected from the experimental animals were likewise cultured on blood agar plates, nutrient broth, and serum broth in order to note the eventual growth of organisms, or bacterial contamination, if any.

Bleeding of horses was performed from the jugular vein. As a rule, both whole blood and citrated blood were collected. Coagulation of the blood was allowed while standing in the refrigerator before the serum was separated. For obtaining plasma, the blood was run into a 3.8 per cent solution of sodium citrate, one-tenth in volume to the blood, as anticoagulant. The smaller animals were bled either by heart puncture or from the ear vein under aseptic conditions.

Extract of organs for subinoculation was prepared by grinding them in a porcelain mortar with the addition of sterile pulverized alundum and physiologic salt solution to make a 10 per cent suspension. This was centrifuged at 3000 rpm for 10 minutes and the supernatant fluid, or its dilutions, was used for inoculation.

Preliminary Experiments

After several successful passages were made in horses by injecting them with infectious anemia virus, their blood was used in preliminary studies of various laboratory tests and to inoculate the following experimental animals: monkeys, hamsters, guinea-pigs, rabbits, and mice.

Monkeys.—As the susceptibility of monkeys had not been sufficiently explored so far, an attempt was made to pass the virus in such animals. Four rhesus monkeys were injected intravenously by Dr. Werner Leemann, who worked in this laboratory in 1948, with virulent blood drawn from Horse 1 while it had a marked fever reaction. Temperatures of the monkeys were taken twice daily and the animals were kept under close observation in order to note the development of eventual symptoms. They remained outwardly healthy for two months, and then they were destroyed. Four weeks following injection of the horse blood, whole blood and citrated blood samples were collected from all four monkeys, the serum and plasma were separated and a pool of 30 cc., containing equal parts of serum and plasma, was injected intravenously into a normal horse (Horse 5) in order to find out whether infectious anemia virus was present in the blood of the monkeys.

The horse developed a fever reaction that began the day of injection and lasted for two weeks; during this time the animal did not eat well. The fever was of the intermittent type with a peak of 104.4°F. on the second day following inoculation. The reaction was first considered as due to some other illness coincident with the time of inoculation. But in our opinion, the more plausible explanation of the fever is that it was a response to antibodies against horse protein, which were present in the monkey serum. Obviously, the monkeys had been sensitized by the initial inoculation with horse blood. However, because the fever was of long duration, there arose the question as to whether the virus of infectious anemia may have been present in the monkey blood. There was a slight remission in the fever attack on the fifth and sixth day, but the temperature started to rise again on the seventh day and reached 103.2°F. on the same day. The second part of the fever response, which lasted about a week, may or may not have been due to the action of the virus.

No further symptoms were noted in the horse during two months of additional observation. When subjected to a challenge inoculation with virulent horse blood, the animal exhibited a marked fever response beginning on the 10th day following the challenge inoculation and continuing until the 27th day when the horse was destroyed. Because the symptoms observed in the test horse immediately following the inoculation of monkey blood were not those of a typical infectious anemia and because the horse reacted to challenge inoculation with a virulent virus, the result of the monkey experiment was considered negative.

Hamsters.—In recent years hamsters have been shown to be susceptible to infection with various viruses. Therefore an attempt was made, early in our preliminary experiments, at transmission of the infection to these rodents. Taylor and Dreguss (455) were the first to demonstrate that laboratory strains of human influenza virus can be readily adapted and serially transmitted in the common European hamster (*Cricetus cricetus*) whose natural habitat is on the plains of Central Europe. Later, during the influenza epidemic of 1941, in three out of four throat washings of human patients the virus could be identified and directly isolated through this species of hamster by intranasal inoculation (Dreguss (93)).

For testing hamsters in our work with equine infectious anemia, an experiment was conducted for transmission of the infection to a variant of these rodents, the Syrian or golden hamster (*Cricetus auratus*), which can be raised and maintained under laboratory conditions. Each of two young hamsters received intracerebrally 0.05 cc. of infectious horse serum (Horse 3), while two others each received intra-abdominally 1 cc. of the same horse serum. The animals were kept under observation to note clinical symptoms, and their weight was checked at weekly intervals for several months. One subinoculation was made in hamsters with fresh whole blood of the intra-abdominally injected animals, by this same route, on the 21st day following the initial inoculation.

None of the inoculated hamsters exhibited any sign of illness. They remained vigorous and ate well during two months of close observation in the laboratory, and their gain in weight was similar to that of control animals. The count of the red blood corpuscles of the inoculated hamsters ranged from 7.8 to 8.5 million—when checked two months after inoculation. This corresponds to the normal range of erythrocytes in these animals (131). Four to five months following the original inoculation, all of the hamsters were sacrificed. Except for some alteration in the consistency of the liver (fragility), no abnormal findings were noted.

Guinea-pigs.—Experiments with guinea-pigs were carried out in the same pattern as described for the hamsters, that is, using intracerebral and intra-abdominal routes of inoculation. One cc. of virulent horse serum was administered intra-abdominally, while the intracerebral dosage here consisted of 0.1 cc. of the same. No symptoms were noted during an experimental period of two months in either the initial group, or in the passage animals of the guinea-pig series.

Rabbits.—Although the literature is controversial with regard to the susceptibility of rabbits to the virus of infectious anemia, there are reports indicative of the possibility of adapting the virus to this species. Because of the great importance attached to the eventual success of adaptation, we initiated several experimental series in rabbits with this goal in mind. In the brief account of the preliminary work, only the first and second groups of rabbits will be discussed.

Each of two young rabbits received 3 cc. of virulent virus (horse serum) in the ear vein, while an adult rabbit was injected intracerebrally with 0.1 cc. of infectious serum. Temperature of the animals was taken twice daily and any change in their behavior, appetite, etc., was noted. Body weight was checked twice a week.

The animals did not exhibit convincing symptoms during one month of observation, although the impression was gained that they were less active and that their appetite was sometimes impaired. The temperature readings of the animals varied between 102°* and 104°F., i.e., within the normal range. The highest figures recorded were 104.1° and 104.0°F. on the 8th and 14th day, respectively, following inoculation.

Another set of rabbits (second group) was used to determine whether serum, plasma, or whole blood might better convey the infection to them. Blood was drawn from an infected horse at the peak of the fever reaction, and the serum was separated within two hours. A citrated sample was also collected at the same time and, after slight centrifugation, the supernatant plasma was separated. Half of the citrated blood sample was left uncentrifuged and used, after gentle mixing, for injection.

Two young rabbits were given serum, two received plasma, and one citrated blood; each received 5 cc. in the ear vein. Temperatures were taken and records were kept as outlined above. At intervals erythrocyte counts were made.

The result did not differ materially from that in the rabbits of the first group. It should be noted, however, that all of the rabbits in the second group showed a mild elevation of temperature after the injection, either on the same day, or on the following day, that is, without any incubation period. This mild temperature response which went as high as 105.3°F. in two of them, subsided in three to five days in all of the rabbits. Probably it was due to the use of fresh blood, as it is known that fresh blood has some toxic effect, when injected into a foreign host, possibly on account of the combined effect of foreign protein and complement present in fresh blood. This effect might have been accentuated by the fact that the blood sample was collected at the peak of a febrile reaction in the horse. The lack of incubation period, however, makes it unlikely that the prompt fever response was the result of infection in the rabbits.

During 45 days of further observation, the temperature did not rise above 104°F. in any of the experimental animals. No symptoms were noted and all of the rabbits gained weight during the same period. In Table 13 a part of the results that were noted in two rabbits is presented in order to illustrate the findings in the group. The rest of the animals exhibited similar or smaller deviations from the normal values. As may be seen from Table 13, no anemia or any significant decrease in the number of erythrocytes developed in the experimental rabbits.

---

* For converting temperature readings in Fahrenheit degrees into centigrades (C), see Table 1 on page 18.

Mice.—Throughout our experimental studies that were devised to determine the possibility of transmission and adaptation of the virus to laboratory animals, efforts were mainly concentrated upon adaptation of the virus to mice. Experimental work in this direction was begun during the summer of 1948, and the preliminary findings were briefly referred to in the Bulletins of the Grayson Foundation published in 1948 and 1950.

The reasons and advantages of selecting the mouse for experimental work are obvious. In case of successful adaptation of the virus, mice could be used in great number for large-scale model experiments to study the

TABLE 13

RABBITS INOCULATED WITH INFECTIOUS HORSE BLOOD

Days following inoculation	*Rabbit No. 9 (serum i. v.)*			*Rabbit No. 12 (plasma i. v.)*		
	Temperature F°		*R.B.C. million*	*Temperature F°*		*R.B.C. million*
(Before)			5.2			5.3
1	104.6	104.8	5.6	105.3	105.1	5.4
2	103.9	105.3		104.4	104.8	
3	104.8	104.6		104.6	104.2	
4	104.0	103.7		103.8	104.4	
5	104.4	104.1		103.4	103.7	
6	103.6	104.0		103.5	103.4	
7	103.4	103.2	5.0	103.0	103.2	5.7
14	103.5	102.8	5.6	103.1	102.8	5.0
21	103.7	104.0	4.9	103.4	103.2	5.2
45	103.2	103.4	5.2	103.0	103.4	4.7

infection and, eventually, neutralization tests could be worked out for testing the presence of antibodies in the blood serum of normal, sick, or recovered horses. Throughout these experiments a healthy stock of white (albino) mice was used. They were purchased from a dealer and were maintained on a constant, balanced diet.

Experience with horses indicates that inoculation of the anemia virus into the original host will cause infection by any parenteral route of application, and that success is regularly achieved by injecting the virus directly into the blood stream. Such a mode of transmission seems to be the first choice in attempts to infect laboratory animals. However, the success reported in the literature in connection with the adaptation of certain viruses to a new tissue in the original, or in a newly tested host by repeated "blind" passages, led us to believe that other routes of infection may eventually produce good results and, therefore, must be explored.

Therefore, various routes of infection were tried in the mouse, as well as in the rest of the experimental animals, in the expectation that symptoms or lesions might be produced that would make the recognition of an ensuing infection easier. Thus, intranasal infection, or intracerebral inoculation might lead to lung lesions, or easily recognizable cerebral symptoms, respectively. Such tissue adaptation has been shown in connection with quite different viruses; for instance, rickettsiae of epidemic typhus fever were adapted to grow in the mouse lung, while yellow fever, influenza, and a number of other viruses were made neurotropic in the laboratory by serial intracerebral inoculations. Accordingly, we chose first to explore the intracerebral and intranasal routes for the inoculation of mice with infectious anemia virus.

A group of five adult mice were inoculated intracerebrally in August 1948 by giving to each of them 0.03 cc. bacterially sterile, infectious horse serum. One of the mice was found dead the day following inoculation, apparently as a result of brain injury. The four surviving mice were kept under close observation for four months. They did not show appreciable symptoms except that they did not eat well during the first few weeks, and their weight was always under that of the control mice. When killed and autopsied four months after the inoculation, a somewhat enlarged spleen was found, but no other gross change was noted. In this group no attempt was made to carry the virus in serial passages by the cerebral route.

Mice were also injected intranasally with horse serum, and a few subinoculations were made, in groups of four mice, to explore the possibility of eventual quick adaptation through this route of infection. Rapid passages were done at 4- to 5-day intervals; the mice were killed, their lungs examined, and a saline suspension of the lungs inoculated into a fresh group of mice as mentioned in the description of methods above.

The intranasally injected mice did not manifest symptoms, neither did they produce marked lesions in their lungs, aside from minor changes such as swelling and a few small foci of congestion which did not tend to increase with passages. Similar changes may be noted in mice in early "blind" passages of other viruses; however, the congestion usually increases with the passages and death may occur soon, particularly in the case of pneumotropic viruses, such as human and swine influenza. After completing four passages of infectious anemia in this series, further transfers were abandoned.

The result was interpreted as indicating that either the virus does not lend itself to quick adaptation to the respiratory system of mice, or its quantity and virulence was not sufficiently high in the original inoculum (serum). There was also the possibility that the interval between the passages was not properly chosen. Before the conclusion of the preliminary experiments, plans were made and new series of more detailed investigations were begun in both rabbits and mice, to study the question of adaptation in additional experiments.

Serial Transmission in Rabbits

Although the result of the preliminary work with rabbits was not encouraging, further attempts were made to use this species in our experiments. Several groups of younger and older animals were inoculated intravenously or intraperitoneally with horse serum or plasma known to be fully virulent for horses. Rabbits of mixed breed and of different age groups were tried, usually the albino variety, ranging from the young to full-grown adults. The dosage of serum or blood injected varied from 3 to 10 cc. per rabbit.

In the third series, groups of two or three rabbits were injected, and the temperature reaction of the animals was followed for more than a month. Although no significant temperature rise was observed, passage was attempted twice by using whole blood, or serum of the rabbits for subinoculation on the 14th and 18th days, respectively, following the initial inoculation. This period was selected on account of the usual incubation period before the marked fever response in horses. In this passage series, young rabbits were used; their weight was between two and three pounds at the time of inoculation. None developed a temperature reaching 105°F. during the experimental period. Occasional counts during the first two weeks gave 5.2 to 6.3 million erythrocytes per cu.mm.

In two other series (fourth and fifth group) relatively young but fully grown rabbits were used. They received infectious serum collected from one of our experimental horses exhibiting unusually severe fever attacks; the blood was taken at the peak of the first and the second fever reaction. Again, no fever response was noted in the rabbits, beyond the physiologic range of fluctuation of the temperature. Therefore, this approach to the problem was abandoned for a while. Because of the essentially negative nature of the results, a detailed description of the experiments is omitted.

While these experiments were in progress, Brueckner and associates reported that they were able to transmit serially the virus of equine infectious anemia in rabbits; they noted in some of their rabbits a mild fever response after shorter or longer incubation period that varied considerably (363). Through the courtesy of Dr. A. L. Brueckner, Director of the State Livestock Service in College Park, Maryland, a rabbit passage series was obtained in June 1949. Each of five adult rabbits was inoculated intravenously with 6 cc. of blood from a rabbit in the 18th serial passage. Thus, this group of rabbits represented the 19th passage in the series of subinoculations. Temperatures were taken twice a day, the red blood corpuscles and the white blood cells were counted at about weekly intervals, and the animals were closely observed for symptoms.

In four out of the five rabbits the temperature rose above 105°F. between the 7th to the 10th day following inoculation and in two of them (Rabbit 390 and Rabbit 392) fever was repeatedly observed around the 14th, 21st, and 35th days almost simultaneously. In Rabbit 391 the temperature was 106.7°F. on the 8th day when it was sacrificed and its blood used for subinoculation. The spleen of this animal was moderately enlarged. One rabbit exhibited only one mild fever response; its temperature reached 105.2°F. on the 7th, and 105.0°F. on the 8th day. This animal died on the 29th day for unknown reasons. The parenchymatous organs appeared normal at this time. One additional rabbit (Rabbit 393), the largest and presumably the oldest of the group, did not show any fever reaction during 45 days of observation.

TABLE 14

HEMATOLOGIC RESPONSE OF RABBIT 392 (19TH SERIAL TRANSFER)

Days of infection	*Temperature F°*		*R.B.C.*	*W.B.C.*
1	103.6	103.8	6.500.000	10.700
7	104.2	105.0	4.950.000	11.500
16	104.0	104.2	5.000.000	8.700
21	105.0	103.8	4.400.000	6.000
37	103.6	104.0	5.100.000	17.600
50	105.4	105.6	5.400.000	15.700

The hematologic changes observed in Rabbit 392 are summarized in Table 14. The animal had 6.5 million erythrocytes per cu.mm. on the day of inoculation; this number decreased to 4.4 million by the third week, and this time a moderate leucopenia was noted; previously the white cell count was in the upper normal range. In two more counts within the next four weeks a definite leucocytosis with relative lymphocytosis was noted and, at the same time, the red blood corpuscles increased in number so that part of the earlier loss was regained. Chart 4 illustrates the temperature response of this rabbit (R. 392). Although the type of fever response of the rabbit is different from that of the horse, the repeated fever attacks are suggestive of a subacute type of infection.

In the remaining rabbits, the hematologic response varied. Two of the animals showed increased red cell counts two days following infection (8.1 and 7.0 million, respectively), and a definite drop (to 5.6 and 4.3 million) on the 7th day. During the same time, the early leucocytosis changed to values in the lower normal range. It is noteworthy that these animals (R. 389 and R. 393) produced the least impressive temperature response in the group. In Rabbit 390 a somewhat similar trend was noted

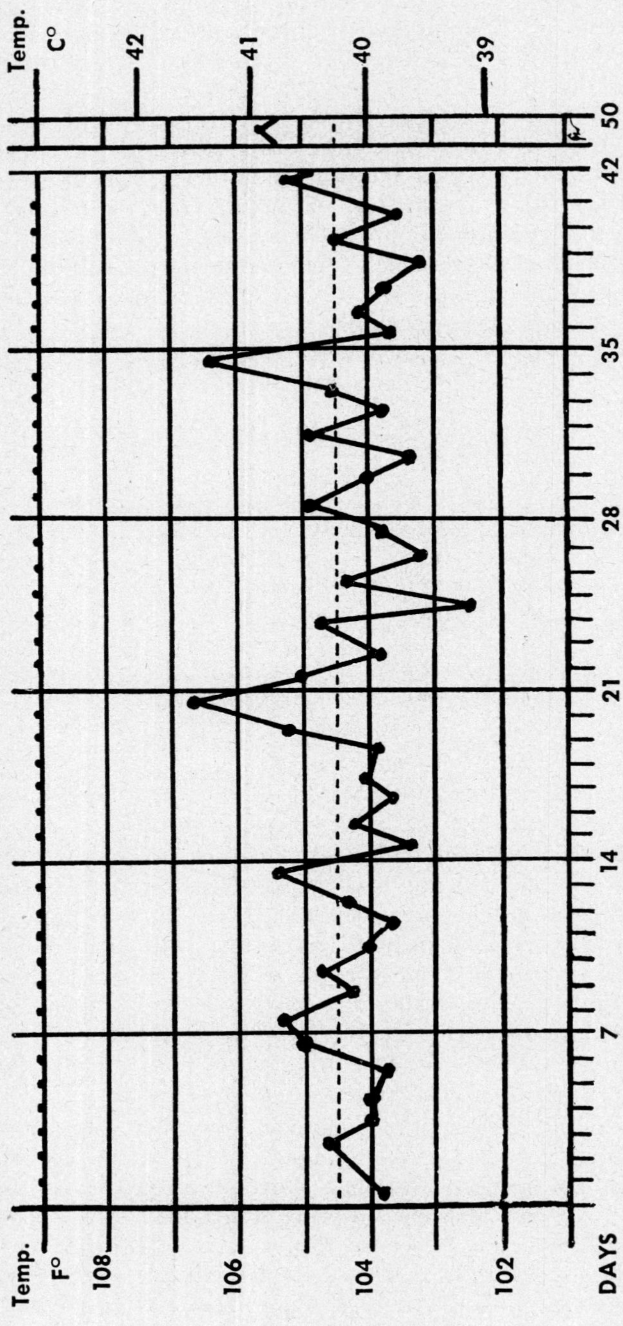

CHART 4.—FEVER RESPONSE OF RABBIT 392 (19TH PASSAGE OF VIRUS)

as in R. 392 but within narrower limits. There was no hematologic change observed in two counts of Rabbit 391.

Subinoculations were made with the blood of Rabbit 391 on the 8th day following its initial inoculation, and with the blood serum of Rabbit 392 on the 22nd day. The technique followed was largely that described by Reagan and co-workers (363).

In two of the rabbits thus injected, poor or no fever response was noted: the temperature reached 105°F. on the 33rd day in only one of them. In two other rabbits receiving blood serum from Rabbit 392, the response was better; one of them had a transient temperature rise on the 20th day, while the other produced a fever response twice within a month, on the 13th and the 20th to 22nd days following inoculation. Some decrease in the number of erythrocytes was recorded in this group but the data are not sufficient to warrant an analysis.

After one more passage in rabbits, it was decided to discontinue the series temporarily. This was partly because we noted that in a control rabbit, which received no injection, similar temperature changes were recorded as in the passage animals. However, it must be admitted that this rabbit was kept in a cage next to the inoculated rabbits, and might have acquired an infection accidentally. Other experiments which were conducted at this time also led to the decision to discontinue the transfer series in rabbits for a while, although the results noted in the 19th serial passage were sufficiently convincing that an infection was present and maintained in the passage series.

Later, two more attempts were made, one to continue the passages with material preserved frozen, and another to initiate a new adaptation series in rabbits by the use of virulent blood drawn from our experimental horses, but the results were not better than in the earlier experiments conducted with the same objective in mind. From this, it would seem that initiating the infection in rabbits with infectious anemia material of equine origin and its successful transfer in rabbits by serial passages is not readily achieved. The reasons governing success or failure are not apparent.

Serial Transmission of the Virus in Mice

In order to extend the scope of investigations intended for transmission of the virus to mice, various passage series were initiated, in October 1948, on the basis of the preliminary experiments. The principle of the serial transfer was utilized as before. A single transfer has, as a rule, no particular value as it may represent only a passive survival of the virus in the new host, without actual multiplication.

Three routes of infection were employed: intracerebral, intraperitoneal, and intranasal. Transfers were made at various intervals to determine the optimum period of time to make the passages. It was thought that very short intervals between the transfers might break down the series, if the virus could not multiply sufficiently within that time; again, an excessively long passage time might destroy the activity of the virus by eventual neutralization through the defense mechanism of the experimental animal. An account will be given here of the series in which the best results were obtained and the results of which were checked by horse inoculation. The details of theoretical interest will be presented elsewhere (96).

Two passage series of intracerebral inoculations with transfers at weekly intervals did not show any evidence of adaptation in six and four passages, respectively. As determined by gross pathologic alterations in the major abdominal organs, better results were obtained in the series of intraperitoneal inoculations carried on in three groups with passage intervals of 5, 7 to 10, and 14 days. Most marked pathologic changes were noted in the group in which transfers were made on the 7th to 10th day following inoculation. Alterations were noted here in the liver, and particularly in the spleen. The spleen was frequently enlarged three to four times the normal size. The parenchyma of the kidney was hemorrhagic in the initial passages. This can probably be explained by the foreign protein effect of horse serum.

In using the intranasal inoculation technique, passages were conducted at 4-day, and again at 8- to 10-day intervals between transfers; in some instances longer intervals were also allowed between passages. Of the several intranasal passage series only those in which the passage material was carried back to horses in subsequent experiments will be outlined. A 10 per cent saline suspension was prepared from both the lung tissue and the nasal mucous membrane of Horse 7 as described under the heading of methods at the beginning of this chapter. After centrifugation at 3000 rpm for one hour, the supernatants were pipetted off and used for intranasal inoculation of two groups of four mice each, giving 0.05 cc. as inoculum. Culture revealed some saprophytes but no pathogenic bacteria in the supernatant fluids. Mice can usually tolerate in their respiratory tract a small number of bacteria comparatively well, if the latter are not specially pathogenic for mice. This is substantiated by the fact that none of the mice thus inoculated died within a week. In order to increase the chances of starting an infection in the new host, superinfection was employed by administering 0.05 cc. of fresh infectious plasma of Horse 9 to each of the mice two days later by the intranasal route.

When the fourth passage of the horse lung series was completed, the mice were killed and a suspension of their lungs was prepared in saline as in previous passages intended for serial transfer by the intranasal route. Two of the mice in this group had an accelerated rate of respiration and showed a definite congestion of their lungs at autopsy. A suspension was also prepared from the spleen of one of the mice in the fourth passage, and transfer was continued through intra-abdominal application of the spleen suspension. In subsequent passages liver, spleen, and eventually the kidneys, were made up for suspension in saline and a mixture was used for injecting the next group of mice. Thus, a straight intranasal series and a combined series were run parallel, the latter being initiated intranasally and continued by the intra-abdominal route.

At the fifth passage in mice following the primary inoculation, a test was made in a normal horse. Lung and spleen suspensions of the passage mice were prepared and after centrifugation the clear supernatant fluids were pooled. Two cc. of the bacterially sterile pool made from the mouse lung and mouse spleen suspensions was intravenously injected to Horse 10 in November 1948 to test the passage materials for presence of the virus.

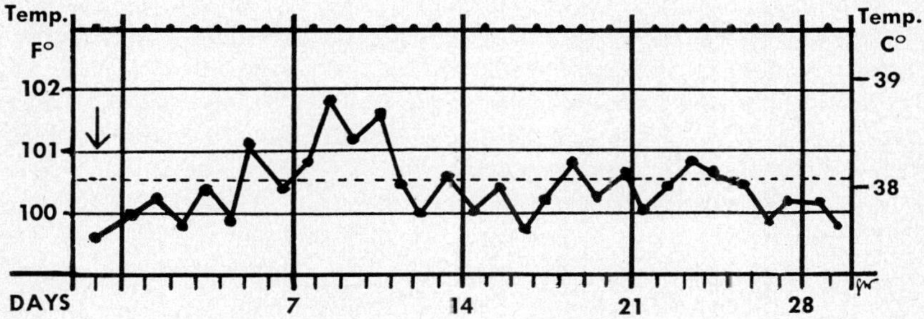

CHART 5.—FEVER RESPONSE OF HORSE 10 TO MOUSE PASSAGE MATERIAL

The test horse was held under close observation for over 50 days following the inoculation of mouse passage material. Temperature was taken twice a day. No marked symptoms were noted, but slight elevations of the temperature were recorded (Chart 5) on the 6th day (101.2°F.), on the 9th to 11th day (101.6° to 101.8°F.), and on the 51st day (101.8°F.). The normal temperature of this horse before inoculation was between 99.5° and 100.5°F. On the 52nd day following the test inoculation with mouse material, the horse was challenged with 5 cc. of infectious horse serum. A typical reaction developed with a fever reaching 105.0°F. on the 16th day after the challenge inoculation, and this was followed by several fever attacks within the next two months. The horse became a chronic case later and remained under observation for more than two years.

Because of the mild fever reaction in the horse following the inoculation of mouse material, it was decided to start mouse passages again with the blood of Horse 10 collected at the peak of the first marked fever reaction. It was thought that this blood sample might contain both a mouse adapted and a horse adapted virus and thus the serial passages would serve as part of an alternate passage series. A similar method had been employed by Baker (10) who successfully adapted the rinderpest virus to rabbits by using the technique of alternate passages in rabbits and the original host.

Accordingly, a passage series was started in mice with citrated blood of Horse 10, giving 0.1 cc. to each mouse by the intra-abdominal route, and it was continued with organ suspensions together with the blood of the mice by the same route for five consecutive passages, making transfers at 6- to 8-day intervals. No symptoms or death occurred during these passages and, except for splenic enlargement, no gross lesions were noted in the mice.

A suspension was prepared from the liver, spleen, and kidneys of mice representing the third passage, and 4 cc. of the supernatant fluid was injected into Horse 15 in February 1949. Not even a mild fever response was noted in six months following the inoculation. When subjected to challenge inoculation with virulent virus, the horse reacted in a delayed fashion and died on the 42nd day following infection. This experiment indicated that a bacterially sterile extract of mouse organs *per se* would not cause a fever reaction in the horse.

Although the horse inoculation tests (in Horse 10 and Horse 15) did not give a final answer, and the result of the challenge inoculations indicated that the horses remained susceptible to a virulent virus, there was a definite suggestion that infectious anemia virus was present in at least one of the mouse passage materials used for injection. This was indicated in Horse 10 by the mild fever response and changes in the blood protein fractions corresponding to those seen in typical cases of infectious anemia. The albumin-globulin ratio of serum (A/G) showed a marked decrease in three weeks following injection with the mouse material; from a preinoculation value of 0.61, it dropped to 0.35 by the 22nd day, indicating the presence of serious systemic reaction. The lack of temperature response in Horse 15 does not rule out the possibility of a latent infection. It is conceivable that, by adaptation to a new host, the equine virus lost considerable virulence for horses. This would explain the mild symptoms in Horse 10 and an eventual latent infection in Horse 15.

Re-transmission of the Virus to Horses

The virulence of the virus, which apparently declined during the mouse passages, was gradually restored by serial transfer in horses. We shall give here an outline of these experiments; for further details, the reader is referred to a publication by one of us (Dreguss (96)).

Horse 34 was inoculated with 2 cc. of serum from Horse 10 collected on the 22nd day following inoculation with the mouse passage material. The result was a mild temperature rise of 101.7°F. on the 4th and 6th day, and a somewhat more pronounced rise on the 16th day with a peak of 102.4°F. No blood sample was taken during the fever reactions; a sample collected 10 days after the second rise showed normal hematologic values except for a mild leucopenia and a marked relative lymphocytosis (55 per cent lymphocytes). This finding was taken as additional evidence that Horse 10 contained in its blood a virus of slight virulence on the 22nd day following inoculation with mouse material.

Two new series of mouse passages by the intraperitoneal and intranasal routes were begun. Fresh blood of Horse 32 was chosen for use as starting

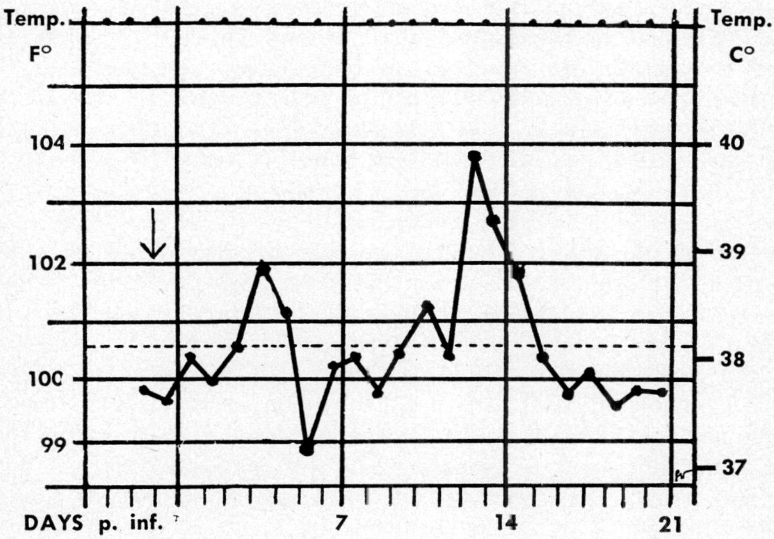

Chart 6.—Fever response of Horse 35
(Second passage of virus at re-transmission to horse)

material to initiate such passages, because this animal was inoculated with blood from Horse 31, which had in turn received blood from Horse 10 taken during the first marked fever attack following challenge inoculation. The blood of Horse 10 at the time of this bleeding presumably carried the virus adapted to both, the horse and the mouse. Consequently, it could be assumed that Horse 32's blood contained both of these theoretical variants of the anemia virus and, therefore, would better lend itself to re-transmission to the mouse.

The passage series in mice with transfers at 9-day intervals, produced suggestive results. In the intraperitoneal series the major abdominal organs were invariably enlarged; in the intranasal group lung lesions of varying intensity were noted and occasionally death occurred, although not regularly; there was no evidence of bacterial contamination

Citrated blood collected from the hearts of mice in the fifth passage of both series (intranasal and intraperitoneal) was pooled with suspensions of the liver and spleen and 4 cc. of the mixture was injected into Horse 36 intravenously. The horse showed a mild fever response on the 18th and 19th day, and again on the 25th and 34th day. Examination of the hematologic values revealed a transient drop of a little over one million in the number of erythrocytes.

Horse 35 was inoculated with 3 cc. of citrated blood taken from Horse 36 on the 8th day following infection. The fever response in Horse 35 was rather typical; a mild response was noted on the 4th and 5th day, and a marked reaction occurred on the 13th day (Chart 6). The full course of the disease was not observed, as both horses were destroyed early because of lack of space in the isolation stables.

In the third horse passage following the mouse passages, two horses were injected with infectious serum of Horse 35 taken 10 days after the marked fever reaction and kept frozen for about a year. Doses of 5 cc. of the same serum were given intravenously to both, Horse 38 and Horse 44. One of the horses exhibited two marked fever reactions, after a prolonged incubation period, which started on the 38th and the 50th days following infection (Horse 38); while the other receiving exactly the same material, showed a definite fever response with a peak of 104.3°F. on the 25th day (Horse 44). The decrease in the number of erythrocytes was 2.5 million in Horse 38, and 1.3 million in Horse 44. Horse 38 showed unusual thirst two weeks after the infection, which lasted for several days; at the same time the blood proteins also manifested changes, but no fever was noted. These were considered as possible indications of a subclinical reaction. The prolonged incubation seems to be related to the fact that both, Horse 38 and Horse 44, had a high level of gamma-globulin in their blood before inoculation (of the two, Horse 38 had the higher value) that usually exerts a delaying influence (see Chapter 9). Both horses were destroyed soon after the fever reaction in order to terminate the experiment. In both animals histopathologic changes typical for infectious anemia were found.

A pool of normal blood taken before inoculation from each of the horses in this series (Horse 35, Horse 36, Horse 38, and Horse 44) was injected into a normal horse. It showed no fever response or any other symptoms in three months, indicating that none of the horses tested carried the virus in its blood before it was infected in this experimental series.

The description of the hematologic and other changes that the virus caused in the mice has been omitted, although this was the subject of a careful study during the experiments designed for serial transmission. It was noted during the first months of the preliminary experiments in 1948 that the survivors of the various passage series did not gain weight as did the control mice of the same age kept on the same diet and same laboratory condition. Erythrocytes counted often revealed as much as 50 per cent decrease as compared with counts on normal mice (409) of the same stock.

As to the result of these studies, it may be briefly mentioned that part of the mice, which were injected with horse blood or passage material from mice, manifested a clear-cut decrease in the number of erythrocytes, amounting to about one or two million as compared with the preinoculation

TABLE 15

HEMATOLOGIC FINDINGS IN PASSAGE MICE

Mouse No.	*Serial Transfer*	*R.B.C. Before Inoculation*	*R.B.C. Decreased to*	*Days Foll. Infection*
M. 161	4th	9,000.000	5,415.000	31
M. 165	5th	9,600.000	5,650.000	18
M. 165			4,700.000	29
M. 166	5th	9,950.000	7,710.000	30
M. 168	5th	9,300.000	8,165.000	21
M. 168			10,350.000	50
M. 241	1st	10,250.000	8,600.000	15
M. 241			9,100.000	28
M. 241			6,250.000	35
M. 252	1st	10,050.000	6,800.000	21
M. 252			7,050.000	42
M. 252			10,200.000	90

values, and often more. This is illustrated in Table 15 by a few figures obtained in this investigation. Some of the mice in the same passage groups, however, did not exhibit significant changes. It was concluded from these experimental studies, to be published in detail elsewhere (100), that hematologic changes in the mouse are not sufficiently regular to suggest their use for the purpose of a practical diagnostic test.

The results of the experiments designed for re-transmission of the virus to horses indicate that the equine infectious anemia virus was successfully transmitted to mice and that it was carried through them in at least five serial passages. During these passages the virus lost much of its virulence for equines, but it was possible to restore the virulence of the virus by repeated horse passages. The gradual return of the virulence for horses is a clear evidence that the virus was not accidentally picked up during the re-adaptation process. This is further confirmed by the horse inoculation test with normal blood samples of the horses used in the experiment. No clear indication was secured as to which of the routes of infection in mice was most effective, since pools were used for testing passage materials and no subdivision, as originally intended, was possible. As may be seen from the description above, the virus—carried in serial transfers through mice and rabbits—causes in these rodents only a mild infection which is not readily recognized in them on the basis of clinical symptoms alone. The possible reasons for this are analyzed in Chapter 9.

*

Many investigators have in the past attempted to transmit the virus of infectious anemia to laboratory animals as well as to some of the domestic animals other than equines. The earliest of such experiments are those recorded in 1906 by Carré and Vallée (58) in their basic study on the malady. They stated that guinea-pigs, rats, rabbits, and mice are not susceptible to the virus, and that dogs, goats, cattle, and sheep also proved to be completely refractory to inoculation with the virus. Other research workers, in addition to making further trials with the animals already mentioned, added more species to the list of animals tested for susceptibility. Such animals were swine (123,191), young cats (593,451), hens and pigeons (405). Later the list was further extended to include the monkey (370,23,279), ferret (370), and even the lion (279). In 1944, Stein and Mott (432) attempted to determine the susceptibility of numerous laboratory and domestic animals to the virus. They concluded that none of the animals tested were susceptible. A brief survey of the literature on the subject may be found in their paper. More recently Morris and Alexander (309), in Washington, tested 14 mammalian and 5 fowl species to determine their suitability for experimental purpose in infectious anemia, with negative result. Their animals included pen-raised dogs, foxes, ferrets, rabbits, cotton rats, albino rats, minks, pigeons, ducks, pheasants, and quails; as well as various species of squirrels, rats, mice, and starlings caught in wild.

It is noteworthy that several experimenters noted transient fever or other symptoms in some of the animals tested, but the experiments were usually discontinued after the blood or tissues of the experimental animal in question failed to produce typical infectious anemia in the horse.

While it is generally agreed that mules and donkeys are susceptible to the virus, there is some divergence of opinion as to whether the virus passaged in horses is equally virulent for the related solipeds. The small African donkey was extensively used in research work by Balozet (13,14) and Martin (279).

Among domestic animals the porcine species is the sole example that has been repeatedly found to be at least partially susceptible to the virus.

Such was the opinion of the Japanese Commission (191) and several other investigators including Habersang (145), Lührs (266), and Kutsche (230); they were able to produce suggestive hematologic and fever responses in young pigs. However, there was some dispute about the validity of their findings (450). Oppermenn and Herrfarth (332) recorded partly successful transmission experiments in young swine later. Köbe (208) noted good results in splenectomized piglets, and re-transmitted the infection to the horse. Král (220) believes that the swine may carry the virus passively if inoculated with it.

The susceptibility of rabbits has been a subject of controversy for some time. Among the first to report positive results with rabbits are Jaffé and Silberstein (189). They injected guinea-pigs, mice, rats and rabbits intramuscularly and intraperitoneally with infectious anemia virus; rabbits were injected also intravenously. Among these, rabbits reacted to the virus, while the rest of the laboratory animals produced negative results. The rabbits exhibited a temperature rise (by 1 to 1.5 C°) on the 6th to 12th day following inoculation and some of them died of the infection. Passages were performed in rabbits but no re-transmission to the horse was attempted. By injecting rabbits with the virus, Oppermann and Lauterbach (333) also recorded favorable results and claimed diagnostic value for them. A great number of publications appeared in the form of doctoral dissertations from the Veterinary College at Hannover, Germany, concerning the suitability of the rabbit for diagnostic inoculation as an experimental test animal in equine anemia. But the interpretations and the conclusions were not accepted by most re-investigators.

In spite of careful analysis and checking by several investigators, the problem of the susceptibility of the rabbit to the anemia virus has remained undecided. Lührs (269) stated that rabbits are of no value in the diagnosis. Schermer and Eigendorf (386) expressed the opinion that the foreign protein effect may be responsible in part for the changes interpreted by others as the criterion of successful transmission in rabbits. Their opinion was based on experimental injections of normal horse serum and normal swine serum to rabbits. Many authors discussed the problem of the diagnostic value of rabbit inoculations; such discussions often included the problem of susceptibility of guinea-pigs as well (187,222,246,332,382,459, 488).

The use of chickens, pigeons, and other fowl species for the purpose of diagnostic test failed to yield any convincing result. Their use was advocated mainly by Oppermann and co-workers (331,334,335); however, the value of histologic alterations resulting from inoculation of horse blood into chickens and pigeons, and their use as a criterion for the decision of positive diagnosis, was strongly disputed by others who considered it doubtful that the changes were caused by the virus of infectious anemia.

Until recently the consensus of opinion was that no laboratory or domestic animal has proven susceptible to the virus of equine infectious anemia, with the possible exception of a slight susceptibility in the case of swine. This certainly appears to be true in the sense that the typical picture of equine infectious anemia with all the characteristics of the disease in the original host has not been produced in laboratory animals, but this is what may be expected in a new host. It is another question, however, whether a laboratory animal could be found which might serve the purpose of experimental studies in the laboratory, after the virus was successfully adapted to it.

Gamaleya (656) reported adapting the virus to rabbits and carrying it through 18 consecutive passages. A very mild disease with a slight febrile reaction was noted and the ninth passage material in rabbits was successfully carried back to a foal. Vaccination was also attempted by the use of rabbit adapted virus. Strangely, the blood of passage rabbits, when injected into horses, which were previously infected with the virus, activated typical symptoms of infectious anemia in them.

As already mentioned, Reagan and co-workers (363,364) similarly succeeded in carrying the virus of infectious anemia up to 20 passages in rabbits, and reported re-transmission of the infection from rabbits to the horse. Our work as outlined above, though incomplete, seems to confirm the presence of the virus in their rabbit transfer series; however, no horse inoculation test was made by us with the rabbit passage material.

Our adaptation experiments in mice (96) were planned on somewhat similar lines but independently from the findings in rabbits. The presence of the virus in mice, at least up to five transfers, was well substantiated by several re-transmission experiments of the virus to the horse, and by regaining its virulence to the original host through serial passages in horses. It could not be decided on the basis of our experiments whether the adaptation to mice was achieved by the alternate passages as described for rinderpest virus by Baker (10), or whether an incomplete virus was first formed and gradually became more complete, and therefore infectious, in the serial passages. The existence of such an incomplete virus has been described and experimentally studied in the case of human influenza virus by von Magnus (272).

The systematic serial passages in our experiments served the purpose of adaptation and also to eliminate the disturbing effect of foreign protein as present in the primary inoculation, since the serial passages are naturally carried out with homologous material. This is all the more desirable in the case of equine infectious anemia, as the mechanism of infection in this disease closely resembles to that of a protein intoxication. (See Chapter 9.)

The important facts brought out by our experiments on mice are that the virulence of the virus for the original host is altered by passages through a new experimental animal, and that the restoration of its virulence may necessitate several passages through the original host (96). Therefore, a potential new experimental animal should not be discarded as useless after an initial inoculation has failed to produce the typical form of the disease, or because the first horse has not exhibited marked symptoms upon an attempt at re-transmission of the virus from the new host. It is by serial passages only that such questions can be decided.

We believe that the possibility of finding a suitable experimental animal for the study of infectious anemia is very close, and that it would be worthwhile to study further the firm adaptation of the virus to rabbits and mice by the technique of serial passages.

CHAPTER 11

CULTIVATION OF THE VIRUS IN CHICK EMBRYOS

It would facilitate the study of infectious anemia enormously, if the virus causing the malady could be cultivated outside of the body of susceptible animals. This has not been possible so far. Successful cultivation of the virus would be desirable for several reasons, but mainly because it might furnish a means for diagnostic test (supplying antigens, etc.), and it might serve as a basis for specific control measures.

Viruses require the presence of living cells for their multiplication. Methods of cultivation that can supply the living cells for this purpose are cultivation 1) in tissue culture, 2) in various kinds of embryonic tissue, for instance in minced chick embryo, or, 3) in the developing chick embryo itself within the egg shell. The latter method has been widely used for propagating a number of mammalian viruses.

Therefore, in 1948, the outline of our work included plans for a preliminary attempt to cultivate the virus by the use of chick embryos. The difficulties met in the experiments for transmitting the infection to animals other than the original host, made a rapid success seem unlikely. It was hoped, however, that methods that had recently led to the successful cultivation of some viruses which previously resisted such attempts might be applicable also to infectious anemia.

As in the experiments designed for the study of transmission to laboratory animals, emphasis was laid on the possibility of adaptation. Thus, "blind" passages were done in a series of embryonated eggs in the hope that the virus would be adapted to the embryonic tissue, producing lesions in them and eventually becoming sufficiently pathogenic to chick embryos as to kill them. We were aware of many difficulties, the worst being the lack of test animals other than the horse. Although it is difficult to judge about the final value of the results we obtained, it is felt that a brief account of the preliminary experiments is warranted.

Routes of Inoculation

Chick embryos in pre-incubated fertile hens eggs were inoculated with infectious material by various routes and at different ages, and serial transfers were made in fresh embryos. The routes customarily used for virus culture in embryonated eggs were tried, that is, inoculation on the chorio-allantoic membrane, into the allantoic cavity, and into the yolk sac, or a combination of these methods. The technique was the one known from work with influenza and other viruses, or rickettsiae, as described in all technical details by Beveridge and Burnet (549). The incubation temperature was 37°C. throughout, before and after inoculation. Survival of the embryos was checked at least once a day by candling the eggs.

In judging the results, the tissues of the inoculated chick embryos were checked for the presence of eventual gross lesions, and the hemagglutination test with chicken red blood cells was routinely made with suspensions made from the tissues and various fluids, mostly the ellantoic fluid of the embryos. For obvious reasons, final horse inoculation test was done in a few cases only. Tests were done as usual for checking bacterial sterility; contaminated material was discarded. Material intended for later test inoculation was preserved in the deep-freezer at –20 to –25° C.

Chorio-allantoic membrane.—In this group, 8 to 10 days old chick embryos were used for inoculation, and transfers were made 4 to 5 days later. The air sac was transferred from the blunt end of the egg to the sidewall of the egg shell by the usual technique. Through a small opening prepared aseptically, 0.1 cc. of inoculum was dripped to the surface of the chorio-allantoic membrane with a tuberculin syringe and a fine 21 gauge needle. The opening of the egg shell was sealed with paraffin. After additional incubation, usually for 2 to 4 days, the eggs were opened with sterile instruments, the membranes were inspected and a 10 per cent suspension of them was made in saline by using powdered alundum for grinding. After centrifugation the supernatant was used for subinoculation, usually in an amount of 0.1 cc. The advantage of this route lies in the eventual success of producing virus lesions on the membrane after proper adaptation.

Allantoic cavity.—In this group 10 to 12 days old chick embryos were used. The material was introduced into the allantoic cavity by inoculation through a small hole made in the egg shell. After additional incubation for 2 to 5 days, allantoic fluid was collected for hemagglutination test and transfer. At the beginning, the transfers were made on the 4th or 5th days. Later, assuming some degree of adaptation, the time of transfer was decreased to 3 days, occasionally to 2 days.

Yolk sac.—Eggs were incubated for 6 to 8 days and then inoculation was made into the yolk sac: a needle of sufficient length was inserted through a hole prepared on the blunt end of the egg to reach about the center of the embryonated egg where the yolk is located. After 5 to 7 days incubation the embryos were removed from the egg and the yolk sac separated. Suspension of the yolk sac in saline (without the bulk of yolk) served for transfers.

In the *combined series* of transfers, early passages were made on the chorio-allantoic membrane. After four or five such transfers, the passage material (membrane suspension) was inoculated into the yolk sac and transfers were continued by the yolk sac technique, a procedure similar to the one successfully used for adapting rinderpest virus (411) to grow in chicken embryos.

Serial Passages in Chick Embryos

For initiating the series of these passages, infectious horse serum or plasma was used; in one instance bone-marrow of an infected horse was utilized.

In the *first group* of the culture series, blood from three bleedings of Horse 22, taken on the 3rd, 10th, and 13th day following infection, was the source of virus. This horse had a marked fever reaction of over 104° F. (40° C.) between the 10th and 15th day. With the three initiating materials and four different passage routes, the first group consisted of 12 different culture series that were run parallel at the same time. Up to 18 serial transfers were made by the chorio-allantoic route, 20 transfers by the allantoic cavity method, and 18 transfers by the yolk sac technique.

In the *second group* the following material was used as first inoculum: a plasma sample of Horse 10 taken at the peak of the first marked fever reaction and stored frozen; a fresh serum sample of Horse 26 taken at the beginning of the fever response 10 days following infection; a suspension of bone-marrow of the same horse that was destroyed on the 11th day. In all inoculations of this second group, except for the initiating injections, 0.1 cc. of a 1:10 dilution of normal horse serum was added to the embryonic transfer material. The serum was obtained from a young, healthy, normal horse and was shown to be free of infectious anemia virus by horse inoculation test.

The routes of inoculation were similar to the first group except that no inoculation was made into the allantoic cavity. The bone-marrow series of Horse 26 and the series initiated with the serum of the same horse were united beginning with the third transfer. The combined chorio-allantoic and yolk sac inoculation series was run as described above. In addition, a rapid passage series was started: after five consecutive passages were done in the series initiated with serum and bone-marrow of Horse 26 by using the chorio-allantoic membrane route, a suspension of the membranes was injected into the yolk sac and transfers were made by means of yolk sac suspension every 24 or 48 hours.

This latter series exhibited some lethal effect in the embryos as early as in the 3rd rapid yolk sac passage; later the mortality reached 80 per cent of the inoculated embryos. Death of the embryos occurred in two to four days after the inoculation. Surprisingly, subinoculation from these embryos would not give as satisfactory result as a yolk sac suspension of an embryo from an egg opened 24 hours following injection while the embryo was alive. Therefore, transfers were made early, while a group of the inoculated embryos was kept longer for recording the lethal effect.

Most of the chick embryos in this series exhibited a clearly noticeable swelling and redness of their skin, often also petechial hemorrhages. Similar changes were occasionally observed in some embryos of the other passage series. As no bacteria could be cultivated in various culture media from such embryos, it was reasonable to assume that a virus was present and passed from embryo to embryo in the series.

It seemed unlikely that, by means of the eggs, some virus of the fowl species was picked up and carried in transfers, since we were unable to increase the virulence in subsequent transfers. The results in which 80 per cent death occurred were not duplicated, and there seemed to be a constant risk of losing the lethal effect in passages to follow. Obviously, a virus originally pathogenic for chickens would not behave this way.

Although some chorio-allantoic membranes in both passage series appeared to be swollen, edematous and congested, no typical focal lesions were observed, as seen in the case of some other viruses adapted to multiply on the membranes.

Test in Horses

Unfortunately, no horse inoculation tests could be carried out in sufficient number to decide the question. This was mainly because the isolation stables were occupied by horses inoculated in immunization experiments. Only a preliminary test in horses was possible for each group of the culture series. It is fully realized that this was insufficient to decide the problem, but we hoped to obtain a lead, at least.

A few horses were injected in succession for obtaining experimental evidence as to whether the virus of infectious anemia was present in the higher transfers of the various culture series. Since individual sampling would have required many horses, pools were used for the purpose of obtaining preliminary information.

Horse 24 received a pool of chick embryo material of the first group of culture series. All inoculation routes were represented in the pool of suspensions made of chorio-allantoic membranes, yolk sacs, and allantoic fluid, ranging from the 7th to the 11th transfer in the various passage series. Horse 24 was inoculated subcutaneously with 10 cc. of the pool. Temperature was taken regularly and frequent bleedings were done. No significant temperature rise was observed in 48 days. At this time the horse received 0.5 cc. of highly virulent virus (Horse 10's plasma) intravenously, and produced a typical fever response with a peak of 105° F. (40.6° C.) on the 13th day following the challenge inoculation.

Although no clinical sign of illness was seen following the inoculation of Horse 24 with chick embryo material, it is noteworthy that the number of red blood corpuscles decreased by one million by the 6th day after inoculation of the culture material. Following a remission, a second drop was noted again on the 20th day with a loss of 1.8 million red blood cells as against the pre-inoculation value. The hemoglobin content of the blood dropped from 12.8 grams per 100 cc. to 10.4 grams on the 8th day, and 10.6 on the 31st day. Similar changes were observed following the challenge inoculation: a loss of 2.3 million red blood cells and 3 grams of hemoglobin occurred in 15 days. In spite of the outcome of the challenge inoculation, there remains a strong suggestion that the chick embryo material contained a virus that was responsible for changes in the blood of the test horse.

For preliminary testing of the second culture group, Horse 27 was intravenously inoculated with 5 cc. of pooled embryonic passage material. The pool consisted of six different suspensions (made of chorio-allantoic membranes and yolk sacs, both from the direct and the combined series) representing the 6th and 8th transfers in the respective passage series, all of which were started with serum and bone-marrow of Horse 26. The test horse exhibited a mild elevation of temperature on the 13th day following inoculation with the embryonic material. Another slight fluctuation of temperature was noted on the 35th through 41st day with readings of 101.4 and 101.8° F. (38.7° C.). Similar rises were repeatedly observed within the next four months; these usually lasted three to five days; sometimes a one-day peak was seen. The red cell count of Horse 27 dropped by 1.7 million by the 14th day, and the loss of hemoglobin was 2.1 grams as against the pre-inoculation value. The loss was 2.1 million red blood cells and 2.9 grams of hemoglobin on the 36th day. A fluctuation between similar values and the normal was noted in the following months, but no definite anemia developed. The total number of white blood cells remained in the lower normal range or exhibited leukopenia, as observed in early months of typical infectious anemia. During the following three months, no symptoms were noted and the minor temperature rises ceased to occur.

The horse was subjected to challenge inoculation eight months following the initial inoculation with culture material; 1 cc. of infectious serum of Horse 10 taken a week before use was given intravenously. The challenge inoculation brought about a temperature rise, milder in character than usual, on the 14th to the 23rd day and this was followed by two marked fever attacks in the next month. A marked drop was noted in the number of erythrocytes and the total number of leukocytes on the 17th day following the challenge inoculation.

The hematologic findings in the test horses, together with the mild recurrent fever reactions noted for five months in the second animal, suggested a subclinical type of infection presumably caused by the virus of infectious anemia present in the egg culture material.

Twice, an attempt was made to decide the question by additional horse inoculation tests, using serum samples of Horse 24 and Horse 27 originally inoculated with egg passage material; samples used for this purpose were collected before the challenge inoculation. One of the new test horses thus injected (Horse 28) with a pool of serum samples of Horse 24, and six weeks later with those of Horse 27, failed to produce evidence of an infection aside from a mild fever response noted on the 9th to the 13th day following the second injection. The same horse remained healthy after it was challenged several times with blood of virus carrier horses. Consequently, the value of this test was questionable.

An additional attempt, two years later, also failed to bring a definite answer. A thoroughbred (Horse 40) exhibited a drop of the red cell count by 3 million on the 30th day following injection with a mixture of serum samples of Horse 24 and Horse 27 stored at refrigerator temperature. Aside from weakness and depression on the same day, no other symptom was observed in this animal, which had to be destroyed on the 35th day for reasons beyond our control. By this time the number of red blood cells in its blood had returned to about normal level. No significant histopathologic changes were noted.

Tests by Hemagglutination and Interference

Hemagglutination tests with chicken red blood cells were carried out with most of the passage material used in these studies, but they did not give any definite result. On a few occasions, positive results were noted with the allantoic fluid or organ suspensions of the embryos, but these were rather inconstant and not always reproducible. Therefore, no detailed account is warranted here.

We sought to reveal the presence of virus in the chick embryo passage series indirectly by the so-called interference phenomenon. Andrewes (6) noted that a virus added to embryonic tissue culture, which was previously inoculated with another related virus, would not multiply at the usual rate; he assumed that this was because the virus inoculated first would interfere with the growth of the second one. Bostick (43) in his experiments used the phenomenon as supporting evidence for indicating the presence of a hypothetic virus in Hodgkin's disease, by causing interference with the growth of influenza *B* virus.

In our experiments, infectious anemia serum or embryonic passage material was first injected either into the allantoic cavity or, more often, into the yolk sac; then, after a few days incubation, an additional inoculation was made into the same eggs, using high dilutions of Newcastle disease virus (allantoic fluid). The growth curve of the latter was checked by virus hemagglutination test (32) in 6, 12, 24 and 48 hours. In the allantoic fluid as well as in the yolk sac suspension of the twice-injected embryos, the titer of Newcastle virus, at 12 hours, was none or significantly lower than in the controls (with no primary inoculation). This observation seemed to confirm the presence of infectious anemia virus, but the interference was not quite clear-cut in higher passages of the series indicating that either the growth of anemia virus diminished with progressive passages, or the phenomenon was not specific. Titration in horses could only decide which of these assumptions is correct.

*

Our preliminary findings were reported to the Scientific Advisory Committee of the Grayson Foundation at the closing of the fiscal year of 1949. This unpublished report is given verbatim below:

> *Cultivation of the Virus in Embryonated Eggs.*—Extensive work was carried out for propagating infectious anemia virus in the chick embryo. Various routes of inoculation and various starting materials have been used. 5 to 11 day old chick embryos were injected with infectious material by the allantoic route, into the yolk sac, and onto the chorio-allantoic membrane. Thousands of fertile eggs were used and serial passages were made up to the 20th subinoculation in eggs.
>
> The first experimental series often showed some changes in the chick embryos that suggested the presence of the virus in some higher passages, however, death of the embryos did not occur regularly. This material, when tested following the 7th egg passage and higher passages by injecting the egg material into a horse, did not give clear evidence of the presence of the virus.
>
> A second egg series was tried with improved and considerably modified technique. Here, more evidence of the propagation was observed and in some passage groups the death rate of the embryos reached 80 per cent. The testing of this egg culture series in horses is under way. At present it can be stated that the horse injected showed very suspect hematological changes in his blood and repeated minor, later stronger elevations of the temperature above normal. The final outcome of this experiment and cross testing of the horse will decide whether or not we succeeded in cultivating the equine anemia virus.

Prior to our experiments, no serious attempt had been made, as far as we are aware, to study the possibility of cultivation of the virus in the case of infectious anemia, aside from some work done by Pinus and Pirog (351) in 1937. Later, the U. S. Bureau of Animal Industry made, in 1950, a brief reference to attempted cultivation in chick embryos though with negative results (462). Because neither of these reports contains closer details about the methods used and the way of testing the culture material for presence of the virus, it is impossible to evaluate the findings. The Bureau stated in the report that a test horse was injected with the culture material; no fever reaction was observed and the animal proved to be susceptible to challenge inoculation with a virulent virus 72 days later.

Our observations upon the chick embryos, together with the response in the test horses, strongly suggest that the virus of infectious anemia was present and multiplied in the serial egg passages. The final experimental proof of this is lacking because it was impossible for us to use sufficient number of horses in testing the culture material on account of the limited facilities to house the experimental animals in screened stables.

If the assumption is correct that the equine anemia virus was present in the egg culture material tested by injection of the first two horses, then a decrease in the virulence of the virus toward the original host is noted; this was manifested by the mild, subclinical response in the test horses. Although there was only a doubtful fever reaction in the first horse (Horse 24) and a mild but suggestive response in the second one (Horse 27), the hematologic values revealed changes identical with those noted in the typical disease, indicating that one can not neglect the changes in the blood and depend upon the fever response alone when judging about the possibility of subclinical infection.

Horse 27 was observed for a long time between the first injection and the challenge inoculation. During the early months of this period it developed repeated mild fever reactions, but did not become progressively anemic as might be expected. This was probably due to adaptation of the virus to the avian species and decrease of its virulence to the horse. A similar observation was made by Jenkins and Shope (192) in connection with the cultivation of rinderpest virus in embryonated eggs.

The conclusion seems to be justified that both horses (H. 24 and H. 27) suffered a mild infection following injection of the cultured virus. On the other hand, if the changes noted in these horses were merely the results of a foreign protein action provoked by a single injection containing a small amount of egg protein—that seems to be unlikely—then a striking analogy must exist between such actions and the mechanism of infection in equine anemia.

The result of the challenge inoculations cannot be utilized to clarify the problem. Positive challenge inoculation in infectious anemia is often interpreted as an evidence against previous subclinical infection. The fallacy of such conclusion is quite obvious, considering the fact that infection is followed by resistance in a small fraction of cases only, while a large majority of infected horses remains more or less susceptible, particularly within the usual time limit of experiments. There is no sound reason to expect immunity following a subclinical infection for, in most instances, not even severe infections would lead to resistance, i.e., solid immunity against re-infection with a virulent virus. In our opinion, based on experimental evidence as discussed in the chapter on pathogenesis, the positive result in a challenge inoculation merely indicates the presence of active virus in the inoculum and, also, that the recipient horse is not a resistant virus carrier; however, it would not reveal whether the infection provoked by the challenge inoculation is a primary one, or represents a superinfection.

The experimental observations as presented above contain suggestive evidence that the virus of infectious anemia was successfully cultivated in embryonated eggs. We believe that a suitable procedure can be completely worked out along lines similar to those presented in the description of our experiments, but it will require much additional experimental work before the problem can be settled.

CHAPTER 12

IMMUNIZATION EXPERIMENTS

One of the main objectives of the present experimental studies was to explore the possibility of developing a practical procedure for preventive immunization. Therefore, investigations aimed in this direction were begun early.

Attempts at immunization have not been lacking in the past, but little or no success was achieved. This may be explained, in part, by the unusual position that this malady occupies among infectious diseases. Although we fully realized that an early success cannot be expected, it seemed worth while to make renewed attempts at immunization along new lines, or on those not thoroughly studied so far, in the hope of gaining at least a clue for future work. First of all, immunization procedures were selected, which would allow the virus to exert a continuous, longer-lasting, or repeated antigenic effect upon the horses thus immunized. Since it is known that one natural attack of infectious anemia does not confer immunity, rather predisposes to renewed attacks within short intervals, it can hardly be expected that appreciable resistance to the virus would develop from a single artificial immunizing stimulus.

After some preliminary studies, we attempted experimental immunization with the virus adsorbed to aluminium hydroxide, and with repeated inoculations of organ suspensions made from tissues of infected horses in the early stage of the disease. Hopes were also attached to the eventual immunizing value of the virus contained in chick embryo cultures or in passage material of laboratory animals, if a successful serial transfer could be achieved.

Adsorption of the Virus to Aluminium Hydroxide

In preliminary studies adsorption of the virus to a suitable adsorbent was studied with the intention of working out a method of immunization based on this principle. In order to find out whether a gelatinous aluminium hydroxide would make partial purification and concentration of the virus possible by adsorbing the virus to it, the following experiments were carried out by Dr. Werner Leemann in this laboratory.

Two horses were injected, one receiving an inoculum corresponding to the active material present in 0.8 cc. of infectious plasma as adsorbed to alum, and the other receiving a small fraction of it, equivalent to 1/5000 cc. of plasma. The above is based on a calculation assuming that practically all virus is adsorbed to and evenly distributed within the alum precipitate, and that no loss of virus would be caused by washing of the gelatinous sediment with physiologic salt solution after adsorption was achieved.

The procedure was as follows: To 10 cc. of infectious plasma of Horse 5, 10 cc. of a buffer solution of pH 4.8 was added (in order to reduce the alkalinity of the aluminium hydroxide), and 5 cc. of a fresh gelatinous aluminium hydroxide preparation (Eimer & Amend). The mixture was kept at 5°C. for 24 hours and was occasionally shaken during this time. Then it was centrifuged at 3,500 rpm for 15 minutes, the supernatant pipetted off and discarded, while the sediment was three times washed and centrifuged with 20 to 25 cc. of physiologic salt solution. There remained about 5 cc. of loose sediment of aluminium hydroxide; 0.5 cc. of this sediment was diluted 10 times with salt solution. Horse 9 simultaneously received 2 cc. of this diluted alum-adsorbate subcutaneously, and 2 cc. intravenously in October 1948.

The loose aluminium hydroxide adsorbate, obtained after the third washing, was preserved in the refrigerator in a sterile vial for a month. Then, again, a ten-fold dilution was prepared with saline, and 0.1 cc. of this was further diluted with physiologic salt solution to give a final volume of 100 cc. One cc. of this final dilution was inoculated intravenously into Horse 11.

Both horses produced typical reactions. In particular, Horse 9, receiving the larger dose, reacted strongly; four marked fever attacks were observed within 2 months and the peak exceeded 106°F. each time.* The experiment was terminated on the 63rd day when the horse was destroyed. Horse 11 first reacted on the 16th day with a marked typical fever attack, and its temperature did not return to normal before the 35th day. It exhibited two additional but milder fever reactions during an experimental period of over three months. Both horses developed considerable anemia with a decrease of about 3 million in the red blood cell count.

It is known that precipitated aluminium hydroxide readily adsorbs colloids and other particulate matter, such as toxins and viruses, at a properly chosen pH. The experiments as outlined above indicated that the virus adsorbed to aluminium hydroxide is not inactivated and will survive for at least a month in the refrigerator while so adsorbed. Furthermore, the typical fever response in both horses, and the fact that the incubation period was not prolonged, indicated that concentration was achieved by means of the adsorption. Without assuming adsorption and concentration, the virus would have been too much diluted for producing even a subclin-

---

* For converting temperature readings in Fahrenheit degrees into centigrades (C°) see Table 1 on page 18.

ical infection. Stein, Lotze and Mott (429), who tested graded dilutions of a virulent virus, reported inapparent, subclinical infection in a horse inoculated with 1 cc. of a serum diluted 1:100,000.

Immunization Experiments with Alum-Adsorbed Virus

There are various immunizing antigens in use against bacterial and virus infections which have been adsorbed to alum precipitate, the advantage being that the aluminium hydroxide suspension can be injected into the subcutaneous tissue and it will form there a "depot" assuring a continuous resorption of the antigenic material. It was thought that a similar type of immunization with infectious anemia virus might induce resistance against subsequent infection. As the preliminary experiments indicated, the virus can be adsorbed and probably concentrated by the use of a precipitated aluminium hydroxide.

We attempted to find out the relative strength of the adsorbed virus through titration in two additional horses by further decreasing the amount of the alum-adsorbate to be injected. This experiment was also intended to test whether an eventual subclinical infection caused by the slowly resorbed virus would render the horses resistant to subsequent infection with a virulent strain.

Horse 12 and Horse 13 both received a fresh preparation of infectious virus adsorbed to aluminium hydroxide as described above. The dilution of the active material present in the inoculum was estimated in equivalents of the original plasma as being about 1:50,000, and 1:2,500,000, respectively. Calculations were made on the same grounds as in the preliminary experiments. One cc. of the properly diluted adsorbate was injected into each of the horses. They did not show symptoms or a typical fever response, although the temperature rose 17 days following inoculation to 101.8F. for one day in the horse receiving the larger dose of the virus; two months later the red blood cell count was decreased by two millions in the same horse. The other animal had an insignificant rise of 101.3F. on the 27th day. Both horses produced a typical reaction after the usual incubation period, when injected two months later with a virulent virus for challenge inoculation; one of them (H.12) died on the 33rd day. The conclusion was that inoculation of the alum-adsorbate containing highly diluted active virus did not confer immunity upon these animals, although one of them suffered, in all likelihood, a mild subclinical infection following the initial inoculation.

As the next step, experiments were devised to determine whether properly inactivated and adsorbed virus could be successfully used for the purpose of immunization. The procedure adopted for the adsorption of virus was in general the same as described above. The only difference was that the virus contained in the infectious serum or plasma was first inactivated by the addition of formalin and that the final precipitate was not markedly diluted before injection, in order to use a sufficiently large amount of inactivated virus for the antigenic stimulus. For each injection a fresh adsorbate was prepared by starting the procedure of inactivation and adsorption at least two months before intended inoculation. Formalin in a dilution of 1:10 was added to 50-100 cc. of fresh infectious horse serum or plasma sufficient to make a final concentration of 0.4 per cent formaldehyde. The formalinized serum was kept for two days at room temperature. After standing two weeks in the refrigerator, adsorption to a fresh gelatinous aluminium hydroxide was carried out, using the same proportions of serum, phosphate buffer, and alum as described above. The mixture was kept in the refrigerator overnight. After this, the adsorbate was washed and finally resuspended with saline to the original volume of blood serum or plasma used in preparation of the material. Thus, a fairly heavy suspension was obtained, each cubic centimeter of which presumably contained the virus present in one cc. of the original infectious material with a marked reduction in the protein and other constituents of the serum or plasma.

The formalinized and alum-adsorbed virus preparation was kept for 30 to 50 days at 5°C. before injection into horses, thus allowing ample time for "attenuation" of the virus. As will be seen, at least a partial inactivation or attenuation was achieved, since the experimental horses did not produce marked clinical symptoms of infectious anemia in spite of the fact that large doses of the vaccine were administered, while a small amount (for instance 0.5 cc.) of the original source material, when given in active form, provoked typical disease with marked symptoms after the regular incubation period.

Two horses were immunized with two and three inoculations of alum-adsorbed virus prepared as described above. Horse 18 received three inoculations at about two-month intervals; 5 cc., 25 cc., and 50 cc. of resuspended alum adsorbate was injected subcutaneously in the cervical region of the animal. A mild temperature response reaching 102.4°F. was recorded on the 35th to 43rd day following the first injection, but no other symptoms were noted. No strong fever attacks followed either this, or the subsequent inoculations. The slight fever response was considered as a possible indication of a very mild infection. The question has arisen whether 1) the additional immunizing doses would bring about a similar or increased reaction, or 2) the animal would resist challenge inoculation, and 3) if so, whether its blood contained active virus before the challenge inoculation, that is, whether or not it became a carrier.

One month following the third immunizing dose, the horse was given 1 cc. of virulent virus intravenously. A somewhat delayed but marked fever response followed; on the 25th day the temperature reached a peak of 105.6°F., the animal appeared sick, became anemic, and exhibited signs of extreme weakness. Thus, the main problem as mentioned above was answered in the negative; that is, the attempt at immunization proved to be a failure in this case.

Horse 21 was immunized with a similar vaccine, but some modifications were introduced in an attempt to obtain better results. A longer "resting" period was allowed after the last immunizing dose, and a challenge inoculation was tried first with a less virulent virus preparation. This horse received two large doses of formalin-inactivated and alum-adsorbed virus, 50 cc. each at 60-day intervals, subcutaneously. The source material used for preparing the vaccine was the same as in the case of Horse 18. From the 17th to 19th day following the first dose of vaccine, a slight temperature response was observed (101.6°F.). Following this slight response, the temperature was elevated on two more occasions, reaching only 101.2°F., and the horse remained outwardly normal.

Seven months following the second immunizing vaccine, a challenge inoculation was attempted intravenously with the serum of Horse 10 collected while this horse was in a balanced chronic carrier stage. No hematologic or fever reaction was noted. When a further challenge inoculation was performed six months later with 0.5 cc. of fully virulent virus, the animal did not show any sign of infection for 5 weeks, and its hematologic values remained normal, but 35 days following the injection a marked fever response was noted. During the next 4 months, several fever attacks followed, which were at first comparatively mild in character, but grew more and more severe later on. This observation was the opposite as compared with the usual course of fever exacerbations seen in animals which were infected without previous treatment. Gradually an anemia developed with a decrease of 3.5 million R.B.C. in four and one-half months, after which the animal was destroyed to terminate the experiment.

Accordingly, this horse seemed to have acquired a relative resistance against infection as a result of immunization. This resistance was apparent when infection was attempted with a less virulent virus. However, the resistance broke down at the second challenge inoculation with a virulent virus after a markedly prolonged incubation period. From the behavior of the individual fever attacks, it would seem that the full susceptibility to the action of the virus was restored gradually with the passing of time. These observations are, in general, contrary to our concept of immunity.

Immunization with Organ Suspensions

In the second group of immunization experiments a mixture of suspensions of various organs of an infected horse was utilized in an attempt to build up resistance to the virus by repeated injections.

The virus present in the organ suspensions was inactivated in order to achieve immunization without clinical infection. While an active virus can be used in minute amounts for immunization, as it will multiply in the recipient following administration, the inactivated virus must be present in sufficient strength and quantity in a vaccine in order to exert proper antigenic stimulus. Observations indicate that the strength of the infectious anemia virus (virulence) reaches its highest point during the first and second fever attack, and from then on a gradual decrease of the virulence can usually be noted. Therefore, we used organs of an infected horse that was destroyed at the peak of the first marked fever reaction. An attempt was first made to immunize a horse with three injections of organ suspension in quick succession. Two other horses received five immunizing doses of such a vaccine, with a long interval inserted.

For obtaining the organ suspensions, Horse 26 was inoculated intravenously with virulent virus and was killed on the second day of the first fever reaction when the temperature reached 105.1°F. Aside from congestion, the internal organs did not show marked gross changes at this early phase of the disease. Samples of the organs were collected aseptically (liver, spleen, lung, kidneys, adrenals, ribs containing red bone marrow, and mediastinal, bronchial, pelvic, splenic, renal, and mesenteric lymph nodes). They were in part used to prepare a vaccine for early application, while the rest were preserved frozen and aliquots of them were used from time to time for preparing new batches of vaccine. To insure a fine distribution of the organ particles, Dr. Gilman—who has done most of the horse inoculations in the immunization series—prepared the suspensions in a Waring blendor, cooled with ice during the operation in order to prevent warming by the heat generated in the process. All manipulations were performed under strictly aseptic conditions.

The first batch of vaccine was made within 24 hours following the killing of Horse 26. A 30 per cent organ suspension, containing about an equal amount of spleen, lymph nodes, bone marrow, and somewhat less of the adrenals, was prepared in saline by means of the Waring blendor. For inactivating the virus in the suspension, formalin was added to a final concentration of 0.4 per cent and the mixture was refrigerated for three days. The first injection was given at this time, while the rest of the formalinized material was refrigerated until the second and third injections were performed.

Horse 25 received subcutaneously three injections of 20 cc. each of this finely dispersed organ suspension at weekly intervals. At the site of the injection a marked inflammation occurred two days following the first injection. This swelling receded in the next three days. A very slight rise of the temperature of questionable significance was seen on the 5th day, while on the 12th day (which was the 5th day following the second immunizing dose) the number of red blood cells dropped by one million, but soon returned to normal. No other change was noted in four weeks when a challenge inoculation was performed by using a virulent virus with positive result. A transient but definite fever reaction was observed on the 12th and 13th days and the R.B.C. count on the 14th day decreased by 2.5

million as against the normal value. Following this, the illness assumed a chronic course with several rather mild fever attacks, which were inter-

TABLE 16

HEMATOLOGIC AND FEVER RESPONSE OF HORSE 25

Date (1950)	*Temperature F°*		*R.B.C. (million)*	*Hemogl. (gram)*	*Hemato-crit*	*W.B.C.*	*Neutr.*	*Eos.*	*Lymph.*
							per cent		
(normal)	99.6	99.4	7.5	13.6	42	8,400	61	3	32
Feb. 18	First inoculation (20 cc. formalinized organ suspension s.c.)								
23	99.6	101.0	7.6	12.9	38	10,300	56	1	35
25	Second inoculation (20 cc. formalinized organ suspension s.c.)								
28	99.4	99.6	7.9	14.0	38	7,800	62	1	36
Mar. 2	99.4	99.8	6.6	12.3	41	8,600	66	2	27
4	Third inoculation (20 cc. formalinized organ suspension s.c.)								
9	99.2	99.8	7.4	13.7	39	8,000	54	0	39
14	99.6	99.8	7.1	13.1	40	8,400	62	0	36
Mar. 16	Challenge inoculation (0.5 cc. virulent virus i.v.)								
21	99.2	99.6	8.0	14.3	46	11,000	60	4	31
28	100.2	102.8	5.3	9.3	26	5,400	80	1	15
30	99.4	100.0	5.0	9.0	26	5,350	66	1	22
Apr. 6	100.2	100.4	7.2	12.1	33	7,700	53	5	27
13	100.0	100.2	6.7	12.4	36	9,350	53	5	35
21	101.2	102.0	6.7	12.9	35	12,250	57	3	26
28	100.2	101.0	5.0	9.5	28	11,900	67	3	19
May 4	101.0	101.8	6.3	10.5	31	7,050	34	1	53
13	103.7	103.4							
15	101.2	101.6	6.4	11.1	33	10.750	56	3	28
23	101.0	101.4	6.6	10.7	32	9,700	65	2	24
June 5	99.8	100.6	5.9	11.6	35	10,850	58	1	30

rupted by long remissions until the horse was destroyed three months after the challenge inoculation.

Some of the pertinent values recorded during the immunization and following challenge inoculation of Horse 25 are given in Table 16.

Two additional animals (Horse 30 and Horse 31) were injected with organ suspensions prepared in a manner similar to that used in the case of Horse 25. Each horse received five doses of the vaccine: the first three inoculations were administered at approximately weekly intervals; then an interval of 75 days was allowed before additional injections were given spacing them two weeks apart. For each immunizing injection a new batch of 30 per cent suspension was made under aseptic conditions by using equal amounts of liver, spleen, lymph nodes, and bone marrow of Horse 26 which were preserved in the frozen state until they were used. The tissues, after addition of saline, were spun in the Waring blendor at 3500 rpm for 30 minutes at refrigerator temperature; then the fine suspension was filtered through a double layer of sterile cheesecloth, and formalin was added to a 0.4 per cent final concentration. After standing three to six days, 20 cc. of this vaccine was given to each of the horses subcutaneously. To assure bacterial sterility, 1000 units of Penicillin were added to 50 cc. of the vaccine.

Experience with Horse 25 demonstrated that inactivation effected by three days' contact with formalin was sufficient to modify the virus to such an extent that it would not produce symptoms of infectious anemia. Total inactivation was not aimed at in these experiments because the literature dealing with similar experiments indicates that a completely killed virus does not influence the susceptibility of the horse in any direction. Therefore, we intended to increase the resistance of our horses against subsequent infection by the use of a virus sufficiently inactivated (attenuated) to be harmless for the animal and still not completely deprived of its ability to act as an antigen. Repetition of the injections was intended to increase the immunizing effect.

Neither of the two horses produced a marked reaction during the process of immunization. However, some slight temperature changes were noted in both of them. Horse 30's temperature rose slightly above 101°F. for a few days starting on the 7th day following the first injection, and similar slight elevations were noted on a few other occasions. But in every other respect, the horse remained healthy. Aside from a decrease of 0.6 million on the 21st day following the first injection, no significant drop was noted in the red blood cell count; however, the sedimentation rate increased considerably after the second and third inoculations.

Horse 31 exhibited a similar behavior of the temperature response; its fever exceeded 102°F. on the 8th day and, while abridged somewhat, it did not return to normal until the 30th day as calculated from the time of the first injection. A few slight but transient elevations were noted later. The number of red cells increased rather than decreased during immunization (against the normal value of 7.6 million per cu. mm.) and no change was noted in the sedimentation rate.

Both horses were subjected to challenge inoculation four weeks after the last immunizing dose of vaccine. Horse 30 received 0.5 cc. of fully virulent virus (serum of Horse 10 preserved frozen), while Horse 31 was given 1 cc. of a serum obtained from a chronic case which has had no symptoms for several months. Both horses reacted to the challenge inoculation, but in different ways. Horse 30 seemed to be fully susceptible to the action of the virulent virus: it produced four marked fever reactions in less than two months, and a definite decrease in the number of erythrocytes (about 2 million) was noted a week after the challenge inoculation. The anemic condition continued until the horse was destroyed.

On the other hand, Horse 31, challenged with less virulent virus, had at first only two minor temperature rises, one on the 8th and one on the 41st day. After a long remission of over a month, the animal started to produce marked and typical fever attacks with prolonged remissions between each of them, until it was destroyed six months following the challenge inoculation. The remarkable fact about this horse is that during this six months no significant drop in the red blood cell count was noted. On the 41st day a decrease by 1 million occurred, but otherwise normal or increased values were recorded (up to 9.8 million per cu. mm.). The sedimentation rate and the hemoglobin values remained within the normal range; the percentage of lymphocytes was increased, the only exception being a value of 26 per cent on the 41st day. During fever attacks, the appetite of the animal was somewhat impaired, but it was always followed by a quick and complete recovery. No other symptoms were apparent. There, again, a gradual increase in the severity of the fever attacks was clearly noted as in the case of Horse 25.

Accordingly, this horse presented an unusual feature of marked fever attacks connected with no anemia. This was due either to the injections of formalinized virus previous to the challenge inoculation, or to using an avirulent virus for challenge inoculation, or possibly to the combination of both. If the horse had not been observed for as long a period, the lack of an early reaction to the challenge inoculation might have been interpreted as a successful immunization against a less virulent virus.

Immunization with Mouse- and Egg-Passage Material

If a virus is successfully adapted to multiply in laboratory animals or in the chick embryo, the possibility of using such a virus for immunization is usually considered, with the hope that an inapparent or mild infection caused by the virus adapted to a new host may eventually build up resistance in the horse against virulent virus strains. Our data are not sufficient to draw definite conclusions in this direction, but the problem presented itself in connection with testing passage materials in horses, after serial transfers were made in mice and cultivation was attempted in chick embryos. Thus, a brief reference to the observations is warranted.

Previous to the mouse passage experiments, Horse 5, which received an initial injection of monkey passage material, produced an accelerated and very strong reaction showing a continuous type of fever response 10 days following the challenge inoculation with an active virus; the temperature of the animal did not return to normal in 18 days, after which the horse was destroyed.

One of two horses receiving a primary inoculation with mouse passage material, became an asymptomatic virus carrier (Horse 10), at least for a while, after exhibiting a typical response and repeated fever attacks following the challenge inoculation with a virulent horse adapted virus. The other horse in this group (H. 15) revealed increased susceptibility rather than immunity and died six weeks after challenge inoculation. The remaining four horses in this series were not subjected to a test with virulent horse adapted strains.

In the group of animals that have been inoculated for evaluation of the experiments devised for cultivation of the virus, Horse 24 and Horse 27, both of which received egg culture material previously, reacted with a typical response to challenge inoculation, although the first temperature rise was milder than usual in Horse 27. An additional horse (H. 28) did not show anemia or any other symptoms following injection of a virulent virus, but we were unable to decide whether this was due to the culture passage virus (2nd transfer in horse), or to several other injections with virus preparations of low virulence received by this animal previously. (For more details of these experiments, see Chapters 10 and 11.)

It seems that injection of passage materials, that presumably contained virus adapted to new hosts, did not confer immunity to the horses. In some instances, such inoculation tended to increase rather than decrease the susceptibility of animals to a virulent horse passage virus.

Neutralization Experiment

It is a general experience in most of the virus diseases that the serum of patients, after they have recovered from an infection, will neutralize the corresponding virus when mixed with the latter *in vitro*. A well-neutralized mixture of immune serum and virus would not, as a rule, cause infection when injected into susceptible experimental animals. The neutralizing capacity of an immune serum is of specific nature; therefore, the test is often used for identification of certain viruses.

While the virus is always present in the serum of sick animals and recovered cases of infectious anemia, specific antibodies have not been clearly demonstrated as yet. Assuming the presence of specific antibodies in the blood fluid of recovered cases, the virus must co-exist with them, possibly in a balanced and well-neutralized form. We made an attempt for testing the neutralizing capacity of the serum obtained from a symptomless virus carrier. This horse proved to be definitely resistant to repeated challenge inoculations with large doses of virulent virus.

Twenty cc. of "immune" serum from the virus carrier (Horse 2) had been maintained at 60°C. for one hour to inactivate any active virus present in it; then it was mixed with one cc. of a known virulent virus (horse serum). The mixture was placed in the refrigerator for 24 hours, then injected into a normal horse. An early and marked fever response was noted which began on the 10th day and lasted for five days. After prolonged remissions two more temperature rises were recorded, but following this no fever was noted during an additional four months of observation and no signs of anemia were noted during the experiment.

It was concluded that no neutralization was achieved in this experiment and that probably no benefit could be expected from passive immunization against infectious anemia by "immune" or "hyperimmune" horse serum.

*

The experiments as outlined above indicate that the virus of infectious anemia can be adsorbed to aluminum hydroxide precipitate and probably concentrated by it. Such an adsorbed virus partly inactivated by formalin, and used in several doses for immunization, made a horse resistant to an active virus of low virulence. The same horse exhibited a mild response, after a definitely prolonged incubation period, when challenged by a fully virulent virus. Thus, a partial immunization was achieved, although the animal was not completely protected against infection.

Repeated injections of organ suspensions containing formalin-inactivated virus seemed to offer partial protection against infection with a virus of low virulence as manifested by prolonged incubation: delayed, but marked fever reactions were noted without ensuing anemia. Similar inoculations provided no protection to horses against highly virulent virus.

It is difficult to interpret the results owing to the fact that the experimental observations could not be extended because the facilities at our disposal were inadequate for handling a sufficient number of experimental horses in properly isolated, screened stables. This much can be said, however, that aside from the slightly increased resistance evoked in a few horses, no satisfactory immunity was apparent, especially not against fully virulent virus strains. This is in agreement with the experience of other investigators, as will be seen by the following brief review of past attempts at immunization.

Carré and Vallée (58) stated in their fundamental study that experiments to produce artificial immunity were in progress at the time of their report. Apparently the results were negative, like those of other early investigators who also made attempts in this direction (338,271,470). After World War I renewed efforts were made in a number of countries with no encouraging results, as for instance by de Kock (210) in South Africa, Lehnert (246) in Sweden, Brunswick (49) in France, and by Mócsy (299) in Hungary.

The problem has been approached from a new angle by French investigators since 1934. Balozet (12,20,21,24) published a series of studies on immunization that he carried out on the small African donkey. Martin infected donkeys with alum-adsorbed virus (277), and also attempted immunization by such a virus with the addition of bile and formalin for attenuation (279). According to Balozet immunization with a properly attenuated virus (what he termed "premunisation") should enable the animal to with stand infection by a virulent strain. He studied a number of chemicals to achieve the best way of attenuation: phenol reduced the virulence (20,22); addition of bile inactivated the virus within a short time (19); glycerine (17,20,21) as well as sodium ricinoleate (24) attenuated the virus; but none of the procedures proved to be satisfactory in making the experimental donkeys resistant to virulent virus. Martin (277) produced clinical infection in seven out of eight asses by a virus adsorbed to aluminium hydroxide, while one of the animals experienced subclinical infection. Addition of bile exerted no influence on the adsorbed virus but formalin inactivated it, giving the animals thus injected a protection against severe symptoms, although not preventing the infection (279).

Velu and co-workers (475) did not note any difference between the susceptibility of normal horses and those immunized with a spleen vaccine inactivated by 0.4 per cent formalin. Later, Mitchell, Humphrey and Walker recorded similar experience (290); their horse, immunized in the same manner, died earlier at challenge inoculation than did the control animal. Stein and Osteen (436) tried many different means of immunization but all of their animals proved to be susceptible when subjected to challenge inoculation. Bankier (30) administered the virus, inactivated by crystal violet, in a dilution of 1:10,000 intradermally; this did not infect the horse but also failed to produce immunity.

Recently, Beller and Traub (37) published cross immunity studies and explained the paradoxical results often following immunization as resulting from antigenic differences among strains of the virus. It must be remembered, however, that the results are just as contrary to expectation when using a single strain as when working with several strains.

It is evident from this brief review of the literature on immunization as well as from our own experience, that methods of immunization, which give fairly satisfactory results in other infectious diseases, have so far failed to bring any appreciable success in infectious anemia. The explanation of this most probably lies in the different manner in which the system of the infected animal reacts to this disease as compared with other virus infections.

In general, infection with the virus of infectious anemia is usually not followed by immunity against repeated infection. Hempel (160) stated as early as 1909 that horses that had apparently recovered from the disease had not acquired immunity but were still susceptible to renewed infection. There is plenty of experimental evidence in the literature to the effect that susceptibility of horses to re-infection is quite common, as reported among many others by Balozet (12,15), Mrowka (313), and Andrievskii (7). Consequently, if a natural attack, as a rule, does not produce immunity, it is difficult to expect protection by an artificial immunization. For the same reason, a serious doubt is cast upon the value of challenge inoculations to indicate whether or not the animal has ever been infected by the virus of infectious anemia.

In addition, it must be stressed that a definite increase in susceptibility of "immunized" animals was often noted (12,21,210,290). Such animals, far from evidencing resistance to test inoculation with an active virus, showed heavier symptoms and died earlier than the control animals. Van Es and co-workers (470) tried to immunize horses by using a mixture of active virus and the serum of a recovered case that exhibited no more infectivity. One horse thus inoculated died within 24 hours. When the same experiment was repeated on two more normal horses, these died in three and five days, respectively. As mentioned in the description of our experiments above, we also have noted evidence of an increased sensitivity in some of the experimental animals at the time of re-inoculation.

All this points in the direction, as discussed in the chapter on Pathogenesis of the infection (page 71), that there is a hypersensitivity component in the mechanism of infectious anemia, and that this is mainly responsible for the lack of success in attempts at immunization. It would seem that one subclinical infection does not serve the purpose of immunization as in other infectious diseases but, rather, causes a sensitization of the animal to subsequent infection. On the other hand, repeated mild infections may, according to the rules of allergy, bring about some desensitization. It is believed that the minor resistance as evidenced against challenge inoculation in our experiments was the result of an initial mild infection combined with partial desensitization by the repeated injections of slightly antigenic material either in the form of a vaccine or as an active virus of low virulence.

Since Carré and Vallée's work (58) it has been known that a small fraction of recovered horses become resistant to subsequent infection (symptomless virus carriers), but by no means all of them behave in the same way. It is quite unfortunate as to the progress in research on infectious anemia that it was often taken for granted, especially since the publication of de Kock (210) in 1920, that all horses will resist re-infection which passed a clinical or subclinical infection by the anemia virus. This led to misinterpretation of the challenge inoculations as to their relative value in deciding whether an experimental animal has been infected in the past, or not. It is obvious from all that has been said above that a positive response noted in a challenge inoculation cannot decide this. In our opinion, based on experimental evidence, the solid resistance occasionally seen in virus carriers is due to successful desensitization on the part of the animal's body, rather than to an active immunity in the usual sense.

If an artificial immunization against infectious anemia is to lead to any success in the future, probably it has to follow a pattern of desensitization, as evidenced by the resistant virus carriers and slightly suggested in one or two of our experiments outlined above. Whether a solid resistance against infection can be achieved without producing new virus carriers remains to be seen.

Chapter 13

HISTOPATHOLOGY

The following description of the pathologic alterations due to infectious anemia is based upon necropsy studies of 18 horses destroyed at different stages of the disease. Following a brief outline of the methods used in this study, and a concise summary of the gross changes observed, we shall concentrate in the description mainly on the microscopic alterations as noted in various organs of our experimentally infected horses.

Materials and Methods.—The horses were inoculated with the New Hampshire strain of the infectious anemia virus as the primary inoculum or as the virus applied for challenge inoculation; the animals reacted with typical symptoms as may be seen from the references made to many of them in previous chapters of this monograph. No horses are included here that were injected only with experimental material of uncertain virus content. The animals ranged in age from 2 to 19 years and were of both sexes; after a period of observation varying from a few weeks to several months, they were considered in good health before infection.

As outlined in the description of symptomatology (Chapter 3), the disease process may be divided into three stages—acute, subacute, and chronic—as has been done by previous investigators. However, it is understood that there is no distinct line of separation between the acute and subacute, or the subacute and chronic stages. Chronic cases are considered in two groups, that is, cases with recurrent fever attacks, and balanced or asymptomatic virus carriers.

The acute cases consist of horses that died or were killed during the first few fever attacks, three or less in number; the average duration of the disease in these horses was 17 days from the beginning of the symptoms. Animals killed at the peak of the first or second fever attack are considered separately from those destroyed in the post-febrile period following the third fever attack. The subacute cases consist of those that had four or more fever attacks and were destroyed 41 to 90 days following inoculation with a virulent virus. The chronic cases are 1) those with four to eight recurrent fever attacks occurring at approximately monthly intervals, and 2) a balanced or asymptomatic virus carrier with no fever attacks during the last few months of existence, but exhibiting 26 recurrent fever attacks previously during an observation period of more than two years. The chronic cases were destroyed 63 to 800 days after the primary inoculation.

It is beyond the scope of this report to consider pathologic differences that exist between the alterations noted in animals following the primary and the challenge inoculation.

Necropsies were performed as soon as possible after death. Sections were taken from the major organs of the body and fixed in the following solutions: Zenker's fixing fluid, 10 per cent aqueous and alcoholic formalin, and Bouin's fixing solution. Paraffin sections were used. Stains employed were hematoxylin and eosin, Giemsa, Hitchcock's and Ehrich's method of malachite green and acridine red for differentiation of plasma cells and Foot's modification of Bielschowsky's reticulum stain. Special histochemical techniques included the Feulgen method as applied by Stowell and the periodic acid leuko-fuchsin method as employed by Hotchkiss. Perl's ferrocyanide reaction for hemosiderin was utilized as well as Mallory's hemofuscin method.

The histologic material that forms the basis of the present analysis was collected during the tenure of our experimental studies and the microscopic slides were prepared by the staff of the Department of Pathology, School of Veterinary Medicine, University of Pennsylvania. Some of the slides with special staining were made available by Dr. Steven C. Mohos.

Gross Pathology.—Animals killed at the peak of the first or second fever attack displayed the following gross changes: mottling of the liver, enlarged splenic and mesenteric lymph nodes, splenomegaly and, least frequently, roughening of the mitral and tricuspid valvular surfaces. Horses destroyed in the post-febrile period following the third fever attack showed the following gross changes in order of frequency: organ hemorrhages (splenic, renal, intestinal, cardiac, pulmonary, nasal, and sublingual), and enlarged splenic and mesenteric lymph nodes. The gross alterations in subacute cases were, in order of frequency: subcutaneous edema, emaciation, mottling of the liver, lymph node enlargement, hepatomegaly, and renal hemorrhages.

The gross changes in chronic cases with recurrent fever attacks were: mottling of the liver, organ hemorrhages (splenic, intestinal, cardiac, pulmonary), subcutaneous edema, hepatomegaly, splenomegaly, and roughening of the cardiac valvular surfaces. In a symptomless virus carrier no gross pathologic changes were noted.

Considering all cases together, in various stages of the disease, the most frequently encountered gross alterations were: mottling of the liver, organ hemorrhages, and lymph node enlargement. Gross hepatic alterations were most apparent in the experimental animals killed during or shortly after a fever attack.

Microscopic Alterations in the Acute Phase

The most significant and consistent changes are seen in the liver (Figs. 7, 8, 9, 11). The normal hepatic architectural pattern has been conspicuously disrupted by degeneration and necrosis of the hepatic cells (Figs. 7, 8), hemosiderosis (Fig. 9), and lymphocytic infiltration (Figs. 9, 11). The main infiltrating cell type, which has been termed by others variously the lymphoid cell, the mononuclear cell, and the histiocytic cell, will be

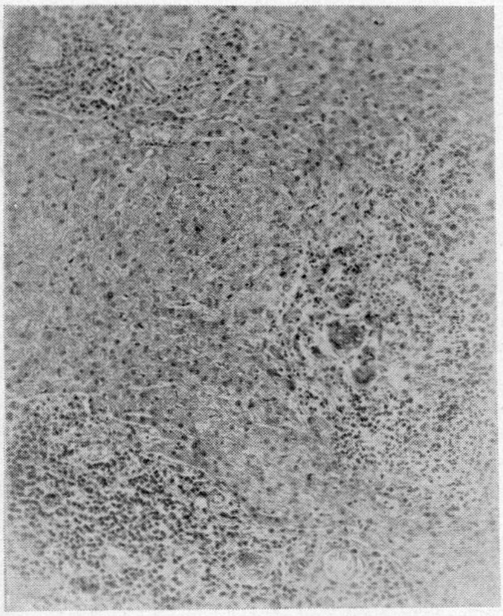

FIG. 7. Focal necrotic areas in the liver; infiltration of lymphocytes and eosinophils. Bile ducts may be noted as landmarks. (Horse 46, Hematoxylin-eosin, 100x.)

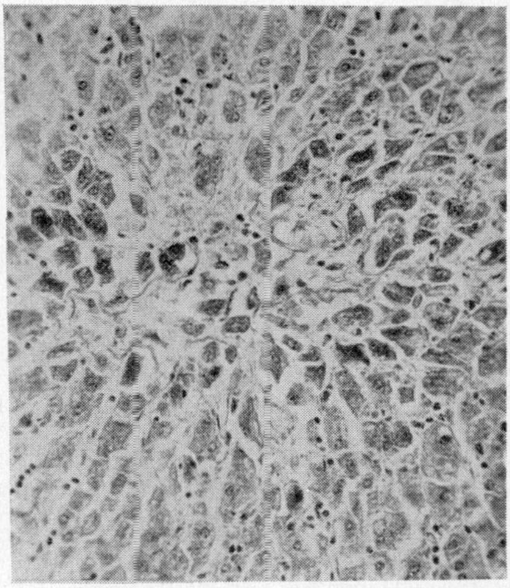

FIG. 8. Central necrosis of the liver. The hepatic cells near the central vein have been destroyed. (H. 7, Hematoxylin-eosin, 200x.)

Microphotographs by Dr. J. W. Mills

treated in more detail in a separate publication (258). It may be said here that we consider it to be a lymphocyte which appears in both mature and immature forms.

Degeneration of the hepatic cells takes the form of fatty metamorphosis and hydropic degeneration. Both the central and peripheral portions of the liver lobule are involved in the necrotic process. Frequently it is difficult to determine the location of the necrotic area because the process destroys all landmarks.

Associated with areas of necrosis are great numbers of macrophages, which together with Kupffer cells and liver cells contain large numbers of hemofuscin granules. The granules stain red with Mallory's hemofuscin stain, black with Wilder's reticulum stain, but fail to stain with hematoxylin and eosin. Hemosiderin is found in Kupffer cells and free macrophages, but it is small in quantity except in the acute cases that have had longer periods of incubation. There is an increase in the number of reticulo-endothelial cells lining the sinusoids.

Lymphocytes are seen infiltrating the portal triads and surrounding necrotic areas. Blood vessels are partly or completely laden with lymphocytes and macrophages. Infiltration of a great number of eosinophils in association with lymphocytes were seen around areas of necrosis in two acute cases, one of which had an incubation of over three weeks and had anaphylactic-like reaction following inoculation with the virus (Fig. 2).

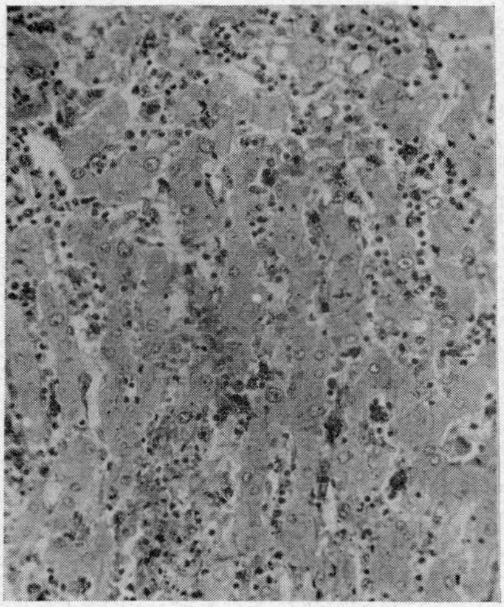

FIG. 9. Hemosiderosis and cellular infiltration of the liver. Hemosiderin is contained largely within the Kupffer cells. (H. 3, Hematoxylin-eosin, 200x.)

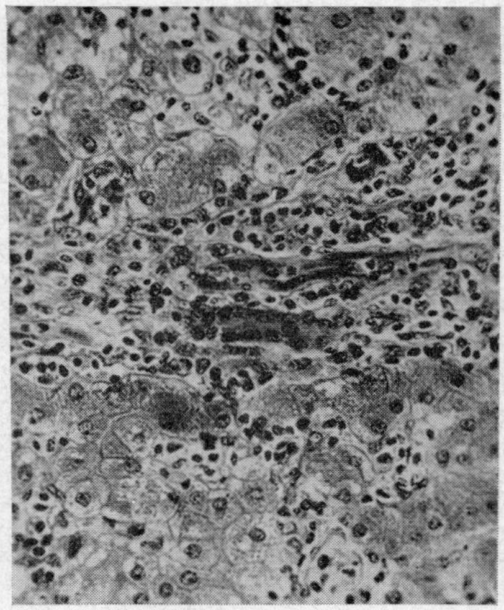

FIG. 10. Proliferation of the bile ducts, represented by two cords of deeply stained cells. (H. 21, Hematoxylin-eosin, 280x.)

Microphotographs by Dr. J. W. Mills

The splenic architecture is partially or almost completely obscured by great numbers of erythrocytes, many of which are undergoing disintegration. Hemosiderin and other unidentified pigments are abundant. Many small focal hemorrhages appear in the capsule and adjacent tissue.

The lymph node alterations consist of lymphoid hyper-plasia and infiltrations of the following cell types: macrophages, some of which contain hemosiderin, eosinophils, and plasma cells (Figs. 3, 4, 19).

In the kidney, the most regular change is that of the lymphocytic infiltration, which is most prominent near glomeruli and around blood vessels (Figs. 5, 6, 17).

In the heart, the most consistent alterations are lymphocytic and neutrophilic cell infiltrations (Fig. 13); cardiac muscle degeneration; and necrosis. In some cases eosinophils were also noted among the infiltrating cell types. Less frequent are the valvular changes, leucocytic and Anitschkow cell infiltrations. In the lungs, the blood vessels contain in their lumens numerous macrophages laden with hemosiderin.

Microscopic Alterations in the Subacute Phase

The hepatic lesions are similar to those described in the acute phase. The most consistent alterations are: degenerative, necrotic and regenerative changes of the hepatic cells, proliferation of bile ducts, hemosiderosis, and lymphocytic infiltration. Hydropic degeneration and fatty metamorphosis involve the liver cells not altered by necrosis. Fatty degeneration is more pronounced around areas of necrosis. The necrotic process appears to have no predilection for any one portion of the liver lobule. Approximately one out of every three lobules has undergone partial necrosis.

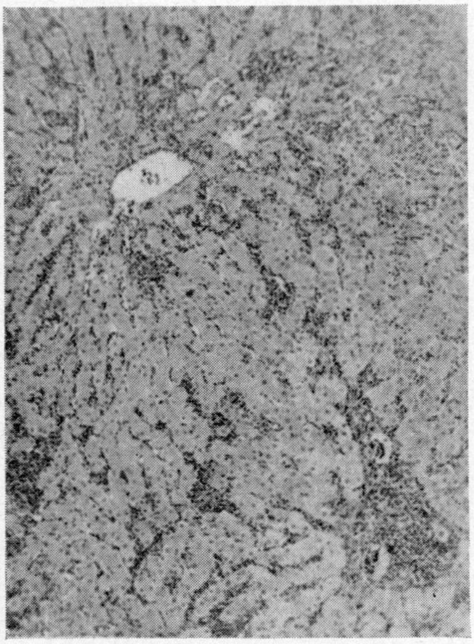

FIG. 11. Cellular infiltration and endothelial cell proliferation in the liver. Endothelial cells, plasma cells, lymphocytes, and polymorphonuclear neutrophils in the sinusoids. (Horse 1, Hemat.-eos., 125x.)

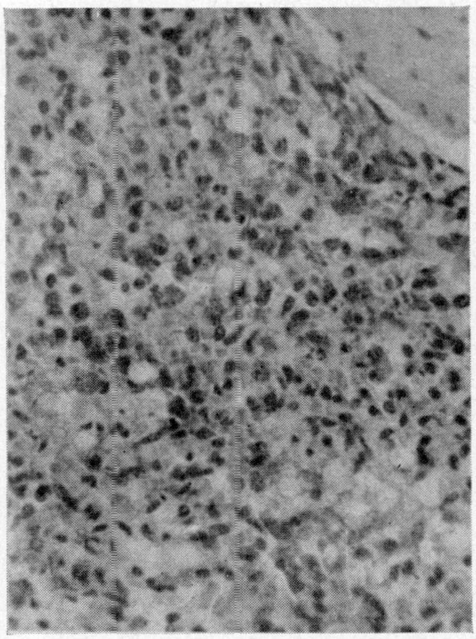

FIG. 12. Infiltration of eosinophils and other inflammatory cells in the spleen. In upper right corner part of a trabecula. (H. 21, Hematoxylin-eosin, 475x.)

Microphotographs by Dr. S. C. Mohos

Only in reparative changes does this phase vary from the acute. Regeneration of liver cells is most apparent at the periphery of the lobules. Newly formed liver cells stain deeply acidophilic and their nuclei are hyperchromatic. Frequently groups of newly formed liver cells take the form of acini or tubules that are not easily distinguishable from newly formed bile duct tubules (Fig. 10).

Hemosiderosis is marked. Kupffer cells are heavily laden with the pigment, and free macrophages are enlarged by the engulfed hemosiderin. The free hemosiderocytes are found in the central veins, sinusoids, periportal spaces, and in necrotic areas. There is a noticeable increase in the number of Kupffer and endothelial cells lining the liver sinusoids.

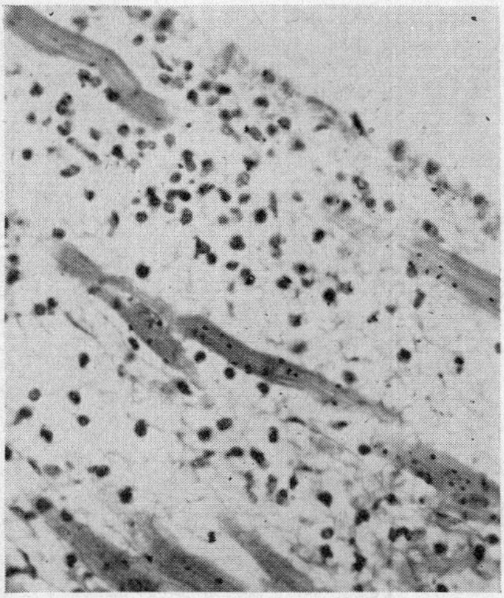

FIG. 13. Cellular infiltration of the endocardium by polymorphonuclear neutrophils and lymphocytes. (H. 7, Hematoxylin-eosin, 475x.)

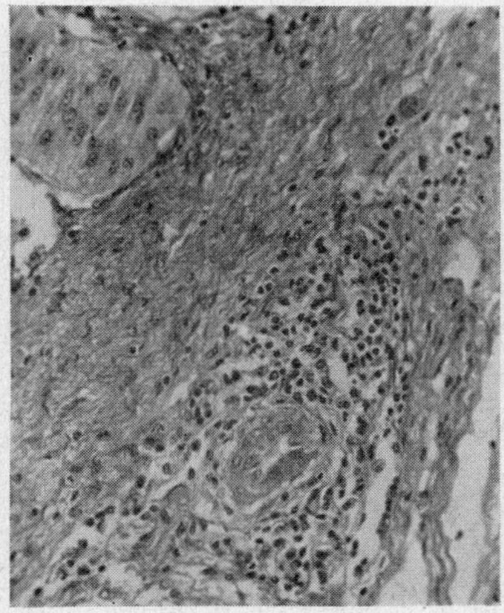

FIG. 14. Perivascular infiltration of the adrenal capsule. A small vessel is surrounded by lymphocytes. (H. 3, Hematoxylin-eosin, 240x.)

Microphotographs by Dr. J. W. Mills

The lymphocytic infiltration is intense. Lymphocytes, both mature and immature forms, are commonly seen between the endothelium of the sinusoids and the hepatic cords, in areas of necrosis, in the connective tissue of the portal triads and in the perilobular connective tissue, as well as packing blood vessels and sinusoids. Together with the hemosiderin laden macrophages, the lymphocytes frequently replace areas in which hepatic cells have been completely obliterated. With Wilder's reticulum stain it can be seen that there is an increase in the recticulum fibrils around the central vein and sinusoids of the majority of the liver lobules.

The splenic changes consist of a marked reduction in hemosiderin content and in the number of erythrocytes as compared with the findings in the acute phase.

Common lymph node alterations are: small focal hemorrhages and hemosiderosis. The pigment is partly extracellular and partly engulfed by macrophages. Proliferation of endothelial cells as well as a few inflammatory cell types are frequently seen (Fig. 19). The argentophil structure remains essentially unaltered (Fig. 20).

The following renal changes exist in the majority of cases classified as subacute: infiltrations of lymphocytes and plasma cells are prominent around Malpighian corpuscles and around blood vessels. The glomeruli are more cellular and frequently fill Bowman's space completely. There

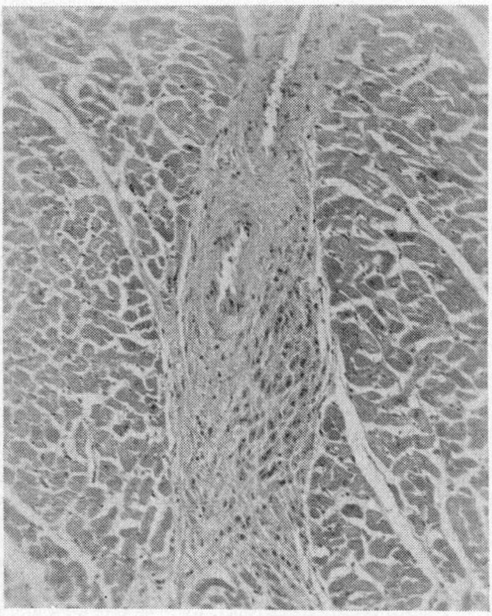

FIG. 15. Vascular lesion in the heart. Proliferation of connective tissue surrounding an arteriole in the myocardium and infiltration of mononuclear and multinuclear cells. (H. 1, Hematoxylin-eosin, 300x.)

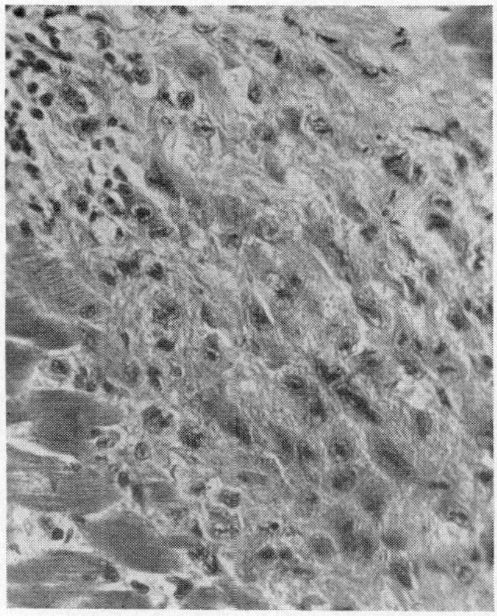

FIG. 16. Cardiac histiocytes ("Anitschkow" cells) in the heart in longitudinal and cross section. A higher magnification of an area adjoining Fig. 15. (H. 1, Hematoxylin-eosin, 475x.)

Microphotographs by Dr. J. W. Mills

are cellular adhesions between the glomerular loops and Bowman's capsule. The capillary loops are almost bloodless. The argentophil framework of the loops is more prominent and Bowman's capsule is thickened. There is a light deposition of hemosiderin pigment in the reticulo-endothelial cells and occasionally in the parenchymal cells of the convoluted tubules. Regressive changes in the tubules are most prominent in the convoluted ones. Tubular cells are seen in various stages of necrosis and many are desquamated. In the medulla there is interstitial edema, lymphocytic and plasma cell infiltrations, as well as scattered foci of necrosis. The intima and adventitia of the renal arterioles are edematous. There is fibroblastic proliferation in the adventitial coat.

The arterioles and capillaries of the adrenal are surrounded by lymphocytes and plasma cells (Fig. 14).

Consistent cardiac findings are: myocardial muscle degeneration and necrosis, fibrinoid degeneration of connective tissue, cell aggregates of lymphocytes, Anitschkow or Aschoff cells, neutrophils and eosinophils.

Hyaline degeneration and necrosis of cardiac muscle fibers occur as scattered focal lesions. Fibrinoid degeneration involves the interstitial and perivascular connective tissue (Fig. 15). The existence of fibrinoid degeneration is determined by its metachromatic staining ability, as well as its positive reaction to Schiff's and to the periodic acid leukofuchsin reagents.

Accumulations of lymphocytes, Aschoff cells, single and multi-nucleated, neutrophils and eosinophils are frequently seen in association with areas of perivascular fibrinoid degeneration and thus resemble the Aschoff body pathognomonic for rheumatic fever (Fig. 15). The above cell types are also found interstitially, but apparently not in association with blood vessels (Fig. 16). Not all the above cell types are present in each lesion, however; the lymphocytes and the Aschoff cell are by far the most constant.

The cardiac blood vessels most often altered are the arterioles. The changes in order of frequency are: infiltration of lymphocytes and Aschoff cells, edema of the adventitia and media, intimal hyalinization and fragmentation of the internal elastic lamina. The cardiac lesions resembling those of rheumatic fever will be recorded in greater detail in a separate publication (99).

The endothelial cells of the pulmonary arterioles and capillaries contain hemosiderin. The lumens of these vessels are partially or completely filled with macrophages containing hemosiderin.

Microscopic Alterations in the Chronic Stage

Chronic with Recurrent Fever Attacks.—Animals grouped under this classification and destroyed during or shortly after a fever attack exhibited hepatic lesions identical in character, though less extensive, than are noted in the subacute phase. Horses killed at a period from 15 to 20 days after the last fever reaction did not exhibit the same hepatic lesions; that is, necrosis was absent and either little or no indication of regenerative changes remained.

In those animals destroyed during or shortly after a fever reaction, the alterations are: degenerative, necrotic and regenerative changes of the hepatic cells, proliferation of bile ducts, hemosiderosis and infiltration of lymphocytes and plasma cells. The normal liver pattern has been extensively altered in that the liver parenchyma has been replaced by fat vacuoles, mature and immature lymphocytes, plasma cells, and hemosiderin laden macrophages. In an occasional case numerous erythrocytes are seen replacing the necrotic parenchyma.

Chronic cases that were killed 15 to 20 days after their last fever reaction exhibited a marked lymphocytic infiltration and a definite hemosiderosis. In addition varying degrees of hepatic parenchymal regeneration and bile duct proliferation are occasionally seen (Fig. 10).

The splenic changes are: a noticeable reduction in hemosiderin content and lymphoid hypoplasia. The lymph follicles are small and reduced in number. Eosinophils and other inflammatory cells are occasionally seen

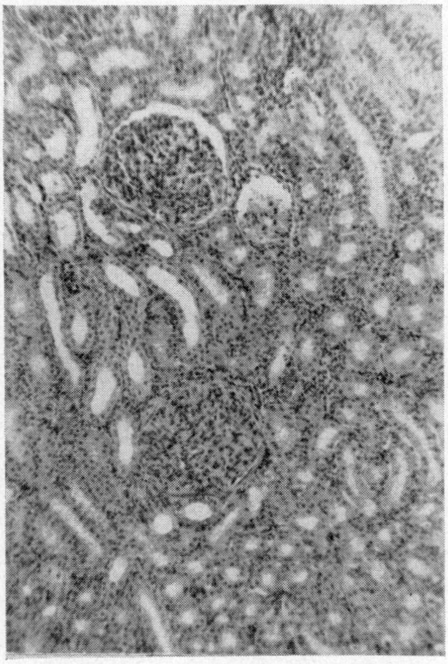

FIG. 17. Periglomerular and interstitial round cell infiltration and proliferation of endothelium of the capillary loops. Adhesions between the capillary tufts and Bowman's capsule. (H. 21, Hematoxylin-eosin, 125x.)

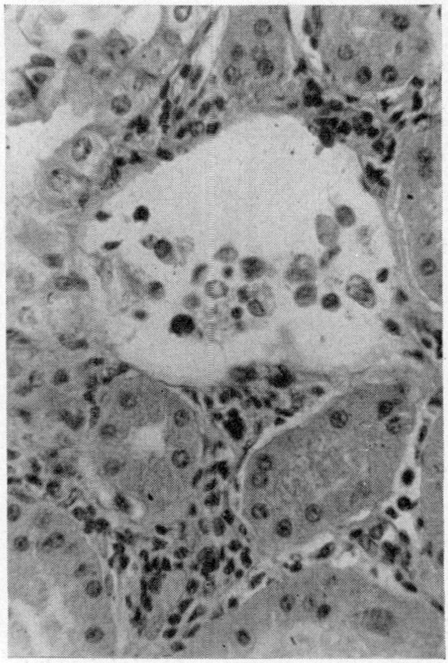

FIG. 18. A distended lymphatic vessel in the kidney containing various cells. Between the tubules are lymphocytes and fibrocytes. Tubular changes are minimal. (H. 21, Hematoxylin-eosin, 565x.)

Microphotographs by Dr. S. C. Mohos

(Fig. 12). Consistent lymph node changes are proliferation of reticuloendothelial cells, hemosiderosis, the presence of numerous plasma cells, and multinucleated giant cells (Figs. 4, 21, 22). The germinal centers are enlarged. Hemosiderin pigment is partly extracellular and intracellular within macrophages. Numerous macrophages contain a phagocytized material not as yet identified. The multinucleated giant cell has a homogeneous, acidophilic staining cytoplasm, with from two to eight vesicular nuclei located at the periphery of the cell (Fig. 22).

Common renal findings are: lymphocytic infiltration, increased cellularity of glomerular loops, thickening of Bowman's capsule, degenerative changes in the cells of the convoluted tubules, hyaline tubular casts, and hemosiderosis (Figs. 5, 6, 18). Foci of lymphocytes are observed near Malpighian corpuscles and blood vessels. Occasionally such foci resemble lymph follicles, having a light staining center that contains immature forms of lymphocytes (Figs. 5, 6, 17).

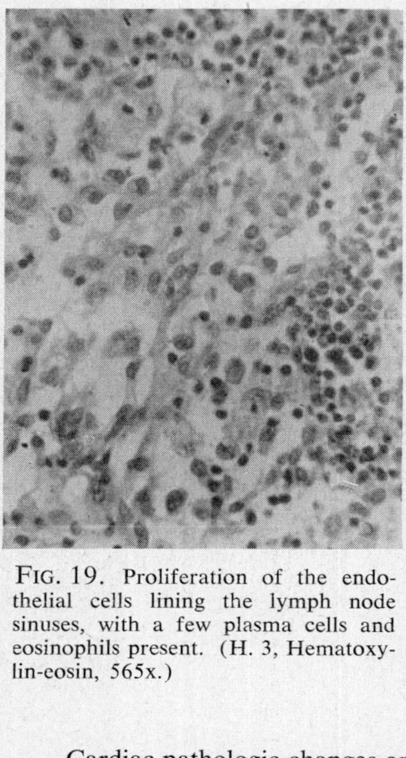

FIG. 19. Proliferation of the endothelial cells lining the lymph node sinuses, with a few plasma cells and eosinophils present. (H. 3, Hematoxylin-eosin, 565x.)

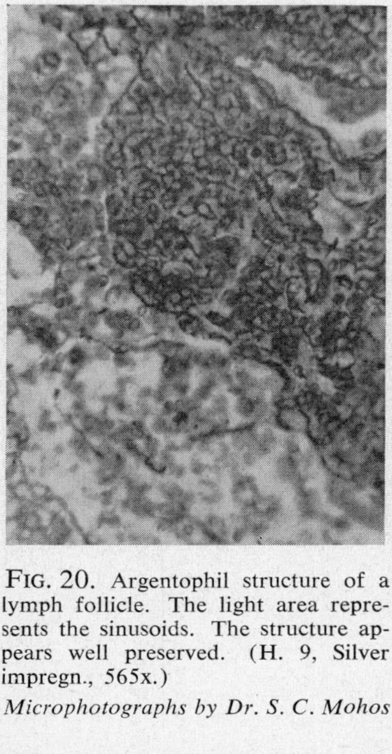

FIG. 20. Argentophil structure of a lymph follicle. The light area represents the sinusoids. The structure appears well preserved. (H. 9, Silver impregn., 565x.)

Microphotographs by Dr. S. C. Mohos

Cardiac pathologic changes are comparable to those of subacute cases, with the exception that myocardial necrosis was absent in all the hearts studied (Fig. 1). Myocardial degeneration, in the form of hyaline degeneration, fibrinoid collagen degeneration, and aggregates of lymphocytes and Aschoff cells are occasionally observed. Valvular alterations were similar to those observed in the acute phase.

Chronic Balanced or Asymptomatic Carrier.—The liver alterations are: fatty metamorphosis, lymphocytic infiltration, hemosiderosis, fibrosis, and bile duct proliferation. The fatty changes are concentrated in the periphery of the lobules. Lymphocytic infiltration is predominantly periportal and perilobular. Hemosiderin is present in small quantities in free and fixed macrophages throughout all lobules. Wilder's reticulum stain demonstrates an increase in reticulum about the central vein and sinusoids of the liver. Increased amounts of collagenous connective tissue are noted periportally and perilobularly. The perilobular bile ducts are increased in number.

Splenic changes consist of lymphoid hypoplasia and sparse hemosiderin. The lymph node architecture is partially obscured by mature and im-

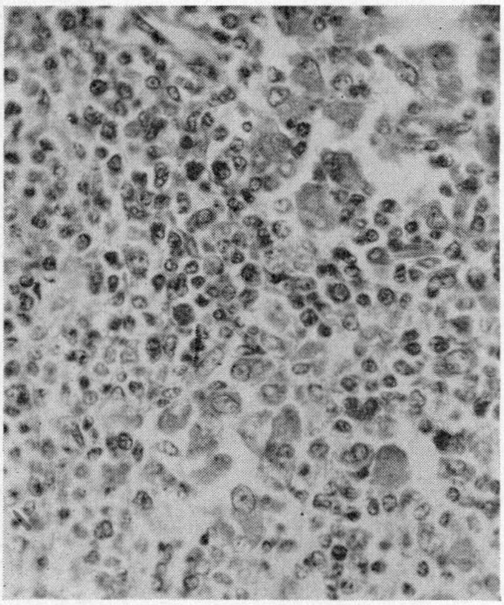

FIG. 21. Plasma cells in a hepatic lymph node. Many plasma cells, both mature and immature, are present. (H. 11, Hematoxylin-eosin, 475x.)

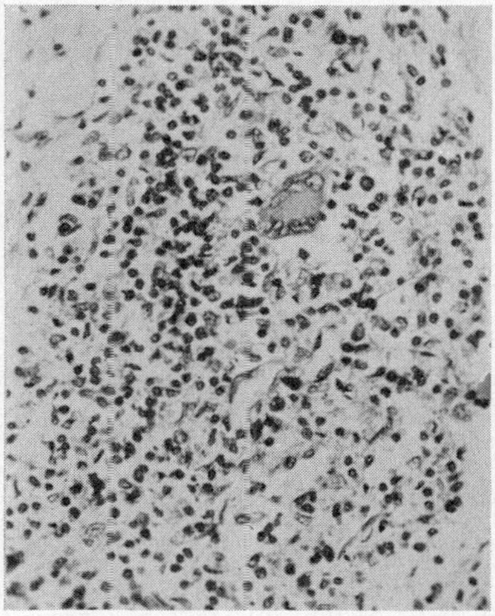

FIG. 22. Giant cell in a hepatic lymph node. A large multinucleated giant cell in the same lymph node as in Fig. 21. (H. 11, Hemat.-eos., 475x.)

Microphotographs by Dr. J. W. Mills

mature forms of lymphocytes and plasma cells, and numerous macrophages containing hemosiderin, fat vacuoles, and other unidentified material (Fig. 4).

The main renal alteration is a lymphocytic and plasma cell infiltration that appears in scattered foci throughout the kidney.

In the lungs, macrophages laden with hemosiderin and lymphocytes fill the alveolar capillaries and larger pulmonary vessels in whole or in part.

*

Certain gross pathologic alterations have been associated with equine infectious anemia from its earliest recognition. The general body changes of emaciation, anemia, edema and jaundice were noted by those first describing the malady in 1843 (68, 78, 256). Petechial hemorrhages involving many organs, splenic enlargement, alterations in the size, color and consistency of the liver, and lymph node enlargement were noted by Carré and Vallée (56, 57, 58). Similar gross findings have been reported from various parts of the world by numerous investigators studying the disease experimentally produced or in proven field cases. The gross pathologic lesions characteristic of the disease have been treated by Van Es and associates (470) in the United States; Todd and Wolbach (451) in Canada; the Japanese Commission (191) in Japan; deKock (211) in South Africa; Schermer (382) in Germany; Verge (476) in France; Dobberstein (84) and Fortner (115) in Germany; Gindin (139) in Russia; Stein (426) in the United States; Balozet (28) in North Africa; Cassamagnaghi and Cassamagnaghi (62) in South America.

The microscopic findings described by Mack (271) in 1909 were extravasation and degeneration of erythrocytes in the major organs, leucocytic exudation in the vicinity of the vascular walls of the major organs, parenchymatous degeneration and necrosis of the liver, heart and kidneys, pigmentation of the liver and lymph nodes. These are basically the same as those described later by Finzi (111) in France; Todd and Wolbach (451) in Canada; Jaffé (188) in Austria; Mócsy (294) in Hungary; deKock (211) in South Africa; Schermer (382) in Germany; Hjärre (168) in Sweden; Balozet (28) in North Africa; Gindin (139) and Fedorov (110) in Russia; Stein (426) in the United States; and Epstein (107) in South America.

Special studies have been made on the typical histologic alterations in individual organs. The changes in the lungs were studied in detail by Steck and Hauser (423); the heart by Dobberstein and Wilmes (88), Matthiessen and Glasser (283), and Schaaf, Hecke and Bert (379); the kidney by Leinati (248); the central nervous system by Nakamura and associates (319); the spleen by Gindin (138); the liver by Hjärre (168); the lymph nodes by Piening (349); and the bone marrow by Wright (492).

Diagnosis based upon the histologic picture has been considered by Ziegler (496) and Nöller and Dobberstein (322). While gross and microscopic findings may be cumulatively helpful in making a tentative diagnosis (426), none is pathognomonic for the disease, nor are all the typical changes taken together sufficient for a positive diagnosis.

Several systems have been considered as the primary site of viral attack. Most authors are in accord that the red blood cell is primarily affected, with rapid destruction of erythrocytes and subsequent accumulation of break-down products in the spleen. Early in the disease process the spleen becomes overloaded and its function of handling blood pigments exhausted, and consequently the burden is placed on the reticuloendothelial systems of other organs, such as the liver and lymph nodes.

Another site of injury is the capillary endothelium, as indicated early in the disease by the common occurrence and general distribution of petechial hemorrhages. The cause of the increased capillary permeability has been attributed to the direct action of the virus (496), to inflammatory changes in the capillary walls, or to injury by toxic break-down products (138). In response to the injury of the reticulo-endothelial cells and to the increased burden of pigment phagocytosis, the system undergoes proliferation.

The bone marrow has been considered as a site of viral action; however, hyperplasia of the red marrow occurs in any disease after marked destruction of erythrocytes, provided that its power of regeneration is not destroyed. The bone marrow changes, though studied in only a few of our experimental animals, were striking only when the anemia was marked. In such cases, erythrocytic hyperplasia was apparent. The nature of the anemia as seen from examinations of the peripheral blood as well as organ changes is that of a normochromic, normocytic anemia and does not simulate the alterations found in pernicious anemia of man.

The degenerative and necrotic changes that occur in the parenchymal cells of the major organs may be the direct result of viral injury (28), or a result of break-down products of the host tissue primarily altered by the virus (138).

The significance of the cardiac lesions resembling Aschoff bodies, the eosiniophilic cell infiltrations of the liver, spleen, and lymph glands, and the renal alterations as possible allergic manifestations will be considered in a separate publication (99).

In concluding the analysis of the microscopic alterations noted in the organs of our experimental animals infected with the virus of infectious anemia, it may be said that the changes show various phases of an inflammatory process, acute, subacute, or chronic in nature. The alterations reflect, on one hand, the direct systemic response of the infected animals to the invading virus, and, on the other hand, a histologic response indicative of the possibility that an allergic component may be present in the infectious process, particularly in the subacute and chronic phase of the disease, as discussed under the heading of Pathogenesis (Chapter 9).

The injury caused by the virus initiates, as described above, degenerative and necrotic processes around the vascular system of the parenchymatous organs, chiefly the liver. In a later stage of the disease process, infiltration of various inflammatory cells, mainly those of the lymphocytic series, is a prominent feature. In the parenchymatous organs, reparative proliferation of the tissues takes place with an increase of connective tissue elements that may lead finally to scar formations. As an example of such proliferation, the Aschoff body-like formations may be mentioned which were observed in the heart.

The involvement of the reticulo-endothelial system is marked in cases of longer duration, exhibiting rich proliferation of the cellular elements of the reticulo-endothelium; this reflects an intensified reaction on the part of the defense mechanism in the infected animal. Noting this, particularly in prolonged chronic cases, some investigators suggested the name of "reticulo-endotheliosis" for use instead of that of infectious anemia.

Hemosiderin deposits in the organs are the histologic expression of injury to a large number of red blood corpuscles. Hemosiderosis manifests itself most strikingly in the liver and, to a lesser degree, in the spleen and the lymph nodes. Anemia, i.e., a more or less marked decrease in the number of the red blood cells, although it is part of the pathologic process and has a considerable clinical significance, is by no means the only important feature of equine infectious anemia. It is rather the inflammatory process in its various phases that characterizes the disease, although neither the gross, nor the microscopic alterations can be considered as specific for the condition.

CHAPTER 14

THERAPY AND CONTROL

Therapy.—For the treatment of equine infectious anemia the cures suggested have been numerous; this is inevitable in the case of an infection that does not respond to any therapy. First many kinds of supporting or symptomatic therapy were tried; then chemotherapeutic treatment was attempted by several investigators. But it seems that all efforts have failed, so far, to find an effective therapy and, in particular, to destroy the virus within the body of the sick animals or virus carriers. Sometimes, one cure or another seemed successful in suppressing symptoms, but in most cases this was very likely due simply to the spontaneous remission that is part of the typical disease.

At the beginning of the chemotherapeutic era, Atoxyl and Trypanblue were among the first drugs to be used by research workers studying infectious anemia. Atoxyl was applied by Francis and Marsteller (123) in 1908, as well as by Dietrich (83) in 1910. The curative effect of Trypanblue was tested by Francis and Marsteller (123) and by Whitehouse (485) in 1911. The results following the use of these two drugs were questionable or negative. Neosalvarsan was also tried for treatment apparently without success (525).

The therapy used in nutritional or various types of secondary anemia in humans was also tried by many investigators. Larsson (237) administered iron, calcium, and phosphorus compounds, but the results were not promising. Gerlach (132) concluded that no therapy was ever successful in his hands. The use of homologous blood in the form of transfusions as well as normal horse serum was reported to give encouraging results. Rózsa (377) noted definite improvement in two-third of a group of infectious anemia horses by giving them transfusions from healthy donors, but one-third of the group did not respond to this treatment. Duvaux (101) found that administration of normal horse serum was quite helpful. Lamarre (233) reported that autotransfusions brought about improvement within 2 to 8 days, while Bailer (524) observed that autohemotherapy was only partly successful. The favorable results may probably be attributed to the stimulating effect of homologous blood on hematopoiesis (54).

The use of nonspecific protein therapy in veterinary medicine was advocated by Fortner (114), but Metzger (286) attempted the treatment of infectious anemia with parenterally administered protein preparations unsuccessfully. Mocsy (299) has seen no curative effect from large doses of normal bovine serum; the same was true for treatment with iodine (Lugol-solution).

Schermer (383) in 1929 suggested the use of treatment similar to the one effective in human pernicious anemia. Following such line in the therapy, Krupski (225) fed infected horses with fresh liver of horses, calves, swine, and cattle in amounts varying from 8 to 26 kilograms. Some favorable results were noted, but they were not lasting. Verge (476) mentioned the parenteral use of Whipple liver extracts, but this procedure did not bring quite satisfactory results either.

Among the numerous pharmaceutic preparations that have been utilized in the treatment of the disease are arsenical compounds, quinine, mercurial preparations, bismuth, antimony, various acids, vitamins, and enzymes. A long list of drugs and chemicals was used in a series of experiments to estimate their therapeutic value by Stein, Osteen, and Mott (437) in 1941. None of the drugs or chemicals tested were found to be effective.

The sulfanilamides were also tested as to their value in the therapy by Gochenour and co-workers (141), but were found to have no specific action on the malady or the virus causing it. Mott, Stein, and Heishman (311) reported in 1946 that penicillin had little or no effect on the course of the disease. While aureomycin has been used successfully in the treatment of some cases of human pernicious anemia by Lichtman, Ginsberg, and Watson (255), and in the acute phase of viral hepatitis by Shaffer and co-workers (407), its use in the treatment of equine infectious anemia has not been reported.

In conclusion it may be said that, at present, we know of no therapeutic agent that has a curative action in equine infectious anemia. Supportive therapy by the use of blood transfusions, homologous serum, and parenteral administration of liver and iron deserve further trial, since several authors have reported favorable or suggestive results following their therapeutic use. We believe that hypersensitivity is responsible, to a great extent, for the severe symptoms; therefore, any treatment that might lower the allergic reactivity in the horse will probably have its place in the symptomatic therapy of the disease even though it cannot ultimately cure the malady by acting on the virus itself.

Control.—The problem of controlling the spread of infectious anemia is as old as the recognition that the disease is infectious. Effective control faces a number of obstacles; the weakest point of control measures is the difficulty of detecting the symptomless virus carriers. Since successful control depends upon the identification and eradication of infected horses, no systematic program can be undertaken until a specific, practical, and inexpensive means of diagnosis of all infected animals is developed (426). The asymptomatic carrier horse probably constitutes one of the most common sources of virus in nature, but the reliable method of detecting such carriers, the horse inoculation test, is costly and time-consuming.

For preventing the spread of infection, various control measures have been suggested. These are designed not only to spare the individual horse owner considerable losses, but also to protect the horse population within a community and this is often of great economic importance (396). Practical measures to serve such a purpose are: 1) reporting all horses suspected of having the disease or carrying the infection, 2) separating them from the ones not affected by the disease, 3) killing either all suspected horses, or at least the proven cases, 4) branding suspected and proven cases if, for some reason, they cannot be killed. It is quite obvious that destroying all proven cases of the infection is, in the final analysis, less expensive than keeping such animals, thus preserving the source of contagion. It has also been proposed to designate some particular regions where chronic cases and carriers can be used for work (371), if the disease is enzootic and widely spread in that area, but unrestricted shipping and export of horses from such regions should be forbidden.

Control measures have been studied and discussed in detail by a number of authors in various countries (36,117,157,172,191,202,275,281, 396,426,476,499). In some countries official government regulations have been adopted for enforcing necessary control measures. Among these are Germany (particularly Prussia), France, Switzerland, Norway, Denmark, Italy, and Slovakia in Europe; Japan in Asia. References related to some of these control regulations can be found under the name of the country in our bibliography. In Germany, official laboratory tests for aiding the diagnosis are performed by central laboratories (668,117,122,729). The *Office International des Épizooties* in Paris (324) proposed measures that could be adopted on an international basis. Recently Flückiger (113) discussed the efforts made in this direction and summarized the suggestions for international collaboration in the matter.

Degen (77), studying the problem of official government control measures in Switzerland, estimated that it cost the government 123,130 Swiss francs in *Baselland* canton alone to take the necessary steps for control during the years of 1930 to 1942. For 306 horses that were destroyed (average value estimated 1000 francs per horse) part-compensation was paid to the owner by the government. Over 29,000 francs of the total government cost mentioned above were used for control measures: investigations, therapeutic trials, autopsies, disinfection of stables. Thus, the average cost of these control measures amounted to 96 francs per horse, while the rest of the sum was spent for compensation.

It is impractical to enumerate all the regulations and suggestions proposed for control. A few examples will suffice.

The Japanese Commission (191) laid down some useful recommendations for practical prevention. According to these, any evidence of the disease should be reported by local officials to the central government office, and competent inspectors should make a physical examination of all horses weekly during the epizootic season and once a month during the rest of the year in regions where infectious anemia is prevalent. Infected animals must be destroyed or isolated, and suspicious cases removed from pastures. If a positive case occurs among a pastured group during the horsefly season, the whole herd should be considered infected. The movement of horses from infected regions must be prohibited. Isolation stables should be located sufficiently distant from the ones used for healthy animals and infected straw, dung, and all such material should be kept in heaps at least for two months and may not be used as manure before the expiration of that period.

Scott (396) discussed the control measures in 1919, when examining the economic importance of infectious anemia in Wyoming, and advocated killing all affected cases immediately—provided the diagnosis is correct—"since many of the infected horses die anyway and the remainder as carriers of the virus become a menace to the rest of the herd". The Japanese suggested setting free recovered cases if they are perfectly free of symptoms, but Scott considers this plan as not entirely safe because, in most cases, the blood of such horses is still virulent. If all affected horses are not killed, he suggested the segregation of sick and well horses by removing the latter to a new, dry pasture at a distance far enough to prevent the passage of biting flies that he clearly has shown in his experiments to be potential transmitters of the virus. The safest isolation is in a barn with openings screened. For reducing the incidence as much as possible, it is important that a careful watch be kept over all horses exposed to the infection (checking the animals' temperature and, eventually, their urine for albumen). Movements and shipment of all horses from an area where an outbreak occurs, must be suspended particularly during the infective season; suspicious cases and chronic carriers should not be moved at any time. Disinfection of stables, though desirable from the sanitary point of view, is considered of little value in preventing the spread of infection.

Serum companies must always be on guard to detect and avert the presence of virus carriers among their production horses, on account of the risk of spreading the infection by the use of preventive and therapeutic horse serum, or other products. Fortner (120) reported that 3000 horses had to be destroyed because of the use of a vaccine (against Borna-disease) made from brain tissue of a horse carrying the virus of infectious anemia. He suggested that strict quarantine measures for the horses be put into effect four months before they are used for serum production, during which time they should be observed closely and temperatures should be taken daily; any suspicious cases should be checked by the horse inoculation test. He also analyzed the problem of differential diagnosis as presented by minor symptoms seen in some of the hyperimmunized serum horses (121). Röhrer and his co-workers (374,376) recently studied the method of "cross-infection" testing in horses which means that pairs of horses are injected with each other's blood. According to them, this procedure would, in most cases, reveal eventual carriers among horses intended for use in serum production. Although they encountered some difficulties in interpreting their results, they reported finding 3 per cent virus carriers among a group of 126 clinically healthy horses by the cross-infection method. The main difficulty lies in the interpretation of mild reactions, since it is not easy to decide whether the donor's blood or the condition of the recipient animal is responsible for the uncertain symptoms.

The United States Bureau of Animal Industry established a safeguard against dissemination of the disease through the use of biological products by requiring that biological supply houses operating under government license heat all antisera prepared from horses at 58° to 59° C. for one hour (426).

Studies of the Bureau of Animal Industry, as described by Stein (426), indicate that the following measures are the most effective means of control: When a definite diagnosis of infectious anemia has been made, one should kill the animal and dispose of the carcass by cremation or deep burial in order to prevent further spread of the infection. If it is not feasible to destroy infected animals, then those known to be diseased and those suspected of being infected should be isolated from healthy animals. The common use on both infected and healthy horses of equipment that may produce skin abrasions or absorb body excretions or secretions, such as bridles, harnesses, saddles, blankets, brushes, and currycombs is to be avoided. Surgical instruments, needles and syringes should be thoroughly sterilized for each animal. Infected mares should not be used for breeding purposes, as they may transmit the disease to their offspring. Animals should not be kept together in small, poorly drained paddocks adjacent to stables and manure dumps. Where premises are badly contaminated, or a number of cases of the disease have developed on certain pastures, it is first advisable to move the animals to new quarters, then plow the ground deeply and fence off the infected area. Horses or mules should not be permitted on such pastures or premises for at least 6 months. There should be maintained good sanitary conditions, fly control, systematic control of intestinal parasites, and a supply of pure, fresh drinking water; under no circumstances should animals be permitted to drink from stagnant pools.

The procedure carried out in New Hampshire, according to the 1948 report of the Chief of the Bureau of Animal Industry (462), for controlling the spread of the infection during the epizootic of 1947 in New Hampshire among a group of thoroughbred horses was as follows:

> An 86-day quarantine was placed on the horses at Rockingham Park and surrounding territory. All sick horses were isolated and placed in an isolation unit. Temperatures of horses at the track stables were taken daily to detect early cases. Flies were controlled by the use of effective fly repellents. Separate drinking and feeding facilities were provided for each horse, and the barns and immediate surroundings were kept in good sanitary condition. All straw, manure, and other refuse from the isolation unit were destroyed by burning. Before the quarantine was lifted the horses that had shown clinical symptoms of the disease were destroyed and the supposedly normal horses were tested by a 40-day horse inoculation test.

For reducing the chances of the spread of infection by insects, either careful screening, or spraying of the stables is recommended with DDT or other insecticides (435). We utilized both of these measures during our experiments.

Reports have been published concerning the successful eradication of the disease from regions where it existed before. Horne (172) stated that strict government control measures added much to practical eradication in Norway. According to Martini (281), such measures were successful in Slovenia. Fairly good success was claimed also as a result of enforcing official control measures in Prussia (202). Although several papers have been published about infectious anemia that was enzootic among small African donkeys in South Africa, the disease is not even mentioned in Henning's book published in 1949 on *Animal Diseases in South Africa.* It would seem that the disease has disappeared since the early experimental studies were performed.

The difficulties of eradicating the disease from a certain area where it has been enzootic for a long time are almost insuperable for the simple reason that tracing all of the healthy-looking symptomless virus carriers is practically impossible without an inexpensive method for detecting such horses. As has been discussed in the chapter dealing with the problem of immunization, preventive vaccination has been studied by many investigators with very little success so far. Thus, it is not included among the list of practicable control measures for the purpose of checking the spread of infection.

CONCLUDING REMARKS

It seems appropriate, in conclusion, to add a few words to what is said in the preceding chapters about the original targets of our experimental studies and the results achieved.

We laid the emphasis in our studies on the experimental aspects. The clinical side of the disease could not be treated equally well, partly for lack of time, and partly because the clinical aspects are better known and described. It is obvious that what is lacking for our better understanding of this malady can be best learned by experimental approach, that is, by the application of methods of investigation developed in recent years for the clarification of similar problems. This explains why, throughout the discussions in this work, preference is given to facts learned by experimentation.

By necessity, the scope of the experimental studies was a modest one, for a great variety of problems had to be explored by a small group. Obviously, a larger group of investigators, representing several experimental fields, could attack more successfully such complex problems as we dealt with. It seemed desirable for us to explore simultaneously as many phases of the problem as possible, although the number of the experimental horses that we were able to handle at the same time was limited. This made it necessary to limit the scope of any given experiment, in order to turn to the exploration of the next problem. Studying one single problem for a long time would have prevented us from looking into a series of diverse questions which all seemed to be important if we wanted to make progress in our investigations. Consequently, several of the problems that we tried to explore experimentally were not studied in sufficient detail, as we were not able to carry them to a firm conclusion during the few years while this experimental work was in progress.

It is felt, however, that in spite of the rather limited extent to which these experiments could be developed, a definite progress was made and several unsolved problems concerning equine infectious anemia came closer to a possible solution.

Our main targets in the experimental studies were attempts at transmission of the infection to small laboratory animals, developing laboratory tests for a quick diagnosis, and eventually finding means of preventive immunization against the disease. The latter two could be best achieved by successful cultivation of the virus outside of the animal's body. As briefly outlined in the corresponding chapters of this monograph, in several phases of our work promising results were recorded which—we believe—may serve as a basis for further attack on the problems.

Systematic experiments conducted to clarify the nature of the pathologic process disclosed the fact, as outlined in Chapter 9 (page 71), that in infectious anemia the primary infection with the virus leads to an allergic state in the infected animal and is not followed by immunity observed in many other infectious diseases. Rather it makes the animal more sensitive to renewed contact with the virus. This explains many strange findings noted by other experimenters as well as by ourselves in studying infectious anemia. It also explains the very limited success noted so far in attempts at preventive immunization. We believe that, even after successful and proven cultivation of the virus, the complicating factor of hypersensitivity present in the infection must be overcome by some device of desensitization before immunization can be achieved.

We are fully aware that in our discussions we often raised more questions than we have answered. It is felt, however, that the weighing of theoretical possibilities may be helpful in future investigations. We are confident that the expansion of our findings regarding the allergic mechanism of the infectious process will contribute to the clarification of the "mystery" of infectious anemia.

This monograph is, naturally, not intended to present the solution to the problems of infectious anemia. It is rather to provide orientation for those problems. Our conclusions in the various chapters are intended to be helpful in formulating opinion on the material presented. As stated in the Foreword, we had the task of bringing together the pertinent information on the subject of infectious anemia and presenting it in concise form. In doing so we divided the material according to subject matter closest to the respective fields of the authors. Dr. Lombard wrote the chapter on Histopathology; she also prepared Chapters 3, 4, and 14 and contributed to the compilation of Chapter 7. For the remaining chapters and for the interpretation of the experimental findings, the senior author has to take the responsibility.

The bibliography at the end of this monograph lists publications up to the end of 1951. For the sake of brevity, we mentioned the most needed references in the discussions of the various chapters. These may well serve for first orientation and may form the basis for further search in the literature on the particular subject. To obtain the full story, the rich material listed in the supplementary bibliography should also be consulted. In reporting developments, we tried to respect priority as much as possible, although our primary object was not to analyze the voluminous literature in detail.

ACKNOWLEDGMENTS

It is our pleasant duty to thank the many friends and colleagues who by their unselfish cooperation helped us in performing our experimental work and compiling the present report about it.

We wish to express our gratitude to the late Dr. Raymond A. Kelser, to whose memory this monograph is dedicated, for his inspiring guidance, understanding, and warmhearted encouragement throughout the many difficult phases of the work. His enthusiasm was always an inspiration to his associates. We are deeply indebted to Dr. Richard E. Shope for his constant interest in our work and for his many useful suggestions both in the experimental work and in the preparation of this monograph. We feel that without his support and understanding this report could not have been prepared.

Our heartfelt thanks are due to Dr. Evan L. Stubbs, head of the Department of Pathology, who obligingly offered to us his help and that of his entire staff in making post-mortem investigations of the experimental horses, and in handling and preparing practically all of the histologic material used in our study. We are grateful to Dr. J. D. Beck, Dr. A. G. Danks, Dr. Th. DeMott, and Dr. W. E. LaGrange for their valuable help and assistance in making the facilities of Bolton Farm available; and to Dr. I. Live and Dr. M. J. Deubler of the Department of Microbiology for various services while we carried out our laboratory work. It is impossible to thank, by name, our many friends and colleagues who willingly helped us during our work, with advice and otherwise, because we would be compelled to list most of the members of the Faculty. We offer our best thanks to them

We are indebted to Dr. John W. Mills, of the Veterinary School, and Dr. Steven C. Mohos of Cornell University Medical College for the fine microphotographs used for illustration of the monograph, and to Dr. Mohos for his comments regarding the interpretation of the microscopic findings.

Finally, we want to express our best appreciation to our co-workers whose names do not appear on the cover of the present report but who made valuable contributions to our experimental work, while they participated in various phases of the study. Our thanks are due to Dr. Werner Leemann of the University of Zürich, Switzerland, to Dr. Arnold R. Gilman, and Miss Jane F. Shirer. Dr. Gilman's well-planned and ambitious work and its findings constitute an integral part of the study. Miss Shirer has been associated with us almost during the whole tenure of our studies, assisting with the experiments and also typing and checking the list of bibliography; her skillful and conscientious work was most valuable. We are grateful to Mrs. Mary McK. Wildermuth of the University of Pennsylvania Press for checking our manuscript and suggesting many improvements and corrections in English.

We are indebted to the Grayson Foundation for sponsoring the project and providing the necessary financial support for the experimental investigation.

LIST OF ABBREVIATIONS

(Journals most frequently quoted in the Bibliography)

Állatorv.Lapok	*Állatorvosi Lapok*
Amer.J.Vet.Med.	*American Journal of Veterinary Medicine* (later *Vet. Med.*)
Amer.J.Vet.Res.	*American Journal of Veterinary Research*
Amer.Vet.Rev.	*American Veterinary Review* (later *J.Am.Vet.Med.Ass.*)
Arch.ges.Virusforsch.	*Archiv für die gesamte Virusforschung*
Arch.Path.	*Archives of Pathology* (*and Laboratory Medicine*)
Arch.Tierheilk.	*Archiv für wissenschaftliche und praktische Tierheilkunde*
Berl.-Münch.Tier.Woch.	*Berliner und Münchener tierärztliche Wochenschrift*
Berl.Tier.Woch.	*Berliner tierärztliche Wochenschrift*
Bull.Acad.Vét.France	*Bulletin de l'Académie vétérinaire de France*
Bull.Off.Intl.Epizoot.	*Bulletin. Office international des épizooties*
Bull.Soc.Centr.Méd.Vét.	*Bulletin et mémoires. Société centrale de médecine vétérin.*
Canad.J.Comp.Med.	*Canadian Journal of Comparative Medicine and Veterinary Science*
Compt.Rend.Acad.Sci.	*Comptes rendus hebdomadaires des séances de l'Académie des Sciences* (Paris)
Compt.Rend.Soc.Biol.	*Comptes rendus hebdomadaires des séances et mémoires de la Société de Biologie* (Paris)
Cornell Vet.	*Cornell Veterinarian*
Deut.Tier.Woch.	*Deutsche tierärztliche Wochenschrift*
Exp.Sta.Rec.	*Experiment Station Record*
Jap.J.Vet.Sci.	*Japanese Journal of Veterinary Science*
J.Amer.Med.Ass.	*Journal of the American Medical Association*
J.Amer.Vet.Med.Ass.	*Journal of the American Veterinary Medical Association*
J.Exp.Med.	*Journal of Experimental Medicine*
J.Immunol.	*Journal of Immunology*
J.Lab.Clin.Med.	*Journal of Laboratory and Clinical Medicine*
Jber.Vet.Med.	*Jahresbericht über die Leistungen auf dem Gebiete der Veterinär-Medizin*
Maanedsskr.Dyrlaeg	*Maanedsskrift for Dyrlaeger*
Monat.Tierheilk.	*Monatshefte für praktische Tierheilkunde*
Monat.Vet.-Med.	*Monatshefte für Veterinärmedizin*
Münch.Tier.Woch.	*Münchener tierärztliche Wochenschrift*
Nord.Vet.Med.	*Nordisk Veterinaermedicin*
Norsk VetTidsskr.	*Norsk Veterinaertidsskrift*
North Amer.Vet.	*North American Veterinarian*
Proc.Soc.Exp.Biol.Med.	*Proceedings, Society for Experimental Biology & Medicine*
Rec.Méd.Vét.	*Recueil de médecine vétérinaire de l'École d'Alfort*
Rev.Gén.Méd.Vét.	*Revue générale de médecine vétérinaire*
Rev.Méd.Vét.	*Revue de médecine vétérinaire*
Schweiz.Arch.Tierh.	*Schweizer Archiv für Tierheilkunde*
Skand.VetTidskr.	*Skandinavisk Veterinärtidskrift*
Tidskr.Vet.-Med.	*Tidskrift for Veterinär-Medicin*
Tierärzt.Rund.	*Tierärztliche Rundschau*
Tijdschr.Diergeneesk.	*Tijdschrift voor Diergeneeskunde*
Vet.Bull.	*Veterinary Bulletin*
Vet.Med.	*Veterinary Medicine*
Vet.Journ.	*Veterinary Journal*
Virchow's Arch.Path.Anat.	*Virchow's Archiv f. pathologische Anatomie u. Physiologie*
Wien.Tier.Monat.	*Wiener tierärztliche Monatsschrift*
Z.Infekt.Haustiere	*Zeitschrift für Infektionskrankheiten der Haustiere*
Z.Vet.kunde	*Zeitschrift für Veterinärkunde*

BIBLIOGRAPHY

A) References

(*Throughout the text, numbers in parentheses refer to publications listed below*)

1. Abbondanza, S.: E una leptospirosi l'anemia infettiva dei cavalli della zona risiera Lombardo-Piemontese? Clinica Vet. 1951, **74.** 10

2. Abderhalden, E., und Frei, W.: Ueber das Verhalten des Blutes (Plasma resp. Serum und rote Blutkörperchen) von an perniziöser Anämie erkrankten Pferden gegen Saponin. Arch. Tierheilk. 1910, **36.** 423

3. Akerström, R.: Sublingual hemorrhage in infectious anemia in horses. Nord. Vet.Med. 1951, **3.** 659

4. Alegren, A.: Anémie infectieuse du cheval en Suède. Bull. Off. Intl. Epizoot. 1951, **36.** 312

5. Altara, I.: L'anémie infectieuse des équidés. (Epizootologie de la maladie.) Bull. Off. Intl. Epizoot. 1951, **36.** 232

6. Andrewes, C. H.: Interference by one virus with the growth of another in tissue culture. Brit. J. Exp. Path. 1942, **23.** 214

7. Andrievskii, I.: Immunity in equine infectious anemia. (*In Russian*) Sovyet Vet. 1939, **16.** (No. 8) 25 (abstr.: V.B. **10.** 671)

8. Anginiard: Observations de contagion par infection de l'anhémie idiopathique du cheval. Rapport de la commission. Rec. Méd. Vét. 1859, **36.** 639 Discussion: 1861, **38.** 325, 421

9. Aschoff, L.: Zur Myocarditisfrage. Verhandl. Deut. Path. Ges. 1904, **8.** 46

10. Baker, J. A.: Rinderpest. VIII. Rinderpest infection in rabbits. Amer. J. Vet. Res. 1946, **7.** 179

11. Balozet, L.: Etude clinique et expérimentale de l'anémie infectieuse des équidés au Maroc. Bull. Soc. Path. Exot. 1923, **16.** 525

12. Balozet, L.: Au sujet de l'immunité dans l'anémie infectieuse des équidés. Compt. Rend. Acad. Sci. 1934, **198.** 992

NOTE.—Boldface numbers indicate volume of journal. Abbreviations used when referring to an abstract of original papers:

B.T.W.	*Berliner Tierärztliche Wochenschrift*
B.M.T.W.	*Berliner und Münchener Tierärztliche Wochenschrift*
D.T.W.	*Deutsche Tierärztliche Wochenschrift*
J.A.V.M.A.	*Journal of the American Veterinary Medical Association*
Jber.	*Jahresbericht über Veterinär-Medizin*
M.T.W.	*Münchener Tierärztliche Wochenschrift*
V.B.	*Veterinary Bulletin* (Brit.)
Diss.	designates doctoral dissertation, followed by the name of city where it was submitted as a thesis

13. Balozet, L.: Sensibilité de l'âne Africain à l'inoculation du virus de l'anémie infectieuse. Compt. Rend. Soc. Biol. 1935, **119**. 62

14. Balozet, L.: Effet des passages successifs par les ânes, sur le pouvoir pathogène du virus de l'anémie infectieuse. Compt. Rend. Soc. Biol. 1935, **119**. 65

15. Balozet, L.: Effet de réinoculations, chez l'âne, du virus de l'anémie infectieuse. Compt. Rend. Soc. Biol. 1935, **119**. 160

16. Balozet, L.: Action de certains agents chimiques: éther, chloroforme, fluorure de sodium, phénol, saponine, sur le virus de l'anémie infectieuse. Compt. Rend. Soc. Biol. 1935, **119**. 162

17. Balozet, L.: Action de la glycérine sur la sérum virulent dans l'anémie infectieuse. Compt. Rend. Soc. Biol. 1935, **119**. 282

18. Balozet, L.: Action de la bile sur la virus de l'anémie infectieuse des équidés. Compt. Rend. Soc. Biol. 1935, **119**. 818

19. Balozet, L.: Etudes expérimentales sur l'anémie infectieuse des équidés. II. Action de la bile sur le virus. Arch. Inst. Pasteur Tunis 1935, **24**. 493.

20. Balozet, L.: Etudes expérimentales sur l'anémie infectieuse des équidés. III. Essais négatifs de prémunisation par l'emploi de la rate virulente, glycérinée ou phéniquée. Arch. Inst. Pasteur Tunis 1936, **25**. 272

21. Balozet, L.: Action de la glycérine sur la virulence de la rate dans l'anémie infectieuse. Compt. Rend. Soc. Biol. 1936, **122**. 283

22. Balozet, L.: Action de l'acide phénique sur la virulence de la rate dans l'anémie infectieuse. Compt. Rend. Soc. Biol. 1936, **122**. 285

23. Balozet, L.: Etudes expérimentales sur l'anémie infectieuse des équidés. IV. Essais d'inoculation à d'autres espèces animales. Arch. Inst. Pasteur Tunis 1937, **26**. 27

24. Balozet, L.: Etudes expérimentales sur l'anémie infectieuse des équidés. V. Action du ricinoléate de soude de l'enrobage et de l'inoculation de faibles doses. Arch. Inst. Pasteur Tunis 1938, **27**. 189

25. Balozet, L.: Sur la nature du virus de l'anémie infectieuse. Bull. Acad. Vét. France 1939, **12**. 369

26. Balozet, L.: Résistance du virus de l'anémie infectieuse au rayonnement de la lampe à mercure. Compt. Rend. Acad. Sci. 1939, **209**. 177

27. Balozet, L.: Filtrabilité du virus de l'anémie infectieuse des équidés. Essai de détermination de la dimension des particules du virus. Compt. Rend. Acad. Sci. 1939, **209**. 703

28. Balozet, L.: Anémie infectieuse des équidés (pp. 843-884), in Levaditi, Lépine, et Verge: Les Ultravirus des Maladies Animales. Paris, Montpellier, 1943.

29. Balozet, L., et Aoustin, L.: Premier cas d'anémie infectieuse des équidés observé en Tunisie. Arch. Inst. Pasteur Tunis 1934, **23**. 360

30. Bankier, J. C.: Equine infectious anemia. Attempted vaccination with crystal violet tissue vaccine. Canad. J. Comp. Med. 1945, **9**. 197

31. Bartels: When should infectious anemia be considered as a possible diagnosis. (*In Danish*) Maanedsskr. Dyrlaeg. 1923, **35**. 177

32. Beach, J.: The application of the hemagglutination-inhibition test in the diagnosis of avian pneumoencephalitis (Newcastle disease). J. Amer. Vet. Med. Ass. 1948, **112**. 85

33. Beamer, P., Bloch, E., Warner, L., Brooks, F., Anliker, J., and Knisely, M.: Sludged blood in three young pigs experimentally infected with hog cholera. Amer. J. Vet. Res. 1949, **10**. 111

34. Béghin: Enzootie d'anémie pernicieuse progressive chez les chevaux. Ann. Méd. Vét. 1906, **55**. 692

35. Behrens: Ansteckende Blutarmut und Tuberkulose der Pferde im Regierungsbezirk Hildesheim. Berl. Tier. Woch. 1926, **42**. 260

36. Beller, K., und Schwarzmaier, E.: Untersuchungen über die ansteckende Blutarmut der Pferde. I. Zur Epidemiologie und Diagnostik der ansteckenden

Blutarmut. (Erfahrungen in Hessen über einen Zeitraum von 7 Jahren.) Arch. Tierheilk. 1940, **76**. 24

37. Beller, K., und Traub, E.: Untersuchungen über die ansteckende Blutarmut der Pferde. Immunitätsversuche. Monat. Tierheilk. Neue Folge, 1951, **3**. 193

38. Bichel, J., Bing, J., and Harboe, N.: Another case of hyperglobinemia and affection of the central nervous system. Acta Med. Scand. 1950, **138**. 1

39. Björneboe, M., and Krag, P.: Studies on a complement fixation in hepatitis with liver extract as antigen. Acta Path. Microbiol. Scand. 1947, **24**. 352

40. Blanchard, L., et Vedel, R.: Thromboses veineuses dans le territoire de la veine porte chez les chevaux atteints d'anémie infectieuse. Bull. Acad. Vét. France 1934, **7**. 116

41. Blotner, H.: Anaphylactic shock with hemoconcentration treated intravenously with saline solution. J. Am. Med. Ass. 1942, **118**. 219

42. Bosh'yan, G. M.: Chemistry of blood of horses with infectious anemia. I. (*In Russian*) Veterinariya 1941, **18**. (No. 3) 28 (abstr.: V.B. **12**. 533)

43. Bostick, W.: Virus interference by serially passed Hodgkin's disease extracts in chicken eggs. Proc. Soc. Exp. Biol. Med. 1950, **74**. 519

44. Bouley, H.: Discussion sur le rapport de M. Sanson. Rec. Méd. Vét. 1861, **38**. 421

45. Boyden, S. V.: The adsorption of proteins on erythrocytes treated with tannic acid and subsequent hemagglutination by anti-protein sera. J. Exp. Med. 1951, **93**. 107

46. Brimhall, S. O., Wesbrook, F. F., and Bracken, H. M.: Swamp fever in horses. Report, Minnesota State Board of Health, Vet. Dept. 1900-1903 (p. 264) St. Paul, 1903

47. Browning, J., Rice, R., and Ulrich, C.: Alteration in blood proteins in rheumatic patients. Amer. J. Med. Sci. 1951, **221**. 183

48. Bruger, M., and Oppenheim, E.: The present status of liver function tests, including observations on the newer flocculation procedures. Bull. New York Acad. Med. 1949, **25**. 16

49. Brunswick: Essais d'immunisation par inoculation du complexe: sang virulente et argent colloidal. Rec. Méd. Vét. 1934, **110**. 79

50. deBurgh, P. M., Yu, P. C., Howe C., and Bovarnick, M.: Preparation from human red cells of a substance inhibiting virus hemagglutination. J. Exp. Med. 1948, **87**. 1

51. Burnet, F. M.: The affinity of the Newcastle disease virus to the influenza group. Austral. J. Exp. Biol. Med. Sci. 1942, **20**. 81

52. Burnet, F. M., and Stone, F. D.: The hemagglutinins of vaccinia and electromelia viruses. Austral. J. Exp. Biol. Med. Sci. 1946, **24**. 1

53. Carlström, B., und Hjärre, A.: Die Bedeutung der Fütterung als prädisponierenden Faktors bei der infektiösen Anämie. Dreizehnter Internationaler Tierärztlicher Kongress, Zürich-Interlaken, 1938 (Bd. 1. S. 287). Bern, 1938

54. Carnot, P., et Deflandre, C.: Sur l'activité hemopoiétique du sérum au cours de la régéneration. Compt. Rend. Acad. Sci. 1906, **143**. 383

55. Carpenter, G., Kahler, J., and Reilly, E.: Elevated titers of serum heterophil antibodies in three instances of monocytic leukemia. Amer. J. Med. Sci. 1950, **220**. 195

56. Carré H., et Vallée, H.: Sur l'anémie infectieuse du cheval. Compt. Rend. Acad. Sci. 1904, **139**. 1239

57. Carré, H., et Vallée, H.: Sur l'anémie infectieuse du cheval. Compt. Rend. Acad. Sci. 1905, **141**. 396

58. Carré, H., et Vallée, H.: Recherches cliniques et expérimentales sur l'anémie pernicieuse du cheval (Typho-anémie infectieuse). Rev. Gén. Méd. Vét. 1906, **8**. 593; 1907, **9**. 113

59. Carré, H., et Vallée, H.: Sur l'étiologie de l'anémie infectieuse du cheval. Rec. Méd. Vét. 1916, **92**. 193

60. Carré, H., et Vallée, H.: Sur l'étiologie de l'anémie infectieuse du cheval. Ann. Inst. Pasteur 1916, **30**. 383

61. Carré, H., et Verge, J.: Les anémies infectieuses des animaux domestiques. Bull. Off. Intl. Epizoot. 1935, **10**. 87, Discussion, p. 422

62. Cassamagnaghi, A., and Cassamagnaghi, A.: La anemia infecciosa. Su reconocimiento en los equinos del Uruguay. Rev. Med. Vet. Montevideo 1948, **4**. 772

63. Cavelti, P. A.: Studies on the pathogenesis of glomerulonephritis. I, II, and III. Arch. Path. 1945, **39**. 148; 1945, **40**. 158; 1945, **40**. 163

64. Cavelti, P. A.: Autoantibodies in rheumatic fever. Proc. Soc. Exp. Biol. Med. 1945, **60**. 379

65. Cavelti, P. A.: Studies on the pathogenesis of rheumatic fever. I. Experimental production of autoantibodies to heart, skeletal muscle and connective tissue. Arch. Path. 1947, **44**. 1

66. Cavelti, P. A.: Studies on the pathogenesis of rheumatic fever. II. Cardiac lesions produced in rats by means of autoantibodies to heart and connective tissue. Arch. Path. 1947, **44**. 13

67. Cavelti, P. A.: Pathogenesis of glomerulonephritis and rheumatic fever. In vivo activation of tissue antigens as a result of streptococcic infection and consequent formation of autoantibodies. Arch. Path. 1947, **44**. 119

68. Charlier: Notice sur la maladie épizootique, qui sévit actuellement sur les chevaux du départment de la Marne. Rec. Méd. Vét. 1843, **20**. 153, 236

69. Chase, M. W.: The allergic state. In Dubos: Bacterial and Mycotic Infections of Man. 2nd edition (p. 168). Philadelphia, London, Montreal, 1952

70. Clawson, B. J.: Relation of the "Anitschkow myocyte" to rheumatic inflammation. Arch. Path. 1941, **32**. 760

71. Coburn, A. F.: The plasma proteins in disseminated lupus erythematosus. Bull. Johns Hopkins Hosp. 1943, **73**. 196

72. Cominotti, L.: L'anemia infettiva del cavallo. Clinica Vet. 1913, **36**. 983

73. Craige, A. H., and Gadd, J. D.: The determination and clinical correlation of variations in the calcium, inorganic phosphorus, and serum proteins of horse blood. Amer. J. Vet. Res. 1941, **2**. 227

74. Davidsohn, I.: Heterophile antibodies in serum sickness. J. Immunol. 1929, **16**. 259

75. Davies, G. O.: Gaiger and Davies' Veterinary Pathology and Bacteriology, 3rd ed. (p. 515). London, 1947

76. Davis, G. E.: Complement fixation in yellow fever, in monkey and in man. Amer. J. Hyg. 1931, **13**. 79

77. Degen, W.: Die infektiöse Pferde-Anämie in Kanton Baselland und deren Bekämpfung durch tierseuchenpolizeiliche Massnahmen. Diss. Zürich, 1945

78. Dénoc: De la fièvre typhoide chez le cheval, maladie qui a régné épizootiquement dans quelques contrées du département de la Marne, dans les mois de Novembre et Décembre 1842, et dans le mois de Janvier 1843. Rec. Méd. Vét. 1843, **20**. 328

79. Denzer, B. S.: The coexistence of antibody and antigen in the body. J. Infect. Dis. 1916, **18**. 631

80. Derrick, J. D.: Mercuric chloride test for infectious anemia. Vet. Bull. U. S. Army 1936, **30**. 197

81. Deutsch, H. F., and Goodloe, M. B.: An electrophoretic survey of various animal plasmas. J. Biol. Chem. 1945, **161**. 1

82. Deutsch, H. F., and Nichol, J. C.: Biophysical studies of blood plasma proteins. X. Fractionation studies of normal and immune horse serum. J. Biol. Chem. 1948, **176**. 797

83. Dietrich, W.: Untersuchungen über die Wirkung des Atoxyls bei Pferd und Hund. Deut. Tier. Woch. 1910, **18**. 81

84. Dobberstein, J.: Kritische Betrachtungen zur Pathogenese der ansteckenden Blutarmut des Pferdes. Berl. Tier. Woch. 1934, **50**. 192

85. Dobberstein, J.: L'extension de l'anémie infectieuse des points de vue géographique et géologique. Bull. Off. Int. Epizoot. 1939, **18.** 149

86. Dobberstein, J., und Hemmert-Halswick, G.: Die Verbreitung der infektiösen Anämie nach geographischen und geologischen Gesichtspunkten. Z. Infekt. Haustiere 1940, **57.** 55

87. Dobberstein, J., und Piening, C.: Ueber eine übertragbare Anämie des Rindes und ihre Beziehungen zur Rinderleukose. Berl. Tier. Woch. 1934, **50.** 449

88. Dobberstein, J., und Wilmes, H.: Die Herzveränderungen bei der infektiösen Anämie des Pferdes. Berl. Tier. Woch. 1934, **50.** 161

89. Domansky, F.: A contribution to the hematological diagnosis of infectious anemia and its therapy. (*In Czech*) Cas. Ceskoslov. Vet. 1948, **3.** 493 (abstr.: V.B. **19.** 338)

90. Donatien, A., et Lestoquard, F.: Etiologie des anémies du mouton et de la chèvre. Rev. Vét. Toulouse 1926, **78.** 597, 675

91. Dreguss, M.: Eine einfache titrimetrische und gravimetrische Methode zur Bestimmung von Natrium in biologischem Material. Biochem. Z. 1939, **303.** 69

92. Dreguss, M.: Kisérleti kanyaró. (Experimental measles.) *In Hungarian.* Orvostud. Közlem. 1942, **3.** 741

93. Dreguss, M.: Versuche zum direkten Nachweis des Influenzavirus durch Impfung von Hamstern und Mäusen. Arch. Virusforsch. 1942, **2.** 306

94. Dreguss, M.: Hemagglutination of chicken cells by serum of horses infected with the virus of infectious anemia. (Preliminary report) Vet. Ext. Quart., Univ. Pennsylvania 1949, No. **116,** p. 3

95. Dreguss, M. N.: Mechanism of infection in equine infectious anemia. (To be published)

96. Dreguss, M. N.: Transmission of equine infectious anemia virus to mice. (In preparation)

97. Dreguss, M. N.: Unpublished experimental observations.

98. Dreguss, M., and Farkas, E.: Complement-fixation test for serological studies in typhus fever. Arch. ges. Virusforsch. 1948, **4.** 47

99. Dreguss, M. N., and Lombard, L. S.: Cardiac lesions in experimental horses infected with infectious anemia virus. (To be published)

100. Dreguss, M. N., and Shirer, J. F.: Hematological response of mice to injection of the virus of equine infectious anemia. (In preparation)

101. Duvaux, L. H.: La typho-anémie infectieuse du cheval dans la région de Neufchâteau. Essai de protéin-otherapie. Thése Paris, 1926 (abstr.: Jber. **46.** 1064)

102. Eaton, M. D., Murphy, W. D., and Hanford, V. L.: Heterogenetic antibodies in acute hepatitis. J. Exp. Med. 1944, **79.** 539

103. Edsall, J. T.: The plasma proteins and their fractionation. Advances in Protein Chemistry 1947, **3.** 383

104. Ehrich, W. E., and Harris, T. N.: The site of antibody formation. Science 1945, **101.** 28

105. Eilmann, H.: Zur pathologischen Anatomie und Histologie der ansteckenden Blutarmut und deren Rolle bei der Mischinfektion mit Tuberkulose und Druse der Pferde. Deut. Tier. Woch. 1934, **42.** 505

106. Ekvall, R.: Pernicious anemia of horses in Norrland. (*In Swedish*) Tidskr. Vet.-Med. 1895, **14.** 208 (abstr.: Jber. **15.** 79)

107. Epstein, B.: Anatomia patológica de la anemia infecciosa de los equinos. Rev. Med. Vet. Montevideo 1948, **4.** 808

108. Epstein, E.: Beitrag zur Theorie und Morphologie der Immunität. Histiocytenaktivierung in Leber, Milz und Lymphknoten des Immuntieres (Kaninchen). Virchow's Arch. Path. Anat. 1929, **273.** 89

109. Evans, A. S., and Curnen, E.: Serological studies on infectious mononucleosis and other conditions with human erythrocytes modified by Newcastle disease virus. J. Immunol. 1948, **58.** 323

110. Fedorov, A.: Histopathology of equine infectious anemia. (*In Russian*) Veterinariya 1947, **24.** (No. 6) 8 (abstr.: J.A.V.M.A. **113.** 80)

111. Finzi, G.: Contribution à l'étude anatomo-pathologique et expérimentale de l'anémie pernicieuse (typho-anémie infectieuse) du cheval. Rev. Gén. Méd. Vét. 1911, **18.** 681

112. Florman, A. L.: The agglutination of human erythrocytes modified by treatment with Newcastle disease and influenza virus. J. Bact. 1949, **57.** 31

113. Flückiger, G.: Internationale Bestrebungen zur Erforschung und Bekämpfung der infektiösen Pferdeanämie. Schweiz. Arch. Tierh. 1951, **93.** 768

114. Fortner, J.: Die Grundlagen der unspezifischen Eiweisstherapie. Münch. Tier. Woch. 1922, **73.** 271, 289, 318

115. Fortner, J.: Das klinische und pathologisch-anatomische Bild der ansteckenden Blutarmut der Einhufer. Münch. Tier. Woch. 1938, **89.** 141

116. Fortner, J.: Die ansteckende Blutarmut der Einhufer. Berl. Tier. Woch. **1938.** 1

117. Fortner, J.: Der Stand der Erkenntnisse über die ansteckende Blutarmut der Einhufer. Deut. Tier. Woch. 1939, **47.** 49; Berl.-Münch. Tier. Woch. **1938.** 751

118. Fortner, J.: Diskussionsbemerkungen zum Thema "Ansteckende Blutarmut der Einhufer". Berl.-Münch. Tier. Woch. **1943.** 410

119. Fortner, J.: Ueber das Dauervirusträgertum bei ansteckender Blutarmut der Einhufer. Deut. Tier. Woch. 1944, **52.** 265

120. Fortner, J.: Die ansteckende Blutarmut der Einhufer in den Impfstoffwerken. Berl.-Münch. Tier. Woch. **1948.** 49

121. Fortner, J.: Zur Differentialdiagnose der ansteckenden Blutarmut bei Serumpferden. Berl.-Münch. Tier. Woch. **1950.** 115

122. Fortner, J., und Wittfogel, H.: Ueber den Wert der Blutuntersuchung für die Erkennung der ansteckenden Blutarmut der Einhufer. Z. Infekt. Haustiere 1942, **58.** 61

123. Francis, M., and Marsteller, R. P.: Infectious anemia of the horse. Bull. No. 119, Texas Agric. Exper. Station. Austin, Texas, 1908

124. Francis, M., and Marsteller, R. P.: Some recent experiments on infectious anemia of the horse. Amer. Vet. Rev. 1911, **39.** 132

125. Franklin, M., Bean, W., Paul, W., Routh, J., de la Huerga, J., and Popper, H.: Electrophoretic studies in liver diseases. I-II. J. Clin. Invest. 1951, **30.** 718, 729

126. Fröhner, E.: Ueber perniciöse Anämie beim Pferde. Arch. Tierheilk. 1886, **12.** 383

127. Fröhner, E.: Klinische Untersuchungen über die infektiöse Anämie der Pferde. Monat. Tierheilk. 1919, **29.** 385

128. Fröhner, E., und Bierbaum, K.: Ueber die Resistenz des Virus der ansteckenden Anämie der Pferde gegen Karbolsäure. Berl. Tier. Woch. 1923, **39.** 243

129. Fulton, J. S.: A preliminary report on a test for swamp fever. J. Amer. Vet. Med. Ass. 1930, **77.** 58

130. Gardner, H. T., and Paul, J. R.: Infectious mononucleosis at the New Haven Hospital, 1921-1946. Yale J. Biol. Med. 1947, **19.** 839

131. Gardner, M. V.: The blood picture of normal laboratory animals. A review of the literature, 1936-1946. Journ. Franklin Inst. 1947, **243.** p. 172 (mouse), p. 251 (rabbit), p. 434 (hamster)

132. Gerlach, F.: Infektiöse Anämie bei Serumpferden. Wien. Tier. Monat. 1921, **8.** 159

133. Ghier, L.: Anémie infectieuse et tuberculose du cheval. L'anémie infectieuse peut-elle constituer le milieu favorable au développement de la tuberculose chez le cheval. Thése, Paris, 1933 (abstr.: Jber. **54.** 273)

134. Gilman, A. R.: The hematological response of the horse to the virus of equine infectious anemia. Vet. Ext. Quart., Univ. Pennsylvania 1951, No. **121,** p. 44

135. Gilman, A. R.: The blood sedimentation rate in the horse. Amer. J. Vet. Res. 1952, **13**. 77

136. Gilman, A. R.: Plasma protein changes in equine infectious anemia. Amer. J. Vet. Res. 1952, **13**. 83

137. Gilman, A. R.: A modified cephalin-cholesterol flocculation test for horse serums. Amer. J. Vet. Res. 1952, **13**. 191

138. Gindin, A. P.: Histopathology of the spleen and its role in the pathology of equine infectious anemia. (*In Russian*) Trud. Vsesoyuz. Inst. Eksp. Vet. 1940, **15**. 14 (abstr.: V.B. **16**. 144)

139. Gindin, A. P.: Pathogenesis of equine infectious anemia. (*In Russian*) Rabot. XIII. Plen. Vet. Sekt. Akad. Sel'khoz. Nauk, 1939 (p. 143). Moscow, 1940 (abstr.: V.B. **16**. 188)

140. Glättli, H.: Wird die perniziöse Anämie des Pferdes durch Blutegel übertragen? Schweiz. Arch. Tierh. 1937, **79**. 165

141. Gochenour, W. S., Stein, C. D., and Osteen, O. L.: Sulfanilamide in the treatment of infectious anemia. Vet. Med. 1939, **34**. 424

142. Guillot, G., et Guilhon, J.: La cholestérinémie dans l'anémie infectieuse expérimentale du cheval. Compt. Rend. Soc. Biol. 1934, **117**. 320

143. Gulland, G. L., and Goodall, A.: Pernicious anemia. A histological study of seventeen cases. J. Path. Bact. 1905, **10**. 125

144. Gutman, A. B.: The plasma proteins in disease. Advances in Protein Chemistry 1948, **4**. 155

145. Habersang: Experimentelle Uebertragung der infektiösen Anämie der Pferde auf das Schwein. Monat. Tierheilk. 1920, **30**. 171

146. Habersang: Chronischer Gelenkrheumatismus beim Pferd Monat. Tierheilk. 1920, **30**. 177

147. Hagan, W. A., and Bruner, D. W.: The Infectious Diseases of Domestic Animals. 2nd ed. (p. 830). Ithaca, New York, 1951

148. Hällfors, A.: Infectious anemia in Finland. (*In Swedish*) Finsk VetTidskr. 1931, **37**. 267; 1933, **39**. 84

149. Hamerski, E.: Equine infectious anemia. (*In Polish*) Rozprawy Biol. 1935, **13**. 202 (abstr.: B.T.W. **1938**. 706)

150. Hammersland, H. L., Herrin, H. S., and Haynes, C. F.: A study of the blood in horses infected with infectious anemia. J. Amer. Vet. Med. Ass. 1938, **93**. 320

151. Hanger, F. M.: The flocculation of cephalin-cholesterol emulsions by pathological sera. Trans. Ass. Amer. Physicians 1938, **53**. 148

152. Hansen, H. E.: An experimental case of swamp fever. Vet. Med. 1931, **26**. 89

153. Hansen, M., Todd, A., Kelley, G., and Hull, F.: Studies on the hematology of the thoroughbred horse. I. Mares in foal. Amer. J. Vet. Res. 1950, **11**. 296

154. Hartley, G., and Lushbaugh, C. C.: Experimental allergic focal necrosis of the liver. Amer. J. Path. 1942, **18**. 323

155. Heath, L. M.: Research on swamp fever or infectious equine anemia. Report Vet. Dir. General for 1931, Appendix 4. Pathol. Div. Dept. Agricult. Canada. Ottawa, 1931.

156. Hecke, F.: Der diagnostische Wert der Sublimatprobe bei der ansteckenden Blutarmut der Pferde. (Zur Erwiderung von Oppermann auf meine diesbezügliche Arbeit.) Arch. Tierheilk. 1934, **68**. 151

157. Hecke, F.: Verbreitungsweise und Bekämpfung der ansteckenden Blutarmut der Pferde. (Eine kritische Uebersicht über den gegenwärtigen Stand der Forschung.) Deut. Tier. Woch. 1934, **42**. 403

158. Heizmann: Vier Fälle von paralytischer Lumbago als Begleitsymptom von infektiöser Anämie der Pferde. Berl. Tier. Woch. 1918, **34**. 274

159. Heller, Jacobson, and Kolodny: A modification of the hemagglutination test for rheumatoid arthritis. Proc. Soc. Exp. Biol. Med. 1949, **72**. 316

160. Hempel, J.: Beitrag zur Kenntnis der ansteckenden Anämie der Pferde. Z. Infekt. Haustiere 1909, **5**. 381

161. Hillebrand, E.: Pyrifer, sein Einfluss auf das Blutbild gesunder Pferde und seine diagnostische Verwendbarkeit bei der ansteckenden Blutarmut des Pferdes. Diss. Berlin, 1937 (abstr.: V.B. 8. 662)

162. Hillmer, F.: Die Verwendbarkeit der Sublimatprobe in den Pferdebeständen der Heeresverwaltung zur Ermittlung von Pferden mit ansteckender Blutarmut. Z. Vet.kunde 1935, **47**. 65

163. Hink, J. H., and Johnson, F. F.: The occurrence in human plasma fractions of the antibodies to *H. pertussis*. J. Immunol. 1950, **64**. 39

164. Hirst, G.: The agglutination of red cells by allantoic fluid of chick embryos infected with influenza virus. Science 1941, **94**. 22

165. Hirst, G.: The quantitative determination of influenza virus and antibodies by means of red cell agglutination. J. Exp. Med. 1942, **75**. 49

166. Hirst, G.: Adsorption of influenza hemagglutinins and virus by red blood cells. J. Exp. Med. 1942, **76**. 195

167. Hirst, G.: Adsorption of influenza virus on cells of the respiratory tract. J. Exp. Med. 1943, **78**. 99

168. Hjärre: Die Leberveränderungen bei der infektiösen Anämie des Pferdes. Münch. Tier. Woch. 1936, **87**. 26

169. Hjärre, A., und Berthelsen, H.: Untersuchungen über das weisse Blutbild bei infektiöser Anämie des Pferdes. Dreizehnter Internationaler Tierärztlicher Kongress, Zürich-Interlaken 1938 (Bd. 1. 259). Bern, 1938

170. Hofferber, O.: Verbreitung und Feststellung der ansteckenden Blutarmut der Einhufer unter besonderer Berücksichtigung des Blutbildes. Veröff. Jber. Beamt. Tierärz. Preuss. 1933-1934, II Teil, S. 357

171. Holz, K.: Beiträge zur sogenannten Bornaschen Krankheit (Kopfkrankheit) und der ansteckenden Blutarmut des Pferdes. Z. Infekt. Haustiere 1938, **53**. 161

172. Horne, H.: Infectious anemia in the horse. (*In Norwegian*) Norsk VetTidsskr. 1924, **36**. 257 (abstr.: J.A.V.M.A. **68**. 237)

173. Horstman, D. M., and Tatlock, H.: Cold agglutinins. A diagnostic aid in certain types of primary atypical pneumonia. J. Amer. Med. Ass. 1943, **122**. 369

174. Hoskins, H. P.: Remarks on infectious anemia. J. Amer. Vet. Med. Ass. 1920, **56**. 650

175. Howard, C. W.: Insect transmission of infectious anemia of horses. J. Parasit. 1917, **4**. 70

176. Howe, C.: The influenza virus receptor and blood group antigens of human erythrocyte stroma. J. Immunol. 1951, **66**. 9

177. Hudson, N. P.: Dried infectious monkey serum as antigen in yellow fever complement fixation. Amer. J. Hyg. 1932, **15**. 557

178. Hughes, T. P.: A precipitin reaction in yellow fever. J. Immunol. 1933, **25**. 275

179. Huguenin, B.: Ueber schwere Anämien der Pferde. Schweiz. Arch. Tierh. 1918, **60**. 293

180. Hutyra, F., und Marek, J.: Spezielle Pathologie und Therapie der Haustiere. 3 Auflage (Bd. 1. S. 849). Jena, 1910

181. Hutyra, F., Marek, J., and Manninger, R.: Special Pathology and Therapeutics of the Diseases of Domestic Animals. 5th ed. (Vol. 3. p. 74). Chicago, 1946

182. Ishii, S.: Diagnostic de l'anémie infectieuse du cheval au Japon. Bull. Off. Intl. Epizoot. 1951, **36**. 282

183. Ishii, S., and Nakamura, N.: On the relationship of the so-called "Histiozytäre Zellen" to the anemia from the hematological observation of the infectious anemia of horses. (*In Japanese*) J. Jap. Soc. Vet. Sci. 1935, **14**. 340 (abstr.: V.B. **6**. 331)

184. Ishii, S., Tanaka, K., Kobayashi, K., Akiyama, Y., and Sato, S.: Anemic substance found in serum of horse with equine infectious anemia. III. Findings in a rabbit injected with serum from a diseased horse. (*In Japanese*) Report, Government Exper. Station for Animal Hygiene, No. 21, p. 11. Tokyo, Japan 1949 (abstr.: V.B. **22**. 523)

185. Ishii, S., und Watanabe, S.: Ueber fiebererzeugender Versuch bei der nichtfiebernden Periode des anämischen Pferdes. (*In Japanese*) Mitt. Regierungsinst. Tierseuch, Japan 1935, **15.** 147 (abstr.: Jber. **59.** 564)

186. Jacobs, M. H.: The red blood cell as a chemical reagent. Science 1951, **113.** 473

187. Jaede und Groth: Der Kaninchenversuch bei der infektiösen Anämie der Pferde. Deut. Tier. Woch. 1924, **32.** 342

188. Jaffé, R. H.: Beiträge zur pathologischen Histologie der ansteckenden Blutarmut der Pferde. Virchow's Arch. Path. Anat. 1921, **233.** 334

189. Jaffé, R. H., und Silberstein, F.: Die Uebertragbarkeit der ansteckenden Blutarmut der Pferde auf kleine Laboratoriumstiere. Z. ges. Exp. Med. 1922, **26.** 104

190. (Japan): Equine Infectious Anemia. (*In Japanese*) Edited by the Ministry of Agriculture and Forestry, Livestock Bureau. Vols. 1 and 2 (436 pages, numerous references). Tokyo, 1949

191. Japanese Commission: Report on the Results Obtained by the Special Committee for the Investigation of Infectious Anemia among Horses. Horse Administration Bureau, Tokyo, 1914

192. Jenkins, D. L., and Shope, R. E.: Rinderpest. VII. The attenuation of rinderpest virus for cattle by cultivation in embryonating eggs. Amer. J. Vet. Res. 1946, **7.** 174

193. Kämper: Auszug aus den Berichten über die Pferdeseuchenstation Berlin. Z. Vet.kunde 1923, **35.** 111

194. Keller, F.: Experimentelle und klinische Untersuchungen über Pferde-Anaemien. Diss. Zürich, 1937 (abstr.: Jber. **62.** 502)

195. Kelser, R. A.: Equine infectious anemia. J. Amer. Vet. Med. Ass. 1922, **62.** 319

196. Kelser, R. A.: Mosquitoes as vectors of the virus of equine encephalomyelitis. J. Amer. Vet. Med. Ass. 1933, **82.** 767

197. Kelser, R. A.: Equine infectious anemia in New England. Vet. Bull. U. S. Army 1936, **30.** 193

198. Kelser, R. A.: Equine encephalomyelitis and its control. Proc. Ann. Meeting U. S. Livestock Sanit. Assoc. 1941 (p. 22), Chicago, 1942

199. Kelser, R. A.: Adaptation of filtrable viruses to different host species and different tissues. Military Surg. 1947, **100.** 289

200. Kelser, R. A.: Equine encephalomyelitis. Ann. New York Acad. Sci. 1947, **48.** 385

201. Kelser, R. A., and Schoening, H. W.: Manual of Veterinary Bacteriology. 5th ed. (p. 589). Baltimore, 1948

202. Kern, W.: Die Entwicklung der veterinärpolizeilichen Anordnungen des Staates Preussen zur Bekämpfung der ansteckenden Blutarmut der Einhufer. Z. Vet.kunde 1940, **52.** 49

203. Kibrick, A. C., and Blonstein, M.: Fractionation of serum into albumin and α-, β-, and γ-globulin by sodium sulfate. J. Biol. Chem. 1948, **176.** 983

204. Kibrick, A. C., and Clements, A. B.: Comparative study of serum albumin-globulin ratio, cephalin-cholesterol flocculation, and thymol turbidity tests for liver function. J. Lab. Clin. Med. 1948, **33.** 662

205. Kinsley, A. T.: Equine infectious anemia. Amer. Vet. Rev. 1909, **36.** 45

206. Klempin: Die Gastruslarven-Anämie und ihre Beziehungen zur perniziösen Anämie der Pferde. Z. Vet.kunde 1918, **30.** 59

207. Knisely, M., Bloch, E., Eliot, T., and Warner, L.: Sludged blood. Science 1947, **106.** 431

208. Köbe, K.: Die Uebertragung der infektiösen Anämie des Pferdes auf das entmilzte Ferkel. Arch. Tierheilk. 1938, **73.** 399

209. de Kock, G.: Notes on the intoxication by Gastrophilus larvae. 5th and 6th Report, Director Vet. Research, Dept. Agric. South Africa (p. 651). Pretoria, 1919

210. de Kock, G.: Further observations on the disease equine pernicious anemia. 7th and 8th Report, Director Vet. Research, Dept. Agric. South Africa (p. 587). Pretoria, 1920

211. de Kock, G.: A contribution to the study of the virus, hematology, and pathology of infectious anemia of equines under South African conditions. 9th and 10th Report, Director Vet. Research, Dept. Agric. South Africa (p. 253). Pretoria, 1924

212. de Kock, G.: Beiträge zur Kenntnis der infektiösen Anämie der Pferde, wie sie in Südafrika beobachtet wird. Z. Infekt. Haustiere 1924, **27.** 30

213. Köpcke: Fieberhafte seuchenartig auftretende Anämie der Pferde. Z. Vet.kunde 1901, **13.** 356

214. Koprowski, H., Richmond, G., and Moore, D.: Electrophoretic study of antiviral sera. J. Exp. Med. 1947, **85.** 515

215. Korotkikh, A. V.: Diagnosis of equine infectious anemia by an allergic reaction. (*In Russian*) Veterinariya 1950, **27.** (No. 12) 16 (abstr.: V.B. **22.** 630)

216. Kracke, R. R.: Diseases of the Blood and Atlas of Hematology. 2nd edition. Philadelphia, London, Montreal, 1941

217. Král, F.: Virus anemia. (*In Czech*) Zverolek. Obzor. 1932, **25.** 81 (abstr.: V.B. **2.** 551)

218. Král, F.: Variability and ultrafiltrability of the virus of equine infectious anemia. (*In Czech*) Zverolek. Rozpr. 1933, **7.** 208 (abstr.: V.B. **4.** 511)

219. Král, F.: La variabilité et ultrafiltrabilité du virus de l'anémie infectieuse du cheval. Rec. Méd. Vét. 1933, **109.** 912

220. Král, F.: L'anémie infectieuse des chevaux. Douxième Congrès International de Médecine Vétérinaire. New York, 1934 (tome **2.** p. 293, Discussion p. 317). Washington, 1935

221. Král, F.: Equine infectious anemia. Vet. Ext. Quart., Univ. Pennsylvania 1949, No. **116**, p. 14

222. Král, F., Macek, K., and Sobra, K.: Anaemia infectiosa equorum. (*In Czech with French, English, and German summary*) Klin. Spisy Vysoké Skoly Zverol. (Brno) 1934, **11.** 25 (abstr.: V.B. **8.** 507)

223. Krauss, S.: Equine infectious anemia in Poland. (*In Polish*) Polskie Arch. Wet. 1951, **1.** 257 (abstr.: V.B. **23.** 79)

224. Krupski, A.: Kritische Bemerkungen zur Frage der Pferdeanämien. Schweiz. Arch. Tierh. 1930, **72.** 468; 1931, **73.** 435

225. Krupski, A.: Zur Behandlung der Anämien des Pferdes mit Leberbrei. Schweiz. Arch. Tierh. 1931, **73.** 122

226. Krupski, A., Grumbach, L., und Leemann, W.: Klinische und bakteriologische Befunde bei der infektiösen Bronchitis und Bronchopneumonie des Pferdes. Beobachtungen über gehäuftes Auftreten einer sekundären Anämie. Bull. Schweiz. Akad. Med. Wiss. 1946, **2.** 209

227. Kubes, V.: Campaña contra la derrengadera y peste boba del ganado caballar en los llanos de Venezuela. (Tres primeros informes sobre sus causas, presentados en los años 1937-38.) Instituto de Investigaciones Veterinarias, Caracas, Venezuela, 1944 (abstr.: V.B. **16.** 438)

228. Kuhn, K.: Die Sedimentierungsgeschwindigkeit der roten Blutkörperchen bei gesunden und kranken Pferden und ihre Bedeutung als Diagnostikum bei der infektiösen Anämie der Pferde. Monat. Tierheilk. 1922, **33.** 193; 1924, **34.** 135

229. Kunkel, H. G., and Hoagland, C. L.: Mechanism and significance of the thymol turbidity test for liver disease. J. Clin. Invest. 1947, **26.** 1060

230. Kutsche, E.: Ein weiterer Beitrag zur Frage der Verwendbarkeit des Schweines als Impftier bei der Feststellung der infektiösen Anämie der Pferde. Monat. Tierheilk. 1920, **30.** 557

231. Laktionov, A. M., Arkhangelskii, N. D., and Kovalevskii, M. F.: The part played by biting insects in the spread of equine infectious anemia. (*In Russian*) Sovvet Vet. 1939, **16.** (No. 2) 13 (abstr.: V.B. **10.** 671)

232. Lamanna, C.: Hemagglutination by botulinal toxin. Proc. Soc. Exp. Biol. Med. 1948, **69**. 332

233. Lamarre, H.: La typho-anémie infectieuse du cheval. Thése, Paris, 1925 (abstr.: Rev. Gén. Méd. Vét. **35**. 503)

234. Lamarre, L.: L'anémie infectieuse du cheval. (Recherches cliniques et expérimentales.) Bull. Acad. Vét. France 1934, **7**. 46

235. Lamarre, L.: Formule leucocytaire dans l'anémie infectieuse du cheval. Bull. Acad. Vét. France 1944, **17**. 79

236. Landsteiner, K., and van der Scheer, J.: On the specificity of agglutinins and precipitins. J. Exp. Med. 1924, **40**. 91

237. Larsson, E.: The symptoms of pernicious anemia. (*In Swedish*) Svensk VetTidskr. 1913, **18**. 391 (abstr.: D.T.W. **21**. 811)

238. Latta, H.: Experimental hypersensitivity in the rabbit. Blood and tissue concentrations of foreign proteins labelled with radioactive iodine and injected intravenously. J. Immunol. 1951, **66**. 635

239. Laurell, B.: Equine infectious anemia. (*In Swedish*) Svensk VetTidskr. 1938, **43**. 29

240. Lay, P.: Chemische und physiko-chemische Untersuchungen des Blutes und Serums normaler und an infektiöser Anämie erkrankter Pferde. Habil. Schrift Hannover, 1929

241. Ledru, E.: Lettre sur les propriétés contagieuses de l'anémie. Rec. Méd. Vét. 1861, **38**. 930

242. Leemann, W.: Die Cadmium-Reaktion nach Wunderly und Wuhrmann im Blutserum vom Pferd. Eine einfache Schnellmethode für die Praxis zur Prüfung der Kolloidstabilität des Serums. Diss. Zürich, 1946

243. Leemann, W.: A simple rapid test for estimation of the colloid content of horse serum with cadmium sulfate. Vet. Ext. Quart., Univ. Pennsylvania 1950, No. **117**, p. 32

244. Lehnert, E.: Serodiagnostic investigations in equine infectious anemia. (*In Swedish*) Skand. VetTidskr. 1924, **14**. 189, 225

245. Lehnert, E.: Practical experiment on the transmission and spread of infectious anemia in horses. (*In Swedish*) Skand. VetTidskr. 1925, **15**. 107

246. Lehnert, E.: Report on studies in infectious anemia of horses during 1923 to 1928. (*In Swedish*) Skand. VetTidskr. 1929, **19**. 205

247. Lehnert, E.: Zur Frage der Bedeutung im Blut normal vorkommender Autoisohamagglutinine für die Blutkörperzerstörung bei gewissen pathologischen Prozessen. Monat. Tierheilk. Neue Folge 1951, **3**. 1

248. Leinati, L.: Beiträge zur Histologie der Nierenveränderungen bei der infektiösen Anämie des Pferdes. Berl. Tier. Woch. 1929, **45**. 17

249. Lemétayer, E.: De la valeur de diverses réactions sérologiques dans le diagnostic de l'anémie infectieuse des équidés. Bull. Acad. Vét. France 1932, **5**. 231

250. Lemétayer, E.: Recherches d'hématologie dans l'anémie infectieuse expérimentale des équidés. Bull. Acad. Vét. France 1933, **6**. 97

251. Lemétayer, E.: La sédimentation sanguine ne peut pas être utilisée pour dépister l'anémie infectieuse chez les chevaux soumis à certaines immunisations. Bull. Acad. Vét. France 1938, **11**. 148

252. Lemétayer, E.: Les polynucléaires dans l'anémie infectieuse des équidés. Bull. Acad. Vét. France 1944, **17**. 218

253. Lemétayer, E.: Recherches sur l'anémie infectieuse expérimentale des équidés. Ann. Inst. Pasteur 1949, **77**. 657

254. Levaditi, C., Lépine, P., et Verge, J.: Les Ultravirus des Maladies Animales (p. 843). Paris, Montpellier, 1943

255. Lichtman, H., Ginsberg, V., and Watson, J.: Therapeutic effect of aureomycin in pernicious anemia. Proc. Soc. Exp. Biol. Med. 1950, **74**. 884

256. Lignée, M.: Mémoire et observations sur une maladie de sang, connue sous le nom d'anhémie hydrohémie, cachexie aqueuse du cheval. Rec. Méd. Vét. 1843, **20.** 30

257. Loginoff, W. P.: Zur Frage des diagnostischen Wertes des Blutaustrittes auf der Schleimhaut der Zunge bei der infektiösen Anämie. (*In Russian*) Sovyet Vet. 1936, **13.** (No. 11) 27 (abstr.: M.T.W. **88.** 176)

258. Lombard, L. S., and Dreguss, M. N.: Histopathological findings in equine infectious anemia (In preparation).

259. Longcope, W. T.: The production of experimental nephritis by repeated proteid intoxication. J. Exp. Med. 1913, **18.** 678

260. Longcope, W. T., and Rackemann, F. M.: The relation of circulating antibodies to serum disease. J. Exp. Med. 1918, **27.** 341

261. Lübke, A.: Zur Diagnose der infektiösen Anämie durch Untersuchung von Zitratblutproben. Deut. Tier. Woch. 1951, **58.** 83

262. Lucas, A.: Etude sur l'anémie infectieuse dans les Vosges. Rev. Path. Comp. 1946, **46.** 97

263. Lucas, A., Andral, L., Bouley, G., Paraf, A., et Quinchon, C.: Importance des facteurs sexuels dans l'anémie infectieuse du cheval. Bull. Acad. Vét. France 1950, **23.** 331

264. Lührs, E.: Die ansteckende Blutarmut der Pferde. Z. Vet.kunde 1919, **31.** 369, 450

265. Lührs: Ist das Wechselfieber der Pferde auf den Menschen übertragbar? Z. Vet.kunde 1920, **32.** 89

266. Lührs: Uebertragung des Wechselfiebers der Pferde auf Schwein. Berl. Tier. Woch. 1920, **36.** 121

267. Lührs: Beiträge zur Frage des Pferdewechselfiebers. (Infektiöse Anämie.) Z. Vet.kunde 1921, **33.** 66

268. Lührs: Das Verfahren "Noltze" als Diagnostikum bei der ansteckenden Blutarmut der Pferde. Veterinärdienst 1923, Sept. S. 9

269. Lührs: Zur Diagnose der ansteckenden Blutarmut des Pferdes mit Hilfe des Kaninchenübertragungsversuches nach Oppermann. Z. Vet.kunde 1925, **37.** 374

270. Mack, W. B.: A study of a serious anemic disease among horses. Amer. Vet. Rev. 1909, **36.** 222

271. Mack, W. B.: Equine anemia. An account of a recent inquiry into the nature and cause of an obscure and fatal disease among horses in eastern Nevada. Bull. No. 68, Agric. Exper. Station, Univ. Nevada. Reno, 1909

272. von Magnus, P.: Propagation of the PR8 strain of influenza A virus in chick embryos. II-IV. "Incomplete" virus. Acta Path. Microbiol. Scand. 1951, **28.** 278; 1951, **29.** 157; 1952, **30.** 311

273. Manninger, R.: Ansteckungsversuche mit dem Virus der ansteckenden Blutarmut der Pferde. Arch. Tierheilk. 1938, **73.** 425

274. Marek, J.: Infectious anemia in Hungary, 1907; quoted by Hutyra and Marek, 1910

275. Marek, J.: A lovak fertözö kevésvérüsége. (Infectious anemia of horses) *In Hungarian.* Állatorv. Lapok 1921, **44.** 109

276. Martin, L.: The recent trend towards a differentiation between allergy and immunity, and the relationship to clinical medicine. Ann. Intern. Med. 1934, **8.** 483

277. Martin, L. A.: Adsorption du virus de l'anémie infectieuse des équidés sur l'hydroxyde d'alumine. Compt. Rend. Acad. Sci. 1939, **208.** 677

278. Martin, L. A.: L'incubation et le premier accès thermique au cours de l'anémie infectieuse expérimentale des équidés. Ann. Inst. Pasteur 1939, **62.** 595

279. Martin, L. A.: L'anémie infectieuse des équidés. I. Recherches sur l'incubation et le premier accès thermique au cours de la maladie expérimentale. II. Données diverses sur le virus anémique. III. Recherches sur le traitement et la prévention de la maladie. IV. Adsorption du virus. Tentatives d'atténuation du virus adsorbé. Arch. Inst. Pasteur Maroc 1940, **2.** 259, 289, 295, 305

280. Martin, L. A.: L'anémie infectieuse des équidés. V. Passages accélérés du virus par un organisme sensible. Ann. Inst. Pasteur 1946, **72**. 489

281. Martini, I.: Le possibilita attuali per una difesa eficiente contro il dilagare della anemia infettiva degli equini. Clinica Vet. 1948, **71**. 102 (abstr.: Wien. Tier. Monat. **37**. 500)

282. Marxer, A.: Die Beziehungen der Gastrophilus-Larven zur infektiösen Anämie. Z. Immun. 1920, **29**. 1

283. Matthiesen und Glässer: Ueber bemerkenswerte Befund an Herz und Gefässen bei der chronischen ansteckenden Blutarmut des Pferdes. Deut. Tier. Woch. 1926, **34**. 95

284. Melnick, D., Burack, E., and Cowgill, G. R.: Development of incompatibilities in dogs by repeated infusions of red blood cells. Proc. Soc. Exp. Biol. Med. 1936, **33**. 616

285. Member, S., Bruger, M., and Chassin, M. R.: Serum cholesterol in horses during immunization with pneumococci. Including a note on the hypercholesterolemia of infectious anemia. J. Immunol. 1940, **38**. 355

286. Metzger: Beiträge zur Pathogenese und Therapie der infektiösen Anämie des Pferdes. Berl. Tier. Woch. 1924, **40**. 283

287. Meyer, K. F.: Equine encephalomyelitis. North Amer. Vet. 1933, **14**. (No. 6) 30

288. Middlebrook, G., and Dubos, R.: Specific serum agglutination of erythrocytes sensitized with extracts of tubercle bacilli. J. Exp. Med. 1948, **88**. 521

289. Miégeville, M.: Du rôle possible de la sangsue dans la pathogénie de l'anémie infectieuse. Rev. Path. Comp. 1926, **26**. 220

290. Mitchell, C. A., Humphreys, F. A., and Walker, R. V. L.: Equine infectious anemia. An outbreak in the Ottawa Valley. Canad. J. Comp. Med. 1944, **8**. 165, 196

291. Mitchell, C. A., and Walker, R. V. L.: Infectious anemia and encephalomyelitis vaccination. Canad. J. Comp. Med. 1943, **7**. 136

292. Miyagawa, Y., Taniguchi, T., Nagao, S., and Takemoto, S.: On the microorganism causing infectious anemia of the horse and its pure cultivation. (Translated from Japanese.) J. Amer. Vet. Med. Ass. 1920, **56**. 642

293. Mócsy, J.: Die Blutkörperchensenkung als diagnostisches Verfahren. Deut. Tier. Woch. 1923, **31**. 207, 224

294. Mócsy, J.: A fertözö kevésvérüség-okozta szöveti elváltozásokról. (Histological changes in infectious anemia.) *In Hungarian.* Állatorv. Lapok 1924, **47**. 1, 17, 35 (abstr.: Jber. **44**. 94)

295. Mócsy, J.: A fertözö kevésvérüség kórjelzéséről. (Diagnosis of infectious anemia.) *In Hungarian.* Állatorv. Lapok 1932, **55**. 157 (abstr.: Wien. Tier. Woch. **19**. 567)

296. Mócsy, J.: Die serologischen Untersuchungsmethoden bei der infektiösen Blutarmut der Pferde. Arch. Tierheilk. 1932, **65**. 451

297. Mócsy, J.: Zur Pathogenese der ansteckenden Blutarmut der Pferde. Arch. Tierheilk. 1932, **65**. 547

298. Mócsy, J.: Ansteckende Blutarmut der Pferde. Zwölfter Internationaler Tierärztlicher Kongress, New York, 1934 (Bd. **2**. S. 282, Diskussion S. 317.) Washington, 1935

299. Mócsy, J.: Immunizálási és gyógyitási kisérletek fertözö kevésvérüségben beteg lovakkal. (Experiments on immunization and cure of horses suffering from infectious anemia.) *In Hungarian.* Állatorv. Lapok 1935, **58**. 58 (abstr.: V.B. **6**. 38)

300. Mócsy, J.: Untersuchungen über die Natur des Anämievirus der Einhufer. Arch. Tierheilk. 1938, **73**. 25

301. Mohler, J. R.: Three diseases of animals which have recently assumed importance to the state sanitarian. Amer. Vet. Rev. 1908, **34**. 198

302. Mohler, J. R.: Swamp fever (infectious anemia) of horses. Ann. Reports, Bureau of Animal Industry, U. S. Dept. Agric. for 1907 (p. 33); for 1908 (p. 225); for 1909 (p. 46); and for 1910 (p. 79). Washington 1909, 1910, 1911, and 1912

303. Mohler, W. M.: Observations on complement-fixation with distilled water-spleen antigen in equine infectious anemia. J. Amer. Vet. Med. Ass. 1936, **88**. 624

304. Moolten, S. E., and Clark, E.: The red blood cell as a vehicle of virus transport. I. Isolation and identification of blood-borne viruses. Trans. New York Acad. Sci. (Series 2) 1952, **14**. 232

305. Moolten, S. E., and Clark, E.: The red blood cell as a vehicle of virus transport. II. Role of blood-borne viruses in autohemagglutination and in hemolytic anemia. Trans. New York Acad. Sci. (Series 2) 1952, **14**. 235

306. Moolten, S. E., and Clark, E.: Viremia in acute hemolytic anemia and in autohemagglutination. Arch. Intern. Med. 1952, **89**. 270

307. More, R. H., and Waugh, D.: Diffuse glomerulonephritis produced in rabbits by massive injections of bovine serum gamma globulin. J. Exp. Med. 1949, **89**. 541

308. More, R. H., Waugh, D., and Kobernick, S. D.: Cardiac lesions produced in rabbits by massive injections of bovine serum gamma globulin. J. Exp. Med. 1949, **89**. 555

309. Morris, J. A., and Alexander, A. D.: Attempts to adapt equine infectious anemia virus to small animals. Cornell Vet. 1950, **40**. 381

310. Moszczenski, Z., und Krupski, A.: Beitrag zur histopathologischen Diagnose der Virus-Anämie. Schweiz. Arch. Tierh. 1943, **85**. 365

311. Mott, L. O., Stein, C. D., and Heishman, J. O.: Penicillin treatment of acute equine infectious anemia. Vet. Med. 1946, **41**. 131

312. Mrowka, F.: Histologische Untersuchungen der Milz bei der infektiösen Anämie des Pferdes. Z. Vet.kunde 1920, **32**. 217

313. Mrowka, F.: Ueber Veränderungen an den roten Blutkörperchen gesunder Pferde nach künstlicher Infektion mit infektiöser Anämie. Arch. Tierheilk. 1935, **69**. 446

314. Mudd, S.: A hypothetical mechanism of antibody formation. J. Immunol. 1932, **23**. 423

315. Müllegger, K.: Das Blutbild nach Anwendung von "Pyrifer". Diss. Wien., 1935 (abstr.: B.T.W. **1937**. 399)

316. Nagao, M.: Ueber die Wiederstandfähigkeit des Virus der infektiösen Blutarmut des Pferdes und der Rekurrensspirochäten gegen die Kälte. (*In Japanese*) J. Jap. Soc. Vet. Sci. 1923, **2**. 127 (abstr.: Jber. **43**. 82)

317. Nagao, M.: Beiträge zur Kenntnis von der pathologischen Veränderungen der roten Blutkörperchen bei derinfektiösen Blutarmut der Pferde. (*In Japanese*) J. Jap. Soc. Vet. Sci. 1924, **3**. 99 (abstr.: Jber. **44**. 94)

318. Nagao, M.: Beitrag zur Pathogenese der Erythrozytenverminderung bei der infektiösen Anämie des Pferdes. (*In Japanese*) J. Jap. Soc. Vet. Sci. 1925, **4**. 151 (abstr.: Jber. **45**. 79)

319. Nakamura, N., Ishii, S., et Watanabe, S.: Etude sur le virus de l'anémie contagieuse du cheval. Observations expérimentales sur la répartition du virus dans plusiers organes au cours de formes évolutives non fébriles de la maladie. Bull. Off. Intl. Epiz. 1938, **16**. 149

320. Neefe, J. R., Stokes, J., Jr., Reinhold, J. G., and Lukens, F. D. W.: Hepatitis due to the injection of homologous blood products in human volunteers. J. Clin. Invest. 1944, **23**. 836

321. Niznansky, F.: Infectious anemia in horses in Czechoslovakia. (*In Czech*) Cas. Ceskoslov. Vet. 1949, **4**. 321 (abstr.: V.B. **20**. 21)

322. Nöller, W., und Dobberstein, J.: Zur Frage der histologischen Diagnose der ansteckenden Blutarmut der Pferde. Berl. Tier. Woch. 1925, **41**. 465

323. Noltze, O.: Die Sedimentierunggeschwindigkeit der roten Blutkörperchen bei der infektiösen Anämie der Pferde als Diagnostikum. Monat. Tierheilk. 1921, **32**. 481

324. (Office International des Epizooties, Paris): Résolutions adoptées dans la 9e session du Comité de l'Office international des Epizooties. I. Rage. II. Maladie d'Aujeszky. III. Peste porcine. IV. Anémies infectieuses. Bull. Off. Intl. Epizoot. 1935, **10**. 453

325. (Office International des Epizooties, Paris): Series of reports on equine infectious anemia by Alegren, Altara, Ishii, Schoening and Stein, Schoop, Steck, and Thiéry. (*In French*), see under the name of authors. Bull. Off. Intl. Epizoot. 1951, **36**. 225-327

326. Oppermann, T.: Infektiöse Anämie als Ursache von gehäuften Abortus bei Stuten und von Fohlensterben. Tierärzt. Rund. 1923, **29**. 578

327. Oppermann, T.: Die Diagnose der infektiösen Anämie des Pferdes. Deut. Tier. Woch. 1923, **31**. 183

328. Oppermann, T.: Die Bedeutung der Leberpunktion bei der infektiösen Anämie des Pferdes. Deut. Tier. Woch. 1929, **37**. 465

329. Oppermann, T.: Der diagnostische Wert der Sublimatprobe bei der ansteckenden Blutarmut der Pferde. (Eine Erwiderung auf den gleichnamigen Artikel von F. Hecke.) Arch. Tierheilk. 1934, **68**. 143

330. Oppermann, T.: Einiges über die ansteckende Blutarmut der Pferde. Deut. Tier. Woch. 1942, **50**. 53

331. Oppermann, Döpelhauer, und Moll: Zur Frage der Spontaninfektion des Huhnes mit dem Virus der ansteckenden Blutarmut des Pferdes. Deut. Tier. Woch. 1929, **37**. 401

332. Oppermann, und Herrfarth: Das Schwein als Versuchtier bei der infektiösen Anämie des Pferdes. Deut. Tier. Woch. 1923, **31**. 131

333. Oppermann, und Lauterbach: Die Diagnose der infektiösen Anämie des Pferdes mit Hilfe des Kaninchens. Berl. Tier. Woch. 1923, **39**. 487

334. Oppermann, und Lauterbach: Der weitere Ausbau der Diagnostik der infektiösen Anämie der Einhufer mit Hilfe der Serologie und des Kleintierversuches. Deut. Tier. Woch. 1928, **36**. 311, 507, 717

335. Oppermann, und Lauterbach: Weitere Beiträge zur Diagnose der infektiösen Anämie des Pferdes mit Hilfe des Hühnerversuchs. Deut. Tier. Woch. 1928, **36**. 735

336. Oppermann, und Ziegler: Infektiöse Anämie der Pferde. In Kolle, Kraus, u. Uhlenhut: Handbuch der Pathogenen Mikroorganismen. 3 Auf. (Bd. 9. S. 77). Jena, Berlin, Wien, 1929

337. Ostertag, R.: Zur Casuistik der perniciösen Anämie beim Pferde. Monat. Tierheilk. 1890, **1**. 127

338. Ostertag, R.: Untersuchungen über das Auftreten und die Bekämpfung der infektiösen Anämie des Pferdes. Z. Infekt. Haustiere 1907, **3**. 1

339. Otto, W.: Beiträge zur Diagnose der infektiösen Anämie der Pferde. Z. Vet.kunde 1921, **33**. 129, 161

340. Panisset, L.: Aperçu de nos connaissances sur le rôle des insectes piquers et suceurs dans la transmission de l'anémie infectieuse du cheval. Rev. Gén. Méd. Vét. 1922, **31**. 191

341. Panisset, L., Carpentier, G., Guillot, G., et Pflieger, C.: Contribution au diagnostic de l'anémie infectieuse du cheval. Bull. Acad. Vét. France 1934, **7**. 282

342. Panisset, L., et Pflieger, C.: Contribution au diagnostic de l'anémie infectieuse du cheval. II. Emploi de la tuberculine. Bull. Acad. Vét. France 1935, **8**. 88

343. Panisset, M.: The blood sedimentation test in the diagnosis of equine infectious anemia. Canad. J. Comp. Med. 1938, **2**. 3

344. Paul, J. R.: Infectious mononucleosis. Bull. New York Acad. Med. 1939, **15**. 43

345. Paul, J. R., and Bunnell, W. W.: The presence of heterophile antibodies in infectious mononucleosis. Amer. J. Med. Sci. 1932, **183**. 90

346. Pentimalli, F.: Ueber chronische Proteinvergiftung und die durch sie bewirkten Veränderungen der Organe. (Experimentelle Untersuchungen) Virchow's Arch. Path. Anat. 1929, **275**. 193

347. Peters, J. T.: Equine infectious anemia transmitted to man. Ann. Intern. Med. 1945, **23**. 271

348. Peterson, O. L., Ham, T. H., and Finland, M.: Cold agglutinins (autohemagglutinins) in primary atypical pneumonias. Science 1943, **97**. 167

349. Piening, C.: Die Veränderungen der Lymphknoten bei der ansteckenden Blutarmut des Pferdes. Berl. Tier. Woch. 1935, **51**. 355

350. Pigoury, L., Borde, R., et Bernard, M.: Intensité du syndrome anémie dans le surra expérimental du cheval. Comparison avec l'anémie infectieuse. Bull. Soc. Path. Exot. 1938, **31**. 622

351. Pinus, A. A., and Pirog, P. P.: Cultivation of the virus of infectious anemia of horses in fowl embryos. (*In Russian*) Sovyet Vet. 1937, **14**. (No. 8) 30

352. von Pirquet, C.: Allergie. Münch. Med. Woch. 1906, **53**. 1457

353. von Pirquet, C.: Klinische Studien über Vaccination und vaccinale Allergie. Leipzig und Wien, 1907

354. von Pirquet, C.: Das Verhalten der kutanen Tuberkulinreaktion während der Masern. Deut. Med. Woch. 1908, **34**. 1297

355. von Pirquet, C.: Das Bild der Masern auf der aüsseren Haut. Z. Kinderheilk. 1913, **6**. 1

356. von Pirquet, C., und Schick, B.: Die Serumkrankheit. Leipzig und Wien, 1905. Serum Sickness (Translated by B. Schick). Baltimore, 1951

357. Portier, et Richet: De l'action anaphylactique de certains venins. Compt. Rend. Soc. Biol. 1902, **54**. 170

358. Ramon, G., et Lemétayer, E.: Sur quelques lésions de l'appareil digestif chez des chevaux ayant succombé à l'anémie infectieuse. Bull. Acad. Vét. France 1931, **4**. 278

359. Ramon, G., et Lemétayer, E.: Pénétration du virus de l'anémie infectieuse des équidés au niveau des plaies et de la conjonctive. Compt. Rend. Soc. Biol. 1934, **116**. 915

360. Ramon, G., et Lemétayer, E.: Essais sur l'anémie infectieuse du cheval. Compt. Rend. Acad. Sci. 1934, **198**. 508

361. Randall, C. C., McVickar, D. L., and Doll, E. R.: A complement fixation test for equine virus abortion. Proc. Soc. Exp. Biol. Med. 1950, **75**. 465

362. Randolph, T. G., and Gibson, E. B.: Blood studies in allergy. II. The presence in allergic disease of atypical lymphocytes and symptoms suggesting the recovery phase of infectious mononucleosis. Amer. J. Med. Sci. 1944, **207**. 638

363. Reagan, R. L., Lillie, M. G., Hauser, J. E., Poelma, L. J., and Brueckner, A. L.: A preliminary report on the propagation of the virus of equine infectious anemia (swamp fever) in rabbits. Proc. Ann. Meeting, U. S. Livestock Sanit. Assoc. in Denver, 1948 (p. 37). Baltimore, 1949

364. Reagan, R. L., Lillie, M. G., Hickman, J. W., and Brueckner, A. L.: Studies of the virus of equine infectious anemia. Amer. J. Vet. Res. 1950, **11**. 157

365. Rice, C. E.: Some factors influencing the selection of a complement fixation method. II. Parallel use of the direct and indirect technics. J. Immunol. 1948, **60**. 11

366. Rich, A. R., and Gregory, J. E.: Experimental evidence that lesions with the basic characteristics of rheumatic carditis can result from anaphylactic hypersensitivity. Bull. Johns Hopkins Hosp. 1943, **73**. 239

367. Rich, A. R., and Gregory, J. E.: Further experimental cardiac lesions of the rheumatic type produced by anaphylactic hypersensitivity. Bull. Johns Hopkins Hosp. 1944, **75**. 115

368. Richters, E.: Die klinische Verwendbarkeit der Lipoidbindungsreaktion nach Meinicke. Z. Vet.kunde 1922, **34**. 112

369. Richters: Die Punktion der Leber bei der ansteckenden Blutarmut der Pferde und ihre diagnostische Bedeutung. Z. Vet.kunde 1929, **41**. 1

370. Richters, C. E.: Erfahrungen der Heeresverwaltung bei der ansteckenden Blutarmut der Pferde. Z. Vet.kunde 1934, **46**. 166

371. Richters, C. E.: Ansteckende Blutarmut der Einhufer. In Gildemeister, Haagen, und Waldmann: Handbuch der Viruskrankheiten. (Bd. 1. S. 618.) Jena 1939

372. Ries, J. N.: Sur la pathogénie et la traitement de l'anémie pernicieuse et infectieuse du cheval. Rec. Méd. Vét. 1906, **83**. 677

373. Röber, E.: Kaninchenpassageversuche mit dem Virus der ansteckenden Blutarmut des Pferdes. Diss. Leipzig, 1924 (abstr.: B.T.W. 40. 251)

374. Röhrer, H., Heinig, A., und Stöhr, P.: Die Anwendung des Kreutzinfektionsversuches in zwei grösseren Pferdebeständen zur Feststellung latenter Fälle von infektiöser Anämie der Pferde. Monat. Vet.-Med. 1950, **5.** 6

375. Röhrer, H., und Quabeck, L.: Untersuchungen über das Vorkommen histopathologischer Veränderungen der ansteckenden Blutarmut in der Leber von Schlachtpferden aus den anämiefreien Regiérungsbezirken Köln und Aachen. Z. Infekt. Haustiere 1939, **55.** 90

376. Röhrer, H., und Stöhr, P.: Der Kreuzinfektionsversuch zur Feststellung der ansteckenden Blutarmut als Quarantänemassnahme für Serumpferde. Monat. Vet.-Med. 1949, 4. 141

377. Rózsa, P.: A lovak fertözö kevésvérüségéröl. (Infectious anemia of horses.) *In Hungarian.* Állatorv. Lapok 1927, **50.** 53, 67, 80

378. Sanson: Rapport sur la communication de M. Anginiard, "Contagion par infection de l'anhémie idiopathique du cheval". Rec. Méd. Vét. 1861, **38.** 325

379. Schaaf, J., Hecke, F., und Bert, F.: Herzmuskelveränderungen bei der ansteckenden Blutarmut der Pferde. Z. Infekt. Haustiere 1935, 47. 178

380. Schalk, A. F., and Roderick, L. M.: The history of a "swamp fever" virus carrier. Bull. No. 168, Agric. Exper. Station, North Dakota Agric. College, 1923

381. Schermer, S.: Die physiologischen Schwankungen verschiedener chemischer und physikalischer Eigenschaften des Pferdeblutes, zugleich ein Beitrag zur Diagnostik der infektiösen Anämie. Deut. Tier. Woch. 1926, 34. 703

382. Schermer, S.: Die histologischen Veränderungen bei der infektiösen Anämie des Pferdes und ihr Vergleich mit denen bei experimentellen Anämien. Arch. Tierheilk. 1927, **55.** 121

383. Schermer, S.: Epikritisches zur infektiösen Anämie. Berl Tier. Woch. 1929, **45.** 509

384. Schermer, S.: Ueber den Wert der Blutuntersuchung bei der infektiösen Anämie. Berl. Tier. Woch. 1934, **50.** 165

385. Schermer, S.: Der Wert der Blutuntersuchung bei der ansteckenden Blutarmut der Pferde und die Grenzen ihrer Leistungsfähigkeit. Berl. Münch. Tier. Woch. **1939.** 389

386. Schermer, S., und Eigendorf, R.: Die diagnostische Bedeutung des Kaninchenimpfversuchs bei der infektiösen Anämie der Pferde. Arch. Tierheilk. 1926, **54.** 299

387. Schermer, S., Eigendorf, R., und Traupe, H.: Hämatologische Untersuchungen bei der infektiösen Anämie und ihre diagnostische Bedeutung. Arch. Tierheilk. 1928, **57.** 445

388. Schindler, R.: Ein Beitrag zur Frage der Bluttransfusion bei Pferden unter besonderer Berücksichtigung ihrer Wirkung auf das Blutbild des Empfängers und der antigen Eigenschaften der Spendererythrozyten. Monat. Vet.-Med. 1949, **4.** 106

389. Schneider, L., und Szathmáry, J.: Ueber die Immunität der neugeborenen Säugetiere. Z. Immun. 1939, **95.** 465

390. Schoening, H. W., et Stein, C. D.: L'anémie infectieuse du cheval aux Etats-Unis. Bull. Off. Intl. Epizoot. 1951, **36.** 260

391. Schoop, G.: Anémie infectieuse des équidés. Bull. Off. Intl. Epizoot. 1951, **36.** 304

392. Schünemann, H.: Ueber die Beeinflussung des Blutbildes des Kaninchens durch wiederholte Infektion mit Virus der ansteckenden Blutarmut des Pferdes. Deut. Tier. Woch. 1926, **34.** 474

393. Schwarzweiss, H., and Tomcsik, J.: Isolation of the heterogenetic "mononucleosis antigen" from the stroma of beef erythrocytes. Proc. Soc. Exp. Biol. Med. 1948, **69.** 558

394. Schwarzweiss, H., and Tomcsik, J.: Beef erythrocyte extracts reacting with hemagglutinins in infectious mononucleosis and in horse serum sickness. Proc. Soc. Exp. Biol. Med. 1949, **72.** 693

395. Scott, J. W.: The transmission of swamp fever. Ann. Report, Univ. Wyoming Agric. Exper. Station, 1913-1914 (p. 180). Laramie, 1914 (Anat. Record 1917, **11**. 540; 1918, **14**. 98)

396. Scott, J. W.: Swamp fever in Wyoming. Economic importance, general characteristics and control. Bull. No. 121, Wyoming Agric. Exper. Station, Univ. Wyoming (p. 91). Laramie, 1919

397. Scott, J. W.: Experimental transmission of swamp fever or infectious anemia by means of insects. J. Amer. Vet. Med. Ass. 1920, **56**. 448

398. Scott, J. W.: Insect transmission of swamp fever or infectious anemia of horses. Bull. No. 133, Wyoming Agric. Exper. Station, Univ. Wyoming (p. 57). Laramie, 1922

399. Scott, J. W.: The experimental transmission of swamp fever or infectious anemia by means of secretions. Bull. No. 138, Wyoming Agric. Exper. Station, Univ. Wyoming (p. 17). Laramie, 1924

400. Seibel: Beitrag zur Kenntnis der ansteckenden Blutarmut. Berl. Tier. Woch. 1933, **49**. 85

401. Semenov, M. A., and Kozlova, E. S.: Lice as vectors of equine infectious anemia. (*In Russian*) Trud. Vsesoyuz. Inst. Eksp. Vet. 1936, **12**. 38 (abstr.: V.B. 8. 26)

402. Sevag, M. G.: Immuno-Catalysis. 2nd ed. Springfield, Illinois, 1951

403. Seyderhelm, K. R., und Seyderhelm, R.: Experimentelle Untersuchungen über die Ursache der perniziösen Anämie der Pferde. Berl. Tier. Woch. 1914, **30**. 610

404. Seyderhelm, K. R., und Seyderhelm, R.: Die Ursache der perniziösen Anämie des Pferdes. Ein Beitrag zum Problem des ultravisiblen Virus. Arch. Exp. Path. Pharm. 1914, **76**. 149

405. Seyderhelm, R.: Ueber die perniciöse Anämie der Pferde. Beitrag zur vergleichenden Pathologie der Blutkrankheiten. Beitr. Path. Anat. 1914, **58**. 285

406. Seyderhelm, R.: Ueber echte Blutgifte in Parasiten der Pferde und des Menschen und ihre Beziehung zur perniziösen Anämie. Münch. Tier. Woch. 1917, **68**. 533, 553

407. Shaffer, J. M., Farquhar, J. D., Stokes, J., and Sborov, V. M.: Studies on the use of aureomycin in hepatic disease. I. Aureomycin therapy in acute viral hepatitis. Amer. J. Med. Sci. 1950, **220**. 1

408. van der Scheer, J., Wyckoff, R. W. G., and Clarke, F. H.: The electrophoretic analysis of several hyperimmune horse sera. J. Immunol. 1940, **39**. 65

409. Shirer, J. F.: The normal erythrocyte count in the white laboratory mouse. (In preparation)

410. Shope, R. E.: The swine lungworm as a reservoir and intermediate host for swine influenza virus. I-IV. The demonstration of masked swine influenza virus in lungworm larvae and swine under natural conditions. J. Exp. Med. 1941, **74**. 41, 49; 1943, **77**. 111, 127

411. Shope, R. E., Griffiths, H. J., and Jenkins, D. L.: Rinderpest. I. The cultivation of rinderpest virus in the developing hen's egg. Amer. J. Vet. Res. 1946, **7**. 135

—Shope, R. E., Maurer, F. D., Jenkins, D. L., Griffiths, H. J., and Baker, J. A.: Rinderpest. IV. Infection of the embryos and the fluids of developing hens' eggs. Amer. J. Vet. Res. 1946, **7**. 152

412. Slagsvold, L.: Serodiagnostic investigation of infectious anemia of the horse. (*In Norwegian*) Norsk VetTidskr. 1925, **37**, 65 (abstr.: J.A.V.M.A. **68**. 236)

413. Sokolowski: Ansteckende Blutarmut. Berl. Tier. Woch. 1932, **48**. 623

414. Stadler, T.: Investigations on equine infectious anemia in Sweden. (*In Swedish*) Skand. VetTidskr. 1917, **7**. 55, 77, 137, 159

415. Steck, W.: Studien über die infektiöse Anämie der Pferde. I. Statistik der Schadensfälle in Kanton Bern. Schweiz. Arch. Tierh. 1937, **79**. 368

416. Steck, W.: Die klinische Diagnose der Anaemia infectiosa equorum. Schweiz. Arch. Tierh. 1943, **85**. 431

417. Steck, W.: Studien über die infektiösen Anämie der Pferde. III. Auftreten von Zungenblutungen und Ausbreitung der Infektion. Schweiz. Arch. Tierh. 1946, **88**. 61

418. Steck, W.: Streptokokkenanämie und Valléesche Krankheit. Eine kritische Betrachtung. Schweiz. Arch. Tierh. 1948, **90**. 165

419. Steck, W.: Untersuchungen über die Ursachen des regionalen Auftretens der Valléeschen Krankheit (infektiösen Anämie) der Pferde. Schweiz. Arch. Tierh. 1951, **93**. 313

420. Steck, W.: Recherches sur l'anémie infectieuse des chevaux. Bull. Off. Intl. Epiz. 1951, **36**. 327

421. Steck, W.: Recent studies on equine infectious anemia. Report, 14th International Veterinary Congress in London, 1949 (Vol. **2**. p. 319). London, 1952

422. Steck, W., et Fortner, J.: Au sujet de l'anémie infectieuse des équidés. Rapport concernant un voyage d'études aux Etats-Unis. Bull. Off. Intl. Epizoot. 1952, **38**. 695

423. Steck, W., und Hauser, H.: Lungenbefunde bei der infektiöser Anämie der Pferde. Schweiz. Z. Path. 1948, **11**. 365

424. Steffan, H.: Das Herz bei inneren Erkrankungen des Pferdes. II. Mitteilung: Infektiöse Anämie. Elektro- und phonokardiographische Untersuchungen. Arch. Tierheilk. 1934, **68**. 328

425. Stein, C. D.: The history and distribution of equine infectious anemia in the United States. Vet. Med. 1941, **36**. 410

426. Stein, C. D.: Equine infectious anemia, or swamp fever. In: Keeping Livestock Healthy, Yearbook of Agriculture, U. S. Dept. Agric. 1942 (p. 392). Washington, 1942

427. Stein, C. D., and Gates, D. W.: The neutralizing effect of antiserum from recovered carriers of equine infectious anemia on the virus of the disease. Vet. Med. 1950, **45**. 152

428. Stein, C. D., Lotze, J. C., and Mott, L. O.: Transmission of equine infectious anemia by the stablefly, *Stomoxys calcitrans,* the horsefly, *Tabanus sulcifrons* (Macquart) and by injections of minute amounts of virus. Amer. J. Vet. Res. 1942, **3**. 183

429. Stein, C. D., Lotze, J. C., and Mott, L. O.: Evidence of transmission of inapparent (subclinical) form of equine infectious anemia by mosquitoes (*Psorophora columbiae*) and by injection of the virus in extremely high dilution. J. Amer. Vet. Med. Ass. 1943, **102**. 163

430. Stein, C. D., Lucker, J. T., Osteen, O. L., and Gochenour, W. S.: Studies on the possible role of endoparasites in the transmission of infectious anemia. J. Amer. Vet. Med. Ass. 1939, **95**. 536

431. Stein, C. D., and Mott, L. O.: Studies on congenital transmission of equine infectious anemia. Vet. Med. 1942, **37**. 370

432. Stein, C. D., and Mott, L. O.: Susceptibility of animals other than solipeds to infectious anemia. Vet. Med. 1944, **39**. 408

433. Stein, C. D., and Mott, L. O.: Equine infectious anemia in brood mares and their offspring. Vet. Med. 1946, **41**. 274

434. Stein, C. D., and Mott, L. O.: Suspected equine infectious anemia in man. Vet. Med. 1946, **41**. 385

435. Stein, C. D., and Mott, L. O.: Equine infectious anemia in the United States with special reference to the recent outbreak in New England. Proc. Ann. Meeting, U. S. Livestock Sanit. Assoc. (p. 37) 1947

436. Stein, C. D., and Osteen, O. L.: Studies on immunization in equine infectious anemia. Amer. J. Vet. Res. 1941, **2**. 344

437. Stein, C. D., Osteen, O. L., and Mott, L. O.: Chemotherapeutic studies of infectious anemia of horses. Vet. Med. 1941, **36**. 306

438. Stein, C. D., Osteen, O. L., Mott, L. O., and Shahan, M. S.: Experimental transmission of equine infectious anemia by contact and body secretions and excretions. Vet. Med. 1944, **39**. 46

439. Stein, C. D., Osteen, O. L., Mott, L. O., and Shahan, M. S.: Action of chemical and physical agents on the virus of equine infectious anemia. Amer. J. Vet. Res. 1944, **5**. 291

440. Steinbrüchel: Ein Beitrag zur Klärung der Frage der Uebertragbarkeit von ansteckender Blutarmut. Z. Vet.kunde 1920, **32**. 315

441. Stokes, J., Henle, G., Drake, M., and Henle, W.: The use of a skin test in studies of viral hepatitis. Trans. Ass. Amer. Physicians 1950, **63**. 122

442. Stubbs, E. L., and Furth, J.: Transmission experiments with leukosis of fowls. J. Exp. Med. 1931, **53**. 269

443. Svanberg, O.: Soil and vegetation in relation to the local occurrence of anemic conditions in northern Sweden. A preliminary report. (*In Swedish*) Lantbrukshögskolans Annaler (Uppsala) 1934, **1**. 209 (abstr.: V.B. **6**. 126)

444. Swingle, L. D.: The transmission of swamp fever in horses. Ann. Report, Wyoming Agric. Exper. Station 1912-1913 (p. 93). Laramie, Wyoming

445. Taylor, R. M., and Dreguss, M.: Serial passage of the human influenza virus in the European hamster (*Cricetus cricetus*). Proc. Soc. Exp. Biol. Med. 1940, **43**. 100

446. Theiler, A., and Kehoe, D.: Infectious or pernicious anemia of equines in South Africa. 3rd and 4th Report, Director Vet. Research, Dept. Agric. South Africa (p. 217). Pretoria 1915

447. Thiéry, J. P.: L'anémie infectieuse des équidés. Bull. Off. Intl. Epiz. 1951, **36**. 225

448. Thorshaug, N.: Equine infectious anemia in Norway, its incidence and control. (*In Norwegian*) 4. Nord. Vet. Mötet, 1933 (p. 343). Helsinki, 1934 (abstr.: V.B. **5**. 268)

449. Tiselius, A., and Kabat, E. A.: An electrophoretic study of immune sera and purified antibody preparations. J. Exp. Med. 1939, **69**. 119

450. Titze, C.: Zur Uebertragung der infektiösen Anämie des Pferdes auf das Schwein. Monat. Tierheilk. 1920, **30**. 569

451. Todd, J. L., and Wolbach, S. B.: The swamp fever of horses. Report, Vet. Director, Dept. Agric. Canada (p. 157). Ottawa 1911

452. du Toit, P. J.: Gastruslarven und infektiöse Anämie der Pferde. Monat. Tierheilk. 1920, **30**. 97

453. Tomcsik, J.: Die Polysaccharide als heterogenetische Antigene. Schweiz. Z. Path. 1945, **8**. 345

454. Tomcsik, J., and Schwarzweiss, H.: Nature of the heterogenetic hapten reacting with hemagglutinins in horse serum sickness. Proc. Soc. Exp. Biol. Med. 1948, **69**. 562

455. Torrance, C. C.: A note on immunologic reactions associated with equine infectious anemia. Amer. J. Vet. Res. 1940, **1**. 63

456. Torrance, F.: Malarial fever in horses in Manitoba. Proc. Amer. Vet. Med. Assoc. 1902 (p. 282). St. Paul, Minn. 1902

457. Torrance, F.: Report on "swamp fever" in horses. Report, Minister Agric. Canada for 1902 (p. 135). Ottawa, 1903

458. Traub, E., Walbrecht, H., und Schafer, W.: Komplementbindungsversuche bei der ansteckender Blutarmut der Pferde. Berl.-Münch. Tier. Woch. **1941**. 134

459. Traupe, H.: Ueber die Alkoholresistenz des Virus der infektiösen Anämie der Pferde, wie über die Spezifität des Kaninchen-Impfversuchs. Diss. Berlin 1926 (abstr.: Jber. **47**. 966)

460. Trautwein, K., und Schmidt, W.: Ansteckende Blutarmut bei Fohlen. Z. Infekt. Haustiere 1940, **56**. 174

461. Treffers, H. F.: Some contributions of immunology to the study of proteins. Advances in Protein Chemistry 1944, **1**. 70

462. (United States of America): Equine infectious anemia. Reports, Chief of the Bureau of Animal Industry, U. S. Dept. Agric. Washington, 1948 (p. 47); 1949 (p. 40); 1951 (p. 40); and 1952 (p. 53)

463. Urbach, E., and Gottlieb, P. M.: Allergy. 2nd ed. (p. 139). New York, 1949

464. Urbain, A., Vallée, M., Guillot, G., et Quentin, M.: Sur la réaction de Fulton appliquée au diagnostic de la typhoanémie des équidés. Bull. Acad. Vét. France 1931, 4. 389

465. Vallée, H.: Sur la typho-anémie infectieuse. Bull. Soc. Centr. Méd. Vét. 1907, 61. 526

466. Vallée, H.: Sur l'anémie infectieuse du cheval. Presse Méd. 1925, 33. II, 1465

467. Vallée, H., et Carré, H.: Sur la nature infectieuse de l'anémie du cheval. Compt. Rend. Acad. Sci. 1904, 139. 331

468. Vallée, H., et Carré, H.: Nature infectieuse de l'anémie du cheval. Rev. Gén. Méd. Vét. 1904, 4. 105

469. Van Es, L.: Swamp fever in horses. Ann. Report, North Dakota Agric. Exper. Station, 1906 (p. 48). Fargo, 1907

470. Van Es, L., Harris, E. D., and Schalk, A. F.: Swamp fever in horses. Bull. No. 94, North Dakota Agric. Exper. Station (p. 257). Fargo, 1911

471. Van Es, L., and Schalk, A. F.: Notes on parasitic anaphylaxis and allergy. Bull. No. 125, North Dakota Agric. Exper. Station (p. 151). Fargo, 1917

472. Van Es, L., et Schalk, A. F.: Sur la nature anaphylactique de l'intoxication parasitaire. Ann. Inst. Pasteur 1918, 32. 310

473. Vaughan, J. H., Bayles, T. B., and Favour, C. B.: The response of serum gamma globulin level and complement titer to ACTH therapy in Lupus erythematosus disseminatus. J. Lab. Clin. Med. 1951, 37. 698

474. Velu: Les anémies pernicieuses du cheval au Maroc et les diagnostics biologiques. Bull. Soc. Centr. Méd. Vét. 1921, 74. 263

475. Velu, H., Zottner, G., Faure, L. et Sarthou: Essais de vaccination contre l'anémie infectieuse des équidés par virus formolé. Bull. Acad. Vét. France 1934, 7. 155

476. Verge, J.: L'anémie infectieuse des équidés. Maladie de Vallée. Rec. Méd. Vét. 1933, 109. 797

477. Waldenström, J., Pedersen, K. O., Harboe, N., and Sonck, C. E.: Ultracentrifugation, electrophoresis and viscosometry of serum proteins. I. Lymphogranuloma venereum. Acta Med. Scand. 1951, 141. 195

478. Wall, S.: On the histological alterations in the liver and kidneys, in pernicious anemia in horse (Infectious anemia in horse). Acta Path. Microbiol. Scand. 1934, Suppl. No. 18, p. 225

479. Wallenstein, W. L., Brueckner, A. L., and Poelma, L. J.: "Rh" and isoimmunizations in thoroughbred horses. Proc. Ann. Meeting, Amer. Vet. Med. Assoc. in Milwaukee, Wisconsin, 1951 (p. 104)

480. Watson, T. W.: Equine relapsing fever. Amer. Vet. Rev. 1896, 20. 196

481. Weidlich, N.: Untersuchungen zur Feststellung der ansteckenden Blutarmut der Pferde, zugleich ein Beitrag zur Erkennung diese Seuche. Prag. Arch. Tiermed. 1932, 12. 149

482. Weidlich, N.: Beitrag zum Vorkommen der ansteckenden Blutarmut der Pferde in der Slowakei. Berl.-Münch. Tier. Woch. 1942. 242

483. White, A., and Roberts, S.: Influence of the adrenal cortex on plasma protein formation and utilization. In Youmans: Plasma Proteins (p. 340). Springfield, Illinois, 1950

484. White, P. D.: Heart Disease. 4th ed. (p. 359) New York, 1951

485. Whitehouse, A. W.: Trypan-blue in infectious anemia. Amer. J. Vet. Med. 1911, 6. 686

486. Wiener, A. S.: Origin of naturally occurring hemagglutinins and hemolysins: A review. J. Immunol. 1951, 66. 287

487. Wirth, D.: Beiträge zur Kenntnis der infektiösen Anämie der Pferde. Monat. Tierheilk. 1918, 29. 97

488. Wittfogel, H.: Der Wert des Meerschweincheninfektionsversuches für die Erkennung der ansteckenden Blutarmut der Einhufer. Z. Infekt. Haustiere 1938, 53. 148

489. Wittfogel, H.: Ueber den Cholesteringehalt des Blutserums mit ansteckender Blutarmut behafteter Pferde. Z. Infekt. Haustiere 1938, 54. 135

490. Wittfogel, H.: Ueber die Formolgelatinierungreaktion als Hilfsmittel zur Feststellung der ansteckenden Blutarmut der Einhufer. Z. Infekt. Haustiere 1939, 55. 175

491. Wolfe, D., Kornfeld, L., and Markham, F.: Simplified indirect complement-fixation test applied to Newcastle disease immune avian serum. Proc. Soc. Exp. Biol. Med. 1949, 70. 490

492. Wright, L. H.: A comparative study of the long bones in infectious equine anemia and other conditions. J. Amer. Vet. Med. Ass. 1920, 56. 444

493. Wright, L. H.: Iron content of the blood and spleen in infectious equine anemia. J. Agricult. Res. 1923, 26. 239

494. Zeller, H.: Klinische, pathologisch-anatomische histologische und serologische Befunde bei 50 chronischen Fällen von ansteckender Blutarmut des Pferdes. Z. Infekt. Haustiere 1924, 26. 67

495. Zenkner, J., Kolodziejska, H., and Jastrzebski, D.: Equine infectious anemia. (*In Polish*) Wojsk. Przegl. Wet. 1938, 9. 5 (abstr.: V.B. 9. 87)

496. Ziegler, M.: Vergleichende histologische Untersuchungen über die infektiöse, perniziöse und chronische progressive Anämie des Pferdes. Zugleich ein Beitrag zur Frage ihrer einheitlichen Aetiologie und ihrer Pathogenese. Z. Infekt. Haustiere 1923, 24. 242, 261; 1924, 25. 1

497. Zimmerman, H. J., Heller, P., and Hill, R. P.: Extreme hyperglobulinemia in subacute hepatic necrosis. New Engl. J. Med. 1951, 244. 245

498. Zschokke, E.: Progressive perniciöse Anaemie der Pferde. Schweiz. Arch. Tierh. 1883, 25. 11, 17; 1886, 28. 293

499. Zwick, W.: Les anémies infectieuses et particulièrement l'anémie infectieuse des chevaux. Bull. Off. Intl. Epizoot. 1935, 10. 151

500. Zwick, W.: Anémies infectieuses en Yougoslavie. Bull. Off. Intl. Epizoot. 1935, 10. 341

B) SUPPLEMENTARY BIBLIOGRAPHY

501. Abderhalden, E., und Buchal, W.: Weiterer Beitrag zur Feststellung der perniziösen Anämie der Pferde. Arch. Tierheilk. 1911, 37. 309

502. Abderhalden, E., und Weil, A.: Ueber das Verhalten des Blutes (Plasma bzw. Serum und rote Blutkörperchen) von an perniciöser Anämie und Rotz erkrankten Pferden gegen Saponin. Arch. Tierheilk. 1912, 38. 243

503. Abelein, R.: Beiträge zur infektiösen Anämie der Pferde. Diss. Leipzig, 1919 (abstr.: M.T.W. 70. 389)

504. Acres, G. H.: Infectious anemia or swamp fever. Amer. Vet. Rev. 1909, 34. 525

505. Agrinskii, N. I., and Filatov, P. V.: Liver biopsy in horses. (*In Russian*) Veterinariya 1946, 23. (No. 1) 35 (abstr.: V.B. 19. 275)

506. Akulov, A. V.: Pathological anatomy of equine infectious anemia. (*In Russian*) Veterinariya 1940, 17. (No. 2) 148 (abstr.: V.B. 15. 187)

507. Albrecht, H.: Beiträge zur Technik der Blutuntersuchung mit besonderer Berücksichtigung der Sublimatprobe (Horgan, Bennett, Kenny, Fulton). Diss. Hannover, 1933 (abstr.: Jber. 54. 359)

508. Alikaev, V. A., and Kulakov, G. E.: Variations in the acid-base equilibrium in horses with chronic infectious anemia. (*In Russian*) Veterinariya 1941, 18. (No. 1) 21 (abstr.: V.B. 12. 533)

509. Andersen, C. W.: Pernicious (infectious) anemia of horses. (*In Danish*) Maanedsskr. Dyrlaeg. 1920, 32. 129

510. Andreev, K. P.: Clinical and epizootic characteristics of concurrent equine infectious anemia and piroplasmosis. (*In Russian*) Veterinariya 1945, **22**. (No. 4-5) 15 (abstr.: V.B. **18**. 457)

511. Andreev, K.: Epidemiology of equine infectious anemia. (*In Russian*) Veterinariya 1947, **24**. (No. 2) 7 (abstr.: V.B. **20**. 585)

512. Andrievskii, I. I.: On the duration of quarantine for equine infectious anemia. (*In Russian*) Trud. XV Plen. Vet. Sekt. Akad. Sel'khoz. Nauk, Moscow. 1939 (Diseases of horses) 1941, p. 33 (abstr.: V.B. **15**. 323)

513. Andrievskii, I. I.: Abortion in mares affected with equine infectious anemia. (*In Russian*) Sovyet Vet. 1940, **17**. (No. 4) 21 (abstr.: V.B. **11**. 22)

514. Angenstein, R.: Beiträge zur infektiösen Anämie der Pferde. Diss. Hannover, 1922 (abstr.: Jber. **43**. 79)

515. Arendt, W.: Eignet sich Pferdemuskelfleisch zur Herstellung chirurgischen Nahtmaterials? Zbl. Chirurgie 1936, **63**. 370

516. Arnez, J.: Das Blutbild bei der Kachexie des Pferdes. Monat. Tierheilk. 1920, **30**. 265

517. Asselmann, A.: Kaninchenimpfversuche mit Blut von sporadisch kranken, in der Sublimatprobe positiv reagierenden Pferden. Diss. Hannover, 1939 (abstr.: Jber. **66**. 218)

518. Atta, A.: Beitrag zur Kenntnis der infektiösen Anämie der Pferde. Diss. Berlin, 1918 (abstr.: Jber. **38**. 72)

519. Auermann, B.: Versuche über die Empfänglichkeit von Jungschafen für das Virus der infektiösen Anämie der Pferde. Diss. Hannover, 1936 (abstr.: D.T.W. **45**. 611)

520. Avramenko, G. D.: The viability of the virus of equine infectious anemia in hay under different methods of preservation. (*In Russian*) Trud. XV Plen. Vet. Sekt. Akad. Sel'khoz. Nauk, Moscow, 1939 (Diseases of horses) 1941, p. 30 (abstr.: V.B. **15**. 323)

521. Baars, G.: Zur infektiösen Anämie der Pferde. Deut. Tier. Woch. 1921, **29**. 224

522. Bachfall, A.: Zur Frage der Spezifität des Noltze'schen Sedimentierungsverfahrens zur Diagnose der ansteckenden Blutarmut. Diss. Berlin, 1923 (abstr.: D.T.W. **32**. 347)

523. Bailer, R.: Verbreitung und Verlauf der "ansteckenden Blutarmut" der Pferde in Deutschland nach dem Kriege unter besonderer Berücksichtigung der Jahre 1924 und 1925. Berl. Tier. Woch. 1927, **43**. 473

524. Bailer, R.: Verbreitung und Verlauf der ansteckenden Blutarmut der Pferde in Deutschland während der Jahre 1926 und 1927. Berl. Tier. Woch. 1929, **45**. 661

525. Bailer, R.: Verbreitung und Verlauf der ansteckenden Blutarmut der Pferde während der Jahre 1928 bis 1930. Berl. Tier. Woch. 1932, **48**. 649

526. Balks, F.: Versuche über Abtötung des Virus der infektiösen Anämie des Pferdes durch 2-prozentige Karbol(säure)lösung. Diss. Hannover, 1925 (abstr.: D.T.W. **34**. 823)

527. Ballah, J. R.: Report on swamp fever. Ann. Report, Dept. Agric. Saskatchewan, 1907 (p. 223) Regina, Canada, 1908

528. Ballot, A.: Deux entéro-toxémies du cheval: la typho-anemie et la méningo-encéphalite infectieuse. Rec. Méd. Vét. 1947, **123**. 153

529. Balozet, L.: Etudes expérimentales sur l'anémie infectieuse des équidés. I. Arch. Inst. Pasteur Tunis 1935, **24**. 258

530. Balozet, L.: Inoculation du virus de l'anémie infectieuse des équidés à d'autres espèces. Compt. Rend. Soc. Biol. 1937, **124**. 1150

531. Balozet, L.: L'immunité dans l'anémie infectieuse des équidés. Cahiers Méd. Vét. 1937, **7**. 133

532. Balozet, L., et Pernot, P.: Deuxième cas d'anémie infectieuse des équidés observé en Tunisie. Arch. Inst. Pasteur Tunis 1935, **24**. 307

533. Bankier, J. C.: Equine infectious anemia. Attempted cross immunity experiments. Canad. J. Comp. Med. 1946, **10**. 274

534. Basset, J.: Fièvre typhoide du cheval et anémie infectieuse. Compt. Rend. Soc. Biol. 1919, **82**. 1262

535. Basset, J.: Fièvre typhoide du cheval et anémie infectieuse. Bull. Soc. Centr. Méd. Vét. 1919, **72**. 442

536. Basset, J.: La fièvre typhoide du cheval (Pferdestaupe, pink eye) avec diverses considérations sur les suivantes maladies infectieuses du cheval: pneumonie, bronchite, anémie. Rev. Méd. Vét. 1941, **92**. 5, 49

537. Bauer: Verbreitung und Verlauf der ansteckenden Blutarmut der Pferde während der Jahre 1931-1934. Berl. Tier. Woch. 1936, **52**. 597

538. Baumann, R.: Ueber die Ausbreitung der ansteckenden Blutarmut der Pferde in der Ostmark. Wien. Tier. Monat. 1940, **27**. 33

539. Beck, A.: Anaemia infectiosa. (*In Hungarian*) Állatorv. Lapok 1917, **40**. 230 (abstr.: Jber. **37**. 88)

540. Beck: Die ansteckende Blutarmut der Einhufer. Berl.-Münch. Tier. Woch. **1939**. 591

541. Bederke, O.: Beiträge zur Diagnose der infektiösen Anämie der Pferde. Monat. Tierheilk. 1921, **32**. 385

542. Bedford, G. A. H.: Notes on the species of Gastrophilus found in South Africa. 5th and 6th Report, Director Vet. Research, Dept. Agric. South Africa (p. 627). Pretoria, 1919

543. Beebe, W. L.: Swamp fever. Second Ann. Report, Minnesota State Livestock Sanit. Board (p. 49). St. Paul, 1905

544. Behnke: Die Feststellung der ansteckenden Blutarmut der Pferde. Z. Infekt. Haustiere 1932, **41**. 141

545. Beller, K.: Stand und Bedeutung der Virusforschung für die Tierheilkunde. Monat. Tierheilk. Neue Folge 1949, **1**. 1

546. Beller, K., und Traub, E.: Untersuchungen über die ansteckende Blutarmut der Pferde. II. Uebertragungsversuche. Arch. Tierheilk. 1942, **77**. 411

547. Benthien, W.: Infektiöse Anämie des Pferdes. Berl. Tier. Woch. 1917, **33**. 524

548. Bettkober: Beitrag zur Kenntnis der infektiösen Anämie der Pferde. Berl. Tier. Woch. 1919, **35**. 21

549. Beveridge, W. I. B., and Burnet, F. M.: The Cultivation of Viruses and Rickettsiae in the Developing Egg. Med. Res. Council Spec. Rep. Series No. 256. London, 1946

550. Bierwagen, D.: Weitere Beiträge zur Diagnose der ansteckenden Blutarmut der Pferde mit Hilfe des Kaninchenversuchs. Diss. Hannover 1935 (abstr.: Jber. **58**. 198)

551. Biesterfeld, J.: Ist die infektiösen Anämie der Pferde auf Hühner und Tauben übertragbar? Tierärzt. Rund. 1926, **32**. 134

552. Bigot: L'anémie pernicieuse du cheval au Maroc. Persistance du virus chez les animaux guéris. Bull. Soc. Path. Exot. 1923, **16**. 300

553. Blanchard, L., et Vedel, R.: Sur la typho-anémie du cheval. Bull. Acad. Vét. France 1933, **6**. 110

554. Blaska, J.: Die therapeutische Wirkung der Jod-Kupfer-Natrium-präparate und der Rinderleber bei infektiöser Anämie. (*In Czech*) Diss. Brno, 1935 (abstr.: Jber. **60**. 302)

555. Blum, J.: Die infektiöse Anämie des Pferdes. Schweiz. Arch. Tierh. 1930, **72**. 419

556. Bolle, W.: Makroskopische Herzbefunde bei Einhufern mit infektiöser Anämie. Arch. Tierheilk. 1934, **68**. 42

557. Bolle, W.: Makroskopische Befunde an der Pulmonalarterie bei Einhufern mit infektiöser Anämie. Arch. Tierheilk. 1939, **74**. 94

558. Bolliger, A.: Zur Therapie der infektiösen Anämie der Pferde. Schweiz. Arch. Tierheilk. 1945, 87. 291

559. Bonhuis, J.: Vergleichende Untersuchungen zwischen Sublimatprobe und Takatareaktion. Diss. Hannover, 1938 (abstr.: D.T.W. 47. 188)

560. Borchers, F.: Ueber die Resistenzbreite der Erythrozyten bei Anämiepferden. Diss. Berlin, 1922 (abstr.: Jber. 41-42. 147)

561. Bornemann: Ein Fall von perniziöser Anämie bei einem fünfjährigen Pferde. Berl. Tier. Woch. 1893. 181

562. Bornholdt, W.: Untersuchungen über die Einwirkung des Virus der infektiösen Anämie der Pferde auf Erythrozyten gesunder Kaninchen in vitro. Diss. Hannover, 1925 (abstr.: Tier. Rund. 32. 384)

563. Bosh'yan, G. M.: Colorimetric test for diagnosis of equine infectious anemia. I. (*In Russian*) Sovyet Vet. 1940, 17. (No. 10) 19 (abstr.: V.B. 12. 533)

564. Bosh'yan, G. M.: Colorimetric test for diagnosis of equine infectious anemia II. (*In Russian*) Veterinariya 1941, 18. (No. 1) 12 (abstr.: V.B. 12. 533)

565. Bosh'yan, G. M.: On infectious anemia of horses. (*In Russian*) Veterinariya 1950, 27. (No. 6) 8 (abstr.: J.A.V.M.A. 118. 263)

566. Bosnic, L.: Equine infectious anemia in Yugoslavia. (*In Croatian*) Vet. Arhiv. 1936, 6. 417 (abstr.: V.B. 7. 424)

567. Boulin: De la médication arsenicomercurielle en thérapeutique vétérinaire et son emploi dans la septicémie hémorrhagique ovine, et dans la typhoanémie infectieuse du cheval. Bull. Soc. Centr. Méd. Vét. 1912, 66. 616

568. Boussard, C. H. E.: La prophylaxie de la typho-anémie infectieuse des équidés. Rec. Méd. Vét. 1927, 103. 60

569. Boussard, C.: La typho-anémie infectieuse des équidés. Conférence tenu à Nancy, 1933. Rev. Gén. Méd. Vét. 1935, 44. 344

570. Braun: Bösartige Anämie bei Pferden. Münch. Tier. Woch. 1910, 54. 230

571. Braunschweig, C.: Untersuchungen über die Resistenzbreite der Erythrocyten bei mit infektiöser Anämie behafteten Pferden. Tierärzt. Rund. 1926, 32. 367

572. Brickman, G. J.: Malarial fever of horses. (*In Swedish*) Svensk VetTidskr. 1906, 11. 120

573. Brocq-Rousseu, D.: La réaction de Makimura. Rev. Path. Comp. 1939, 39. 772

574. Brown, T. M., Wichelhausen, R. H., Merchant, W. R., and Robinson, L. B.: A study of the antigen-antibody mechanism in rheumatic diseases. Amer. J. Med. Sci. 1951, 221. 618

575. Brunklaus, J.: Therapeutische Versuche an Kaninchen über die Einwirkung des Wismutpräparates "Olbisol" auf das Virus der ansteckenden Blutarmut. Diss. Hannover, 1939 (abstr.: Jber. 66. 108)

576. Brunschwick, M., et Davesne, J.: La formol-leuco-gélification dans le diagnostic de l'anémie infectieuse du cheval. Compt. Rend. Soc. Biol. 1937, 125. 333

577. Buchal: Beiträge zur Kenntnis der perniciösen Anämie der Pferde. Diss. Berlin, 1911 (abstr.: Jber. 31. 150)

578. Bumüller, E.: Untersuchungen über eine Vereinfachung des diagnostischen Kaninchenversuches bei der ansteckenden Blutarmut des Pferdes. Diss. Hannover, 1937 (abstr.: Jber. 63. 166)

579. Burghardt: Blutgruppen beim Pferde. Z. Vet.kunde 1933, 45. 33

580. Bürgi, O.: Ansteckende Blutarmut, Virusanämie der Pferde. Schweiz. Arch. Tierh. 1949, 91. (Nov.) S. 41

581. Burke, R. W.: The relation of Monadina to pernicious anaemia, equine and human. Vet. Journ. 1890, 30. 175

582. Burke, R. W.: Malarial fever among horses in India. Vet. Journ. 1890, 30. 393; 1890. 31. 15

583. Burkhardt, W.: Wie wirkt sich die parenterale Einverleibung des Virus der infektiösen Anämie der Pferde auf den histologischen Befund der Leber tuberkulöser Meerschweinchen aus? Diss. Hannover, 1931

584. Busse, F.: Versuche an Kaninchen über das Verhalten des Virus der infektiösen Anämie in entzündlichen Infiltraten. Diss. Hannover, 1938 (abstr.: D.T.W. 47. 189)

585. (California): Investigation of diseases of animals at the California Station. Report, California Agric. Exper. Station (p. 240) 1923

586. (Canada): Rep. Vet. Dir. General, Dept. Agric., 1933 (p. 54). Ottawa, 1933

587. (Canada): Report, Science Service, Dept. Agric., 1946 (p. 19, 80). Ottawa, 1946

588. Carlé: Ein Beitrag zur infektiösen Anämie der Pferde. Berl. Tier. Woch. 1918, **34**. 83.

589. Carré, H., et Vallée, H.: Sur l'anémie infectieuse du cheval. Rev. Méd. Vét. Toulouse 1905, **62**. 783

590. Carré, H., et Vallée, H.: Rapport sur l'anémie infectieuse du cheval. Bull. Off. Renseign. Agric. 1905, p. 1075

591. Cernyak, V. Z.: Tongue, macroscopic and histologic changes of the tongue in equine infectious anemia. (*In Russian*) Sovyet Vet. 1937, **14**. (No. 6) 31

592. Chamber, E. E.: Three field cases of infectious equine anemia. Vet. Med. 1941, **36**. 310

593. Charlton, G. A.: Swamp fever. Ann. Report, Dept. Agric. Canada, Prov. Saskatchewan, 1906 (p. 146). Regina, 1907

594. Charon, P.: Note sur un cas de typho-anémie infectieuse au 6e cuirassiers à Sainte-Menehould. Bull. Soc. Centr. Méd. Vét. 1907, **61**. 531

595. Chernyak, N., and Ledyaew, A.: Toward a method of determining the resistance of the blood vessels in equine infectious anemia. (*In Russian*) Veterinariya 1948, **25**. (No. 11) 12 (abstr.: J.A.V.M.A. **114**. 169)

596. Chnelewski, P.: Beiträge zur Biologie des Erregers der infektiösen Anämie des Pferdes. Diss. Hannover, 1930 (abstr.: Jber. **50**. 1058)

597. Christi, H.: Beobachtungen über den Verlauf, die Ausbreitung, die Formen und die Therapie der infektiösen Anämie der Pferde. Münch. Tier. Woch. 1932, **83**. 409

598. Cilli, V.: L'anemia infettiva degli equini e i suoi rapporti con le anemie tipo pernicioso dell'uomo. Azione Vet. 1936, **5**. 624

599. Cilli, V.: Studio de un focolaio di anemia infettiva dell'asino in Eritrea. (Considerazioni patogenetiche con le anemie perniciose dell'uomo.) Nuova Vet. 1938, **16**. 179

600. Cilli, V.: Anemia infettiva degli asini ed anemia perniciosa dell'uomo. Fourth International Congress for Comparative Pathology in Rome, 1939 (Vol. **2**. p. 169)

601. Cohrs, P.: Die Erschöpfung des Pferdes. (Zugleich ein Beitrag zur Differentialdiagnose der infektiösen Anämie.) Erste kriegspathologische Mitteilung. Deut. Tier. Woch. 1941, **49**. 277

602. Czekelius, F.: Pathologisch-anatomische und histologische Befunde bei Pferden mit experimenteller ansteckender Blutarmut. Diss. Berlin, 1942 (abstr.: Jber. **70**. 534)

603. Dehner, O.: Unspezifische Tuberkulinreaktionen bei an infektiöser Anämie erkrankten Pferden. Arch. Tierheilk. 1931, **63**. 23

604. Delafond, O.: Recherches sur une maladie du cheval encore peu connue. Rec. Méd. Vét. 1851, **28**. 481, 633, 730, 814; 1852, **29**. 173

605. Delage, B.: Le système lipoprotéidique du sérum au cours de l'anémie infectieuse et de la dourine chez les équidés. Compt. Rend. Soc. Biol. 1938, **128**. 985

606. De Paolis, E.: Su di un focolaio di anemia infettiva riscontrato di un gruppo di muli in una azienda agricola del Foggiano. Profilassi 1942, **15**. 1

607. Detlefsen: Heilung der chronischen Anämie beim Pferd durch Plastoserum. Deut. Tier. Woch. 1934, **42**. 543

608. Detweiler, D. K.: The value of combating acidosis and providing fluid in hemorrhage and shock in the dog. Vet. Ext. Quart., Univ. Pennsylvania 1946, No. **104**. page 3

609. Diessel, A.: Untersuchungen über den Virusgehalt des Harnes von mit ansteckender Blutarmut behafteten Pferden. Diss. Hannover, 1938 (abstr.: Jber. **64.** 470)

610. Dobberstein, J.: Die chronisch-stationäre Anämie der Pferde und die geographische Verbreitung der ansteckenden Blutarmut. Deut. Tier. Woch. 1938, **46.** 458

611. Doerr, R.: Mensch und Tier als Virusträger und Virusausscheider. 5. Die ansteckende Blutarmut der Pferde. In Doerr und Hallauer: Handbuch der Virusforschung (I. Ergänzungsband, S. 161). Wien, 1944

612. Domanski, E., Dobrowolska, D., and Zalewska, E.: The phenomenon of anemia in equine infectious anemia. (*In Polish*) Polskie Arch. Wet. 1951, **1.** 317 (abstr.: Biol. Abstr. **27.** 192)

613. Domansky, F.: Equine infectious anemia. (*In Czech*) Cas. Ceskoslov. Vet. 1950, **5.** 193

614. Donatien, A., et Lestoquard, F.: L'anémie pernicieuse du mouton et de la chèvre. Bull. Soc. Centr. Méd. Vét. 1924, **77.** 386

615. Donner, W.: Beitrag zur Kenntnis der Anämien des Pferdes. Diss. Berlin, 1922 (abstr.: Jber. **41-42.** 148)

616. Dupas, L.: Contribution à l'étude clinique de la typho-anémie infectieuse. Rev. Gén. Méd. Vét. 1910, **15.** 129

617. Eckmeyer: Perniciöse Anämie. Woch. Tierheilk. Viehzucht. 1891, **35.** 380

618. Eichinger, O.: Infektiöse Anämie in Bayern. Münch. Tier. Woch. 1923, **74.** 521, 560

619. Eigendorf, R.: Untersuchungen über die Ermittlung von Virusträgern bei der infektiösen Anämie der Pferde. Diss. Hannover, 1923 (abstr.: Jber. **43.** 79)

620. Eilmann, H.: Die infektiöse Anämie im Kreise Wehlau. Diss. Hannover, 1926 (abstr.: D.T.W. **38.** 395)

621. Eilmann, H.: Infektiöse Anämie bei zwei tuberkulosekranken Pferden und Genese der dabei auftretenden Endokard- und Intimaverkalkungen. Deut. Tier. Woch. 1936, **44.** 195

622. Eisenblätter: Zur infektiösen Anämie des Pferdes. Berl. Tier. Woch. 1918, **34.** 345

623. Ekvall, R.: Pernicious anemia of the horse. (*In Swedish*) Svensk VetTidskr. 1915, **20.** 97

624. Emmerich, P.: Beiträge zur Therapie der infektiösen Anämie des Pferdes. Diss. Hannover, 1923 (abstr.: Jber. **43.** 78)

625. Equine Infectious Anemia. Vols. I and II. (264 and 172 pp.) (*In Japanese*). Published by the Ministry of Agric. and Forestry, Livestock Bureau, Japan. Tokyo, 1949

626. Ernst, D.: Untersuchungen über den Virusgehalt des Fäzes, des Harnes und des Speichels von mit infektiöser Anämie behafteten Pferden. Diss. Hannover, 1924 (abstr.: D.T.W. **32.** 357)

627. Ezovitov, N. B., Marchenko, G. F., Pogodin, A. L., and Dmitriev, K. G.: Differential diagnosis of equine infectious anemia and *Babesia equi* infection. (*In Russian*) Veterinariya 1941, **18.** (No. 2) 104 (abstr.: V.B. **13.** 15)

628. Falcoz, R.: Contribution à l'étude de l'anémie infectieuse des équidés dans la Haute-Marne. Thèse, Lyon, 1943 (abstr.: Rec. Méd. Vét. **119.** 64)

629. Fargel, E.: Das Verhalten des Virus der infektiösen Anämie des Pferdes bei Kaninchenpassagen. Diss. Hannover, 1924 (abstr.: D.T.W. **32.** 429)

630. Faure, L.: Dépistage de l'anémie infectieuse des équidés par le sédimentation. Bull. Acad. Vét. France 1934, **7.** 317

631. Faure, L.: Contribution à l'étude des modes d'infection dans l'anémie infectieuse des équidés. Rev. Vét. Milit. 1935, **19.** 209

632. Faure, L.: Pyodermite et anémie infectieuse des équidés. Rev. Path. Comp. 1936, **36.** 919

633. Favero, F.: Larve di Gastrophilus equi ed haemorrhoidalis e tifo-anemia infettiva del cavallo. Alcune osservazioni alle richerche di K. R. e R. Seyderhelm. Nuovo Ercolani (Milano) 1916, **21**. 4, 17

634. Fedorov, A.: The pathology of the kidneys in equine infectious anemia. (*In Russian*) Trud. XV Plen. Vet. Sekt. Akad. Sel'khoz. Nauk, Moscow, 1939 (Diseases of horses) 1941. (abstr.: V.B. **16**. 45)

635. Fedorov, A. I., and Dobin, M. A.: Histological differential diagnosis of equine infectious anemia and septicaemia. (*In Russian*) Veterinariya 1941, **18**. (No. 3) 31 (abstr.: V.B. **13**. 15)

636. Feers, A. G.: Infectious anemia of horses. Amer. J. Vet. Med. 1918, **13**. 527

637. Feldmann, L.: Untersuchungen über den Virusgehalt des Speichels von mit ansteckender Blutarmut behafteten Pferden. Diss. Hannover, 1937 (abstr.: Jber. **63**. 384)

638. Filatov, P. V.: Arterial and venous pressure in equine infectious anemia. (*In Russian*) Veterinariya 1951, **28**. (No. 3) 40 (abstr.: V.B. **23**. 18)

639. Findlay, G. M.: Variation in Viruses. 25. Infectious anemia. In Doerr und Hallauer: Handbuch der Virusforschung (Vol. **2**, p. 913). Wien, 1939

640. Flower, E. P.: Pernicious anemia (swamp fever). Proc. 13th Ann. Meeting, Interstate Assoc. Livestock Sanit. Boards (p. 162). Chicago, 1909

641. Flückiger, G.: Ueber die Massnahmen der zivilen Behörden zur Bekämpfung der infektiösen Pferdeanämie in der Schweiz. Schweiz. Arch. Tierh. 1943, **85**. 18

642. Flückiger, G.: Zur Erforschung und Bekämpfung der infektiösen Pferdeanämie. Monat. Vet.-Med. 1951, **6**. 462

643. Focken, D.: Therapeutische Versuche bei der infektiösen Anämie des Pferdes. Diss. Hannover, 1923 (abstr.: Jber. **43**. 78)

644. Fomina, A. Y.: Attempts to propagate in rabbits the virus of equine infectious anemia. (*In Russian*) Sovyet Vet. 1939, **16**. (No. 6) 11 (abstr.: V.B. **10**. 759)

645. Fontaine: Beiträge zur Diagnose des Pferdewechselfiebers (ansteckende Blutarmut). Z. Vet.kunde 1921, **33**. 242

646. (France): Arrêté concernant la police sanitaire de l'anémie infectieuse des équidés. Bull. Off. Intl. Epizoot. 1936, **13**. 610

647. (France): Arrêté du 7 décembre 1936 relatif à l'exécution du décret du 21 novembre 1936 ajoutant l'anémie infectieuse des équidés à la nomenclature des maladies réputées contagieuses. Rev. Méd. Vét. 1937, **89**. 56

648. Fricke, O.: Beiträge zur Diagnostik der infektiösen Anämie der Pferde. Diss. Hannover, 1922 (abstr.: Jber. **42**. 148)

649. Friedrich: Die perniciöse Anämie der Pferde. Berl. Tier. Woch. **1908**. 469

650. Frisch, R.: Prophylaktische und therapeutische Versuche bei der infektiösen Anämie des Pferdes, angestellt an Kaninchen. Diss. Hannover, 1924 (abstr.: Jber. **44**. 91)

651. Froehlich: Ein typischer Fall von perniziöser Anämie. Z. Vet.kunde 1916, **28**. 383

652. Führer, H.: Untersuchungen über die Tenazität des Virus der ansteckenden Blutarmut in Pferdeharn. Diss. Hannover, 1939 (abstr.: D.T.W. **47**. 484)

653. Fulton, J. S.: The incidence of swamp fever in Saskatchewan in relation to soil type. J. Amer. Vet. Med. Ass. 1930, **77**. 157

654. Fürbass: Beitrag zur Diagnose und Therapie der infektiösen Anämie des Pferdes. Berl. Tier. Woch. 1932, **48**. 181

655. Furch, K.: Pathologisch-anatomische und histologische Untersuchungen von mit infektiöser Anämie infizierten Kaninchen. Diss. Hannover, 1934 (abstr.: Jber. **56**. 262)

656. Gamaleya, N. F.: Research on the virus of equine infectious anemia. (*In Russian*) Trud. Vsesoyuz. Inst. Eksp. Vet. 1940, **15**. 7 (abstr.: V.B. **16**. 145)

657. Gambarov, G. S.: Contact infection in equine infectious anemia. (*In Russian*) Sovyet Vet. 1940, **17**. (No. 6) 11 (abstr.: V.B. **12**. 532)

658. Gambarov, G. S., and Balitskaya, A. K.: Diagnosis of equine infectious anemia. (*In Russian*) Sovyet Vet. 1940, **17**. (No. 2-3) 46 (abstr.: V.B. **12**. 533)

659. Gates, W. L.: Equine infectious anemia (swamp fever). J. Amer. Vet. Med. Ass. 1940, **96**. 195

660. Gerdemann, J.: Histologische Untersuchungen bei sensibilisierten und mit dem Virus der ansteckenden Blutarmut infizierten Kaninchen. Diss. Hannover, 1939

661. Gerlach, F.: Serumkrankheit bei Rind und Pferd. Z. Immunforsch. 1922, **34**. 75
(abstr.: Jber. **67**. 204)

662. Gerlach, F.: Infektiöse Anämie der Schafe. Wien. Tier. Monat. 1933, **20**. 577

663. (Germany): Gemeinfassliche Belehrung über die ansteckende Blutarmut des Pferdes. Berl. Tier. Woch. 1918, **34**. 276

664. (Germany): Der Wert des Sedimentierungsverfahrens zur Feststellung der infektiösen Anämie. Deut. Tier. Woch. 1923, **39**. 7

665. (Germany): Ansteckende Blutarmut der Pferde. Veröffentlichung des Ministeriums. Deut. Tier. Woch. 1924, **32**. 44; 1926, **34**. 201; 1932, **40**. 78

666. (Germany): Verordnung über die ansteckende Blutarmut der Pferde. Münch. Tier. Woch. 1933, **84**. 600

667. (Germany): Verbreitung und Verlauf der ansteckenden Blutarmut der Pferde während der Jahre 1928 bis 1930. Mitteilung des Reichsgesundheitsamtes. Münch. Tier. Woch. 1934, **85**. 371

668. (Germany): Verordnungen über ansteckende Blutarmut. Reichsgesundheitsblatt 1928, **3**. 36; 1931, **6**. 438; 1936, **11**. 361; 1936, **11**. 541

669. Gerosa, G.: La diagnosi dell'anemia infettiva degli equini. Clinica Vet. 1942, **65**. 212

670. Geweniger: Das Blutbild der infektiösen Anämie der Pferde und sein diagnostischer Wert. Z. Vet.kunde 1929, **41**. 446

671. Giffey, E.: Untersuchungen über den Virusgehalt des Blutes von an infektiöser Anämie erkrankten Pferden. Diss. Hannover, 1925 (abstr.: Jber. **45**. 78)

672. Gilles et Charon: La typho-anémie infectieuse peut-elle être une cause de resolution de vente? Rec. Méd. Vét. 1908, **85**. 242

673. Gindin, A. P.: Biological diagnosis of equine infectious anemia by use of fowls and pigeons. (*In Russian*) Trud. Vsesoyuz. Inst. Eksp. Vet. 1936, **12**. 67 (abstr.: V.B. **8**. 27)

674. Gindin, A. P., Kudryavtsev, A. A., and Ergaev, M. Y.: Some unusual anatomical changes in splenectomized foals affected with infectious anemia. (*In Russian*) Veterinariya 1941, **18**. (No. 2) 38 (abstr.: V.B. **13**. 15)

675. Girg, N. H.: Allergische Reaktionen bei Askaridenbefall des Pferdes. Arch. Tierheilk. 1930, **61**. 235

676. Gmelin, W.: Die Anämie der Pferde. Berl. Tier. Woch. 1927, **43**. 341

677. Gmelin, W.: Ein Beitrag zur Frage der Anämie und Kopfkrankheit der Pferde. Berl. Tier. Woch. 1934, **50**. 529

678. Gochenour, W. S., Stein, C. D., and Osteen, O. L.: Infectious anemia (swamp fever). Farmers' Bull. No. 1819, U. S. Dept. Agric. Washington, 1938

679. Goncharov, N. P.: A chemical test for hemosiderin in the liver and spleen in equine infectious anemia. (*In Russian*) Sovyet Vet. 1939, **16**. (No. 8) 31 (abstr.: V.B. **10**. 759)

680. Goret, P., et Sandor, G.: Etude du système lipo-protéidique du sérum des chevaux atteints d'anémie infectieuse. Bull. Acad. Vét. France 1934, **7**. 383

681. Goret, P., Sandor, G., et Domercq, J.: Etude comparative du système lipo-protéidique du sérum des chevaux atteints d'anémie infectieuse, des chevaux normaux, des chevaux fiévreux et hyperimmunises. Bull. Acad. Vét. France 1935, **8**. 517

682. Goryachev, G. A.: Is equine infectious anemia spread by contact during the chronic stage of infection? (*In Russian*) Sovyet Vet. 1939, **16** (No. 2) 16 (abstr.: V.B. **11**. 22)

683. Gossler, G.: Der Wert des Kaninchenimpfversuches für die Diagnose der infektiösen Anämie des Pferdes. Diss. Hannover, 1934 (abstr.: Jber. **56.** 106)

684. Goubine: Les porteurs et les excréteurs du virus de l'anémie infectieuse du cheval. (*In Russian*) Trud. Vsesoyuz. Inst. Eksp. Vet. 1936, **12.** 30 (abstr.: Rec. Méd. Vét. **113.** 618)

685. Gourvitch, B. M., Oleinik, K. K., and Avromenko, G. D.: The complement fixation test in equine infectious anemia. (*In Russian*) Sovyet Vet. 1936, **13.** (No. 6) 24

686. Gövert, H.: Weitere Untersuchungen über die Diagnose der ansteckenden Blutarmut des Pferdes mit Hilfe der vereinfachten Kaninchenversuches. Diss. Hannover, 1938 (abstr.: Jber. **63.** 384)

687. Gratzl, E., und Traub, E.: Zum Vorkommen von hämolytischen Streptokokken bei den katarrhalisch entzündlichen Erkrankungen der Luftwege des Pferdes. Arch. Tierheilk. 1942, **77.** 347

688. Grayson Foundation: Current research projects. Equine infectious anemia. Bulletin of Grayson Foundation (p. 14). New York, 1948

689. Grayson Foundation: Status of research projects. Equine infectious anemia. Bulletin of Grayson Foundation (p. 12). New York, 1950

690. Greenberg, D. M., and Mirolubova, T. N.: Modifications in the colorimetric determination of the plasma proteins by the Folin phenol reagent. J. Lab. Clin. Med. 1936, **21.** 431

691. Gressner, J.: Histopathological changes of the spleen in infectious anemia. (*In Czech*) Thesis, Brno, 1935 (abstr.: Jber. **60.** 309)

692. Griffin, C. A., and Brose, C. P.: Report of an outbreak of equine infectious anemia with observations on blood changes. J. Amer. Vet. Med. Ass. 1936, **89.** 664

693. Groht, W.: Ueber Blutbefunde bei mit infektiöser Anämie behafteten Pferden, anschliessend prophylaktische Versuche mit B 205 und B 844. Diss. Hannover, 1924 (abstr.: Jber. **44.** 92)

694. Grunert, C. H.: New suggestions on swamp fever therapy. Vet. Med. 1925, **20.** 15

695. Guillot, G., et Caudron, M.: La réaction de Fulton et la réaction au carmin (Chorine). Rev. Vét. Milit. 1939, **23.** 149

696. Gunnemann, F.: Infectious anemia in the Pajala district. (*In Swedish*) Svensk VetTidskr. 1931, **36.** 310

697. Gunnemann, F.: Some experience with pernicious anemia in horse. (*In Swedish*) Skand. VetTidskr. 1939, **29.** 133

698. Gutsche, W.: Die ansteckende Blutarmut. Z. Vet.kunde 1919, **31.** 221

699. Haag, A.: Beitrag zur Diagnose der ansteckenden Blutarmut des Pferdes. Diss. München, 1923 (abstr.: M.T.W. **75.** 1087)

700. Habermalz, F.: Versuche über die Abtötung des Virus der infektiösen Anämie der Pferde im Serum durch Formalin. Diss. Hannover, 1924 (abstr.: D.T.W. **32.** 759)

701. Habersang: Beitrag zur Biologie des Erregers der infektiösen Anämie der Pferde. Monat. Tierheilk. 1921, **32.** 1

702. Habersang: Zur ansteckenden Blutarmut der Pferde. Berl. Tier. Woch. 1924, **40.** 281

703. Habersang, F.: Ist die infektiöse Anämie der Pferde ein unlösbares Problem für die Seuchenbekämpfung? Tierärzt. Mitt. 1937, **18.** 755

704. Habersang: Ueber die Provokation der infektiösen Anämie der Pferde durch SO_2-Gasbehandlung. Monat Vet.-Med. 1950, **5.** 289

705. Hadwen, S.: Notes on swamp fever. J. Amer. Vet. Med. Ass. 1920, **56.** 439

706. Hadwen, S., and Bruce, E. A.: Anaphylaxis in cattle and sheep produced by the larvae of *Hypoderma bovis, H. lineatum* and *Oestrus ovis*. J. Amer. Vet. Med. Ass. 1917, **51.** 15

707. Haferkamp, W.: Untersuchungen über die durch das Virus der infektiösen Anämie im Blutbilde des Kaninchens hervorgerufenen Veränderungen. Diss. Hannover, 1923 (abstr.: Jber. **43.** 79)

708. Hagedorn, T.: Das Verhalten des Huhnes gegenüber dem Virus der infektiösen Anämie des Pferdes. Diss. Hannover, 1923

709. Hagemeister, W.: Infektiöse Anämie. Berl. Tier. Woch. 1923, **39**. 551

710. Hahn, F.: Infektionsversuche am Kaninchen mit dem Virus der ansteckenden Blutarmut der Pferde. Diss. Hannover, 1925 (abstr.: Tierärzt. Rund. **31**. 83)

711. Hallauer, C.: Die Haemagglutination durch Virusarten. In Doerr und Hallauer: Handbuch der Virusforschung (2. Ergänzungsband, S. 141). Wien, 1950

712. Hallauer, C., und Moosbrugger, G. A.: Untersuchungen über das Virus der infektiösen Anaemie der Pferde. Schweiz. Arch. Tierh. 1949, **91**. (Nov.) S. 28

713. Halloran, D.: Infectious anemia. Amer. Vet. Rev. 1911, **38**. 671

714. Haltenhoff, R.: Beitrag zur Diagnostik der infektiösen Anämie des Pferdes. Diss. Hannover, 1922 (abstr.: Jber. **43**. 79)

715. Haltenhoff, R.: Ueber das Wesen der Botelhoschen Probe und ihre Brauchbarkeit für die Feststellung der ansteckenden Blutarmut der Einhufer. Z. Infekt. Haustiere 1937, **52**. 44

716. Haltenhoff, R.: Beitrag zur hämatologischen Differentialdiagnose der ansteckenden Blutarmut der Einhufer. Arch. Tierheilk. 1939, **74**. 85

717. Hansmann, J.: Beiträge zur Senkungsgeschwindigkeit der roten Blutkörperchen bei Pferden. Diss. Leipzig, 1924 (abstr.: D.T.W. **34**. 445)

718. Haring, K.: Untersuchungen am Kaninchen und Pferd über den cutanen Infektionsweg bei der ansteckenden Blutarmut der Pferde wie über die Empfänglichkeit des Schafes für das Anämievirus. Diss. Hannover, 1937 (abstr.: Jber. **62**. 368)

719. Hartmann, W.: Beiträge zur Uebertragung des Pferdewechselfiebers auf den Menschen. Diss. Berlin, 1924 (abstr.: Jber. **44**. 93)

720. Hartwigk, H.: Auswertung an dem für die Diagnose der ansteckenden Blutarmut des Pferdes in den Jahren 1947-1950 (I. Quartal) eingesandten Untersuchungsmaterial. Exper. Vet. Med. (Leipzig) 1950, **2**. 86

721. Hayashi, T.: Biochemical studies of infectious anemia in the horse. VII. (*In Japanese*) J. Cent. Soc. Vet. Med. 1937, **50**. 805

722. Hayashi, T., and Arakawa, T.: Diagnosis of contagious anemia in horses. (*In Japanese*) Jap. J. Vet. Sci. 1938, Sect. II, **4**. 85

723. Heath, L. M.: Research on swamp fever or infectious equine anaemia. Report, Vet. Director, Dept. Agric. Canada, 1931 (p. 70). Ottawa, 1931

724. Hecke, F.: Der diagnostische Wert der Sublimatprobe bei der ansteckenden Blutarmut der Pferde. Arch. Tierheilk. 1934, **67**. 410

725. Heiermann, G.: Untersuchungen über die Abtötung des Virus der infektiösen Anämie des Pferdes im Serum durch Karbolsäure und Chloroform. Diss. Hannover, 1923, 1924 (abstr.: Jber. **44**. 93)

726. Hellich, I. A.: Der Wert des Sedimentierungsverfahrens zur Feststellung der infektiösen Anämie. Berl. Tier. Woch. 1923, **39**. 7

727. Helm, R.: Die künstliche Uebertragung der infektiösen Anämie des Pferdes auf Meerschweinchen und Kaninchen. Arch. Tierheilk. 1924, **51**. 365

728. Helm, R.: Weitere Versuche zur Uebertragung der infektiösen Anämie der Pferde auf Meerschweinchen. Berl. Tier. Woch. 1926, **42**. 37

729. Hemmert-Halswick, A.: Bericht über die in fünf Jahren (1940-1944) für das gesamte Reichsgebiet durchgeführten histologischen Untersuchungen bei Pferden mit Verdacht der ansteckenden Blutarmut. Deut. Tier. Woch. 1951, **58**. 365

730. Henning, M. W.: Animal Diseases in South Africa. 2nd edition. Pretoria, 1949

731. Henning, W.: Beiträge zur Prophylaxie der infektiösen Anämie der Pferde. Diss. Hannover, 1923 (abstr.: Jber. **44**. 95)

732. Himmel, L.: Die ansteckende Blutarmut der Pferde in Preussen und ihre veterinärpolizeiliche Bekämpfung. Berl. Tier. Woch. 1922, **38**. 429

733. Hirato, K., Miura, S., Uweno, Y., and Minowa, H.: Experimental transmission of infectious anemia of horses by horse flies. (*In Japanese with Engl. summary*) Jap. J. Vet. Sci. 1945, **7**. 187.

734. Hirth, H.: Ueber den Wert der amtlichen Blutuntersuchung auf ansteckende Blutarmut und die Möglichkeiten einer Vereinfachung dieser Untersuchung. Diss. Hannover, 1939 (abstr.: Jber. **66.** 138)

735. Hizatullin, K.: The diagnostic value of examination of the optic fundus in infectious anemia of horses. (*In Russian*) Veterinariya 1947, **24.** (No. 9) 17 (abstr.: J.A.V.M.A. **113.** 80)

736. Hjärre, A.: Liver changes in equine infectious anemia. (*In Swedish*) 4. Nord. Vet. Mötet, 1933 (p. 361). Helsinki, 1934

737. Hjärre, A.: Infectious anemia of horses. (*In Swedish*) 50 Ar Skandinaviska Kreatursförsäkringsbolaget 1890-1940 (p. 169). Uppsala, 1940 (abstr.: V.B. **15.** 34)

737a. Hjärre, A., and Berthelsen, H.: Method for fixing neutral-red in supravital stained blood smears. (Diagnosis of equine infectious anemia.) Nature (London) **1937, 140.** 155

738. Hnatek, R.: Ein neues serodiagnostisches Verfahren nach Kenkichi Tagawa bei der infektiösen Anämie des Pferdes. Wien. Tier. Monat. 1924, **11.** 452

739. Hobmaier, M.: Beiträge zur Biologie und Bekämpfung der Gastrusfliege (*Gastrophilus equi*). Monat. Tierheilk. 1919, **29.** 138

740. Hochstein: Infektiöse Anämie. Woch. Tierheilk. Viehzucht. 1907, **51.** 145

741. Hock, R.: Das Vorkommen von autogenem Pigment in den Milzen und Lebern gesunder und kranker Pferde. Arch. Tierheilk. 1923, **49.** 117

742. Hofferber, O.: Ueber die Verbreitung der ansteckenden Blutarmut in Deutschland unter besonderer Berücksichtigung des Seuchenstandes in Preussen. Berl. Tier. Woch. 1936, **52.** 156

743. Hofferber, O.: Ueber Ursache und Wesen der ansteckenden Blutarmut der Einhufer. Deut. Tier. Woch. **1937, 45.** 49

744. Hoffmann, L.: Ueber die Beeinflussung des Blutbildes kleiner Versuchstiere durch das Virus der infektiösen Anämie des Pferdes. Diss. Hannover, 1923 (abstr.: Jber. **43.** 79)

745. Hokamp, G.: Beeinflussung der Resistenzbreite der Kaninchen-Erythrozyten durch das Virus der infektiösen Anämie der Pferde. Diss. Hannover, 1924 (abstr.: D.T.W. **32.** 682)

746. Holz, K.: Beiträge zur Pathologie des Zentralnervensystems. V. Zur Entstehung der Ependymitis granularis des Pferdes. Berl. Tier. Woch. 1937, **53.** 65

747. Holz: Zur Ermittlung des Verdachtes der ansteckenden Blutarmut an Schlachtpferden und Pferdeleichen mit Hilfe der Schwefelammon-Methode. Berl. Tier. Woch. 1937, **53.** 460

748. Holz: Beiträge zur Pathologie des Zentralnervensystems. VIII. Uvulafibrose. Berl.-Münch. Tier. Woch. **1938.** 413

749. Holz: Thrombangiitis obliterans und Ependymitis granularis bei der ansteckenden Blutarmut der Pferde. Berl. Tier. Woch. 1938, **54.** 257

750. Holz, K.: Zur postmortalen Differentialdiagnose der ansteckenden Blutarmut des Pferdes. Z. Infekt. Haustiere 1944, **60.** 287

751. Holz, K., und Grinewitsch, A.: Weitere Untersuchungen über die postmortale Differentialdiagnose der ansteckenden Blutarmut des Pferdes. Tierärzt. Zeit. **1944.** 9

752. Homutov, P.: Recherches sur la pathologie, la physiologie pathologique et la traitement de l'anémie infectieuse du cheval. Bull. Off. Intl. Epizoot. 1936, **13.** 1

753. Höner, L.: Therapeutische Versuche bei der infektiösen Anämie der Pferde. Diss. Hannover, 1923 (abstr.: Jber. **43.** 81)

754. Hooker, S. B.: Human hypersensitiveness to different proteins of horse serum. J. Immunol. 1923, **8.** 469

755. Hörchner: Ueber Erschöpfungskrankheiten der Pferde unter besonderer Berücksichtigung der infektiösen Anämie. Deut. Tier. Woch. 1948, **55.** 216

756. Horn, V., und Boguth, W.: Serumlabilitätsprüfungen bei Haustieren. Deut. Tier. Woch. 1951, **58.** 368

757. Hornyacsek, J.: Beobachtungen über die ansteckende Blutarmut der Einhufer in Niederschlesien in Vergangenheit und Gegenwart. (Vorlesung) Berl.-Münch. Tier. Woch. **1943**. 95

758. Hornyacsek, J.: Die ansteckende Blutarmut der Einhufer in Niederschlesien in Vergangenheit und Gegenwart. Deut. Tier. Woch. **1944**. 153

759. Horstmann, A.: Untersuchungen über die Beeinflussung des Blutbildes bei mit Phenylhydrazin anämiesierten Kaninchen durch Plastoserum "Neu". Diss. Hannover, 1936 (abstr.: Jber. **61**. 568)

760. Huber: Infektiöse Anämie. Mitt. Ver. Bad. Tierärzte 1925, **25**. 37

761. Hubmaier, und Walz: Neuere Beobachtungen über die Diagnose der infektiösen Anämie. Berl.-Münch. Tier. Woch. **1943**. 96

762. de la Huerga, J., and Popper, H.: Estimation of serum gamma globulin concentration by turbidimetry. J. Lab. Clin. Med. 1950, **35**. 459

763. Hummel: Perniciöse Anämie. Arch. Tierheilk. 1899, **25**. 218

764. Hundt, O.: Vermögen die Erreger des Stutenabortus und der Fohlenlähme den Tauben- und Hühnerinfektionsversuch für die Diagnose der infektiösen Anämie der Pferde zu beeinflussen? Diss. Hannover, 1931 (abstr.: Jber. **51**. 1144)

765. Hunold, F.: Weitere Beiträge zur Diagnose der ansteckenden Blutarmut des Pferdes mit Hilfe des vereinfachten Kaninchenversuchs. Diss. Hannover, 1938 (abstr.: Jber. **64**. 469)

766. Hupbauer, A., and Malensek, S.: Equine infectious anemia. (*In Croatian*) Jugoslov. Vet. Glasn. 1935, **15**. 623 (abstr.: V.B. **7**. 175)

767. Hyman, G. A., and Southworth, H.: Hemolytic anemia associated with liver disease. Amer. J. Med. Sci. 1951, **221**. 448

768. Ikeda, T.: Ueber die Nachprüfung der serochemischen Diagnostik von Makimura für infektiöse Blutarmut des Pferdes. (*In Japanese*) J. Jap. Soc. Vet. Sci. 1931, **10**. 269 (abstr.: Jber. **51**. 1052)

769. Isaksson, A., and Jonsson, G.: Liver sampling of horses and cattle for diagnostic purposes. (*In Swedish*) Skand. VetTidskr. 1941, **31**. 87

770. Ishii, S.: On the histopathological studies of infectious anemia of the horse. III. Observations on tissue-iron and siderocytes. (*In Japanese*) Jap. J. Vet. Sci. 1939, **1**. 211 (abstr.: V.B. **10**. 421)

771. Ishii, S.: Siderocyte examination in the diagnosis of equine infectious anemia. (*In Japanese*) J. Jap. Vet. Med. Ass. 1950, **3**. 220

772. Ishii, S., Nakamura, N., and Nobuto, K.: Studies on the histopathological changes in the horse suffering from infectious anemia. IV. Several observations on the ovary. (*In Japanese*) Jap. J. Vet. Sci. 1939, **1**. 315 (abstr.: V.B. **10**. 421)

773. Ishii, S., Nobuto, K., and Tanaka, K.: On the histopathological studies of infectious anemia in horses. On the detection of siderocytes in the blood of vena jugularis and its clinical diagnostic value. (*In Japanese*) Jap J. Vet. Sci. 1940, **2**. 531 (abstr.: V.B. **11**. 857)

774. Ishii, S., Tanaka, K., and Sukawa, Y.: On the anemic substance found in serum of horse affected with infectious anemia (Report 1). (*In Japanese*) Report, Government Exper. Station for Animal Hygiene (No. **20**, p. 157). Tokyo, Japan, 1949

775. Ishii, S., Tanaka, K., Taduchi, E., and Ishihara, T.: On the anemic substance found in serum of horse affected with infectious anemia. (Report 2) Several findings demonstrated in diseased horse. (*In Japanese*) Report, Government Exper. Station for Animal Hygiene (No. **20**, p. 181). Tokyo, Japan, 1949

776. Ishii, S., und Watanabe, S.: Ueber das Leukocytenbild bei der ansteckenden Anämie des Pferdes. (*In Japanese*) Mitt. Regierungsinst. Tierseuch. Japan, 1930, **13**. 1 (abstr.: Jber. **50**. 1059)

777. Ishii, S., und Watanabe, S.: Ueber fiebererzeugenden Versuch bei der nichtfiebernden Periode des anämischen Pferdes. (*In Japanese*) Mitt. Regierungsinst. Tierseuch. Japan, 1935, **15**. 147 (abstr.: Jber. **59**. 564)

778. Ishii, S., und Watanabe, S.: Ueber die Blutplättchen beim anämischen Pferde. (*In Japanese*) Mitt. Regierungsinst. Tierseuch. Japan 1935, **15**. 199 (abstr.: Jber. **59**. 564)

779. (Italy): Per lo studio dell'anemia infettiva dei cavalli (in Lombardia). Azione Vet. 1941, **10**. 164

780. Jacobs: Ein Fall von progressiver perniciöser Anämie beim Pferde. Berl. Tier. Woch. **1892**. 145

781. Jaede, P.: Das normale Blutbild des Kaninchens und seine Beeinflussung durch Injektion von Blut von gesunder und anämiekranker Pferde. Diss. Hannover, 1922 (abstr.: Jber. **43**. 184)

782. Jaffé, R. H.: The reticulo-endothelial system in immunity. Physiol. Rev. 1931, **11**. 277

783. Jakob, H.: Die klinischen Erscheinungen der ansteckenden Blutarmut beim Pferde unter besonderer Berücksichtigung der Differentialdiagnose. Münch. Tier. Woch. 1937, **88**. 217

784. Jalkanen, J.: Atypical cases of equine infectious anemia. (*In Finnish*) Suom. Eläinlääkril.-Finsk VetTidskr. 1944, **50**. 57

785. Janott, H.: Klinische, hämatologische und anatomo-histologische Untersuchungen bei Schlachtpferde, unter besonderer Berücksichtigung anämischer Zustände. Diss. Hannover, 1932

786. Jarmatz: Anämie der Pferde. Z. Vet.kunde 1904, **16**. 68

787. Jäschke, W.: Beiträge zur Diagnose der infektiösen Anämie der Pferde. Diss. Hannover, 1923 (abstr.: Jber. **43**. 79)

788. Jaskowski, L.: Observations on artificial insemination of mares as an auxiliary method of the control of infectious anemia in horses. (*In Polish*) Medycyna Wet. (Warsaw) 1951, **7**. 239

789. Jastrzebski, T., et Szymanowski, Z.: L'anémie contagieuse des chevaux. (*In Polish*) Wiad. Weteryn. (Warsaw) 1929, July (abstr.: Bull. Inst. Pasteur **27**. 947)

790. Jensen, H.: Beiträge zur Diagnostik der infektiösen Anämie der Pferde. Diss. Hannover, 1923 (abstr.: Jber. **43**. 79)

791. Jeppsson, B.: Some remarks on infectious anemia of the horse. (*In Swedish*) Skandinaviska Kreatursförsäkringsbolagets Femarsberättelse för Ar 1945. (p. 86) Uppsala, 1945

792. Jerris, H. B. F.: Infectious anemia? Amer. Vet. Rev. 1911, **40**. 245

793. Jirina, K.: Beitrag zum klinischen Bild der infektiösen Anämie. Berl-Münch. Tier. Woch. **1940**. 591

794. de Jong, D. A.: Chronische Anämie bei Pferden. Deut. Z. Tiermed. 1890, **17**. 212

795. Kalikin, B.: Clinical pathology of equine infectious anemia. (*In Croatian*) Jugoslov. Vet. Glasn. 1935, **15**. 531 (abstr.: V.B. **7**. 175)

796. Kamann, H.: Ueber die Beeinflussung des reticulocytären Blutbildes des Kaninchens durch das Virus der infektiösen Anämie der Pferde. Diss. Hannover, 1931

797. Kamp, F.: Untersuchungen über die Auswertung der Erythrozyten von Anämiekaninchen bei der serologischen Diagnose der infektiösen Anämie des Pferdes. Deut. Tier. Woch. 1926, **34**. 659

798. Kanther, H.: Untersuchungen über Beziehungen zwischen Senkungsgeschwindigkeit der Erythrozyten und dem Verhalten des Albumin-Globulin-Gehaltes des Serums sowie der Sublimatprobe bei gesunden und kranken Pferden. Diss. Hannover, 1937 (abstr.: Jber. **62**. 382)

799. Kasai, K., Miura, S., and Ueda, S.: On the simple inactivation of the infectious anemia virus present in immune serum. Jap. J. Vet. Sci. 1943, **5**. 613

800. Kasai, K., Nobata, R., and Ryu, E.: On the incidence of Streptococcus haemolyticus in normal tonsils of horses and the typing of equine tonsilar streptococci. Jap. J. Vet. Sci. 1944, **6**. 116.

801. Katic, R. V.: Ausscheidung und Uebertragung des Virus der infektiösen Anämie der Pferde und ihre Diagnostik im Lichte der neueren Untersuchungen. (*In Serbian*) Jugoslov. Vet. Glasn. 1940, **20**. 92 (abstr.: Jber. **68**. 378)

802. Kaupp, B. F.: A typical blood picture of pernicious anemia. Amer. Vet. Rev. 1911, **38**. 675

803. Keimer, A.: Passageversuche bei durch Phenylhydrazin sensibilisierten und mit Serum gesunder Pferde injizierten Kaninchen. Diss. Hannover, 1938 (abstr.: Jber. **64**. 362)

804. Kettner, K.: Das Verhalten der Erythrozyten und der Normalamboceptoren im Blute gesunder und kranker Pferde, mit besonderer Berücksichtigung der infektiösen Anämie. Diss. Berlin, 1920 (abstr.: Jber. **39-40**. 147)

805. Keweloh, H.: Therapeutische Versuche bei der infektiösen Anämie des Pferdes, angestellt am Kaninchen. Deut. Tier. Woch. 1926, **34**. 172

806. Kickinger, H.: Die Neufassung der Massnahmen zur Bekämpfung der ansteckenden Blutarmut der Einhufer. Deut. Tierärztebl. 1940, **7**. 67

807. Kinsley, A. T.: Infectious equine anemia. Report, Ann. Meeting, U. S. Livestock Sanit. Assoc. Chicago, 1910 (p. 143)

808. Kipfer, F.: Ueber das Blutbild des Kaninchens nach Injektion von normalen Pferdeserum. Ein Beitrag zur Diagnostik der progressiven perniziösen Anämie des Pferdes nach Oppermann. Diss. Bern, 1928 (abstr.: Jber. **48**. 984)

809. Klempin: Braune Atrophie des Hüftdarmes infolge ansteckender Blutarmut. Z. Vet.kunde 1922, **34**. 151

810. Knisely, M., Bloch, E., Brooks, F., and Warner, L.: Microscopic observations of the circulating blood of nine healthy normal horses, all of which had unagglutinated circulating blood cells and high in vitro sedimentation rates. Amer. J. Med. Sci. 1950, **219**. 249

811. Koch, A.: Untersuchungen über die Diagnostik und Therapie der infektiöse Anämie des Pferdes. Diss. Hannover, 1923 (abstr.: Jber. **43**. 78)

812. Koch, E.: Einige Vorversuche zur Vereinfachung der Diagnose der ansteckenden Blutarmut des Pferdes mit Hilfe des Kaninchenimpfversuches. Diss. Hannover, 1938 (abstr.: Jber. **64**. 469)

813. de Kock, G.: Beiträge zur Kenntnis des Erregers, zur Haematologie und pathologischen Anatomie und Histologie der infektiösen Anämie der Pferde, wie sie in Südafrika beobachtet wird. Diss. Bern, 1923 (abstr.: Jber. **44**. 91)

814. de Kock, Fourie, Quin, Mönnig, Graf, and Kellermann: Anaemia in South African domesticated animals. S. African Med. J. 1935, **9**. 443

815. Koher, F.: Untersuchungen über die Konservierung des Virus der infektiösen Anämie des Pferdes im Taubenkörper. Deut. Tier. Woch. 1925, **33**. 824

816. Koljakoff, Pinus, Worozoff, Pirog, und Afanasewa: Material betreffs der experimentellen Infektion kleiner Versuchstiere mit dem Virus der infektiösen Anämie der Pferde. (*In Russian*) Sovyet Vet. 1936, **13**. (No. 11) 24 (abstr.: M.T.W. **88**. 176)

817. König, K.: Die Verbreitung des Virus der infektiösen Anämie des Pferdes im Körper des infizierten Kaninchens. Tierärzt. Rund. 1926, **32**. 568

818. Kornau, H.: Die Diagnose der ansteckenden Blutarmut des Pferdes mit Hilfe des Impfversuches an sensibilisierten Meerschweinchen. Diss. Hannover, 1939 (abstr.: D.T.W. **47**. 393)

819. Korotkikh, A. V.: Epidemiology of equine infectious anemia. (*In Russian*) Veterinariya 1951, **28**. (No. 6) 32 (abstr.: V.B. **23**. 18)

820. Kossmag, M.: Pferdestaupe (Leuma) oder infektiöse Anaemie? Tierärzt. Rund. 1929, **35**. 702

821. Kovác, V.: Is equine infectious anemia transmissible to sheep? (*In Slovakian*) Zverol. Rozpr. 1938, **12**. 253 (abstr.: Zbl. Bakt. I. Ref. **132**. 523)

822. Kovalevskii, M. F.: Therapeutic treatment of equine infectious anemia. (*In Russian*) Veterinariya 1941, **18**. (No. 1) 18 (abstr.: V.B. **12**. 553)

823. Köves, J., und Hoffmann, F.: Wie lange verweilt das eingespritzte Immunserum im Tierkörper. Arch. Tierheilk. 1941, **76**. 173

824. Kowalski, F.: Untersuchungen über die infektiöse Anämie der Pferde. (*In Polish*) Przegl. Wet. (Lwow) 1924, **37.** 165 (abstr.: Jber. **44.** 93)

825. Kozlova, E., et Semenov, M.: L'état physico-chimique du sang des chevaux atteints d'anémie infectieuse. (*In Russian*) Trud. Vsesoyuz. Inst. Eksp. Vet. 1936, **12.** 13 (abstr.: Bull. Off. Intl. Epizoot. **13.** 986)

826. Král, F.: Sur l'anémie infectieuse. (*In Croatian*) Jugoslov. Vet. Glasn. 1932, **12.** 328 (abstr.: Rev. Gén. Méd. Vét. **42.** 558)

827. Krämer, J.: Untersuchungen über die Wirksamkeit der Kupferlösung nach Fischer bei anämischen Kaninchen. Diss. Hannover, 1937

828. Kramolovsky, R.: Beiträge zur Kenntnis der infektiösen Anämie. Diss. Berlin, 1929 (abstr.: D.T.W. **40.** 232)

829. Krause, C.: Betrachtungen über die ansteckende Blutarmut der Einhufer. Tierärzt. Rund. 1941, **47.** 288

830. Kriwinka, und Král: Ueber infektiöse Anämie beim Pferde. Prag. Tierärzt. Arch. 1934, **14.** 17 (abstr.: Jber. **55.** 276)

831. Krukenberg, F.: Therapeutische Versuche bei der infektiösen Anämie der Pferde, angestellt an Kaninchen. Diss. Hannover, 1925 (abstr.: Jber. **45.** 77)

832. Krupski, A.: Weitere Untersuchungen über die Pferde-Anämien. Schweiz. Arch. Tierh. 1931, **73.** 435

833. Krynitz: Perniziöse Anämie. Z. Vet.kunde 1913, **25.** 469

834. Kubes, V.: Estudios preliminares sobre la "derrengadera" y "peste boba" en la región de los Llanos. Ministerio de Agricultura y Cria 1938 (p. 423) Caracas, Venezuela (abstr.: V.B. **11.** 704)

835. Kubes, V.: Estudio acerca de la existencia de la anemia infecciosa de los equinos en la América del Sur. Su presencia en Venezuela y confusión con la trypanosomiasis caballar, las llamadas, "peste boba" y "derrengadera". Ministerio de Agricultura y Cria 1939. Caracas, Venezuela (abstr.: V.B. **11.** 704)

836. Kübitz: Infektiöse Anämie. Z. Vet.kunde 1918, **30.** 433

837. Kudrjaveew: Veränderungen der Hufe bei den mit infektiöser Anämie befallenen Pferden. (*In Russian*) Sovyet Vet. 1938, **15.** (No. 7) 53 (abstr.: Jber. **66.** 49)

838. Kudryashov, M. V., and Troitskii, I. A.: The retraction of the blood clot as a test for equine infectious anemia. (*In Russian*) Trud. Vsesoyuz. Inst. Eksp. Vet. 1940, **15.** 21 (abstr.: V.B. **16.** 145)

839. Kühdorf, H.: Experimentelle Beiträge zu dem vereinfachten Kanincheninfektionsversuch zwecks Diagnose der ansteckenden Blutarmut der Pferde. Diss. Hannover, 1938 (abstr.: D.T.W. **47.** 188)

840. Kuhns, W.: Isoimmunization in the pig following multiple transfusions of incompatible blood. Proc. Soc. Exp. Biol. Med. 1950, **74.** 685

841. Kuhrmeier, H.: Therapeutische Versuche bei der infektiösen Anämie der Pferde. Diss. Hannover, 1925 (abstr.: D.T.W. **34.** 459)

842. Kulakov, G. E.: Presence of the virus of equine infectious anemia in blood of ruminants. (*In Russian*) Trud. Vsesoyuz. Inst. Eksp. Vet. 1940, **15.** 10 (abstr.: V.B. **16.** 145)

843. Kutii, T., Suto, H., Kawaguchi, H., and Kasai, K.: Experimental studies on the superinfection of *Salmonella abortivo-equina* in horses infected with infectious anemia. Jap. J. Vet. Sci. 1946, **8.** 235

844. Laktionov, A. M., Arkhangel'skii, N. D., and Kovalevskii, M. F.: The role of contact in spreading infectious anemia. (*In Russian*) Sovyet Vet. 1938, **15.** (No. 10) 5 (abstr.: Jber. **66.** 535)

845. Lamarre, H., et Boussard, C.: Essais sur le traitement de la typho-anémie infectieuse des équidés par le Stovarsol. Bull. Soc. Vét. Prat. 1929, **13.** 22

846. Lamarre, L. A.: L'anémie infectieuse du cheval. (Recherches cliniques et expérimentales). Thèse, Paris, 1933 (abstr.: Jber. **54.** 273)

847. Lamarre, L.: Contribution à l'étude de l'anémie infectieuse du cheval. Rec. Méd. Vét. 1933, **109.** 269

848. Lamarre, L.: L'anémie infectieuse du cheval en Haute-Marne. Rev. Path. Comp. 1950, **50**. 728

849. Langenheim, K.: Ueber die Spezifität der Veränderung des Kaninchenblutbildes durch das Virus der infektiösen Anämie. Diss. Hannover, 1925 (abstr.: Tier. Rund. **32**. 366)

850. Larsson, E.: Epizootic anemia of horses and its control. (*In Swedish*) Svensk VetTidskr. 1930, **35**. 180

851. Larsson, E.: Statistics on infectious anemia in the Torps district. (*In Swedish*) Svensk VetTidskr. 1935, **40**. 159

852. Larsson, E.: Beobachtungen bei der infektiösen Anämie der Pferde. Tierärzt. Mitt. 1937, **18**. 655

853. Lauda, E.: Weitere Beiträge zur infektiösen Anämie der Ratte. Zbl. Bakt. I. Orig. 1926, **98**. 522

854. Launois, M. A.: Contribution à l'étude de l'anémie infectieuse du cheval. Thèse, Paris, 1931 (abstr.: Jber. **51**. 1052)

855. Laurencik, P.: Beitrag über die Verbreitung und Bekämpfung der infektiösen Anämie in der Slowakei. Diss. Vienna, 1944 (abstr.: Tier. Rund. **1944**. 244)

856. Law, J.: Textbook of Veterinary Medicine (Vol. **1**, p. 375, Progressive pernicious anaemia or idiopathic anaemia). Ithaca, New York, 1896

857. Leduc, M. E.: Sur un cas de typho-anémie. Bull. Soc. Vét. Prat. 1934, **18**. 198

858. Lehnert, E.: Infektiöse Anämie, ansteckende Blutarmut, beim Pferde. Skandinaviska Kreatursförsäkringsbolaget. Bericht über die fünfunddreissigjährige Tätigkeit der Gesellschaft, 1890-1925 (p. 101) Stockholm, 1925

859. Lehnert, E.: Infectious anemia in the horse. (*In Swedish*) Skandinaviska Kreatursförsäkringsbolaget. Berättelse över bolagets fyrtioarige verksamhet, 1890-1930 (Vol. **2**. p. 46) Stockholm, 1930

860. Lehnert, E.: Ein Beitrag zur Kenntnis der Bluttypen des Pferdes mit Hilfe arteigener, hochwertiger, gruppenspezifischer Isoimmunsera. Uppsala, Sweden, 1939

861. Lehnert, E., and Svensson, S.: The iron percentage of horse blood, especially with respect to infectious anemia in horses. (*In Swedish*) Skand. VetTidskr. 1932, **22**. 21

862. Lemétayer, E.: Recherches sur l'anémie infectieuse expérimentale des équidés. Report, 14th International Vet. Congress in London, 1949 (Vol. **2**. p. 322) London, 1952

863. Lemétayer, E., Nicol, L., Gorard, O., et Corvazier, R.: Variations pondérales dans l'anémie infectieuse des équidés. Bull. Acad. Vét. France 1946, **19**. 276

864. Lerner, J.: Beiträge zur Epidemiologie der ansteckenden Blutarmut der Pferde im Saargebiet. Diss. Hannover, 1933 (abstr.: Jber. **54**. 359)

865. Lestoquard, F., et Ekrem, I.: L'anémie pernicieuse des petits ruminants en Turquie. Rev. Vét. Toulouse 1932, **84**. 11

866. Lgovski, A.: Equine infectious anemia: its genesis, development, and prevention. (*In Russian*) Veterinariya 1949, **26**. (No. 12) 17 (abstr.: V.B. **22**. 186)

867. Lier, A.: Untersuchung über die Wirksamkeit des Präparates 750 D 1 bei der infektiösen Anämie des Pferdes. Tierärzt. Rund. 1926, **32**. 538.

868. Lignières, J.: A propos de la typho-anémie et des pasteurelloses. Bull. Soc. Centr. Méd. Vét. 1908, **62**. 187

869. Lindqvist, C. A.: Case of pernicious anemia in animals. (*In Swedish*) Tidskr. Vet. Med. 1888, **7**. 39

870. Live, I., Sperling, F. G., and Stubbs, E. L.: Further studies on the allergic activity of sonic filtrate of *Brucella abortus*. Vet. Ext. Quart, Univ. Pennsylvania 1946, No. 102, p. 3

871. Lorscheid: Zwei Fälle von perniziöser Anämie bei Militärpferden. Deut. Tier. Woch. 1916, **24**. 419

872. Lübke, A.: Die Bedeutung der Resistenzprüfung für Diagnostik der infektiösen Anämie. Deut. Tier. Woch. 1948, **55**. 65

873. Lucas, A.: Germes de sortie dans l'anémie infectieuse du cheval. Rec. Méd. Vét. 1950, **126**. 595

874. Lückmann, A.: Beiträge zur klinischen Diagnose chronischer Anämien bei Pferden. Diss. Hannover, 1930 (abstr.: Jber. **50.** 1060)

875. Ludewig, J.: Beitrag zum Verhalten der Gitterfasern des Pferdes unter spezieller Berücksichtigung der infektiösen Anämie. Diss. Hannover, 1935 (abstr.: Jber. **57.** 551)

876. Ludwig, H.: Wismutbehandlung bei ansteckender Blutarmut der Pferde. Berl. Tier. Woch. 1925, **41.** 650

877. Ludwig: Ueber Erschöpfungskrankheiten der Pferde unter besonderer Berücksichtigung der infektiösen Anämie. Deut. Tier. Woch. 1947, **54.** 41; 1948, **55.** 218

878. Lührs: Wissenschaftliche Kriegserfahrungen in der Tierseuchen Bekämpfung. 3. Die ansteckende Blutarmut der Pferde. Z. Vet.kunde 1920, **32.** 185

879. Lührs: Die Erkennung der ansteckenden Blutarmut der Pferde. Mitt. Deut. Landw. Ges. 1922, **37.** 263

880. Lührs: Ansteckende Blutarmut. Z. Vet.kunde 1922, **34.** 329

881. Lührs: Die Diagnose der ansteckenden Blutarmut nach Oppermann. Veterinärdienst 1924, (Jan.-Feb.) 143

882. Lührs: Tätigkeitsbericht des Heeres-Veterinär-Untersuchungsamtes für das Jahr 1924. Z. Vet.kunde 1925, **37.** 201

883. Lukin, J. B., and Semenov, V. V.: Diagnostic value of clinical symptoms in infectious anemia of horses. (*In Russian*) Sovyet Vet. 1938, **15.** (No. 10) 11 (abstr.: Jber. **66.** 272)

884. Lutsch, E.: Untersuchungen über das Vorkommen von histologischen Veränderungen der infektiösen Anämie in der Leber von Schlachtpferden aus Luxemburg. Diss. Hannover, 1942 (abstr.: D.T.W. **51.** 177)

885. Lutsch, E.: Die Sternzellenhämosiderose in der Leber bei Schlachtpferden aus Luxemburg. Arch. Tierheilk. 1943, **78.** 316

886. Mack, W. B.: A fatal anemic disease among horses. Proc. Amer. Vet. Med. Assoc. 1909 (p. 307). Philadelphia, 1910

887. Mack, W. B.: Equine anemia investigations in Nevada. A clinical study. Report, Ann. Meeting U. S. Livestock Sanit. Assoc. in Chicago, 1910 (p. 137) Chicago

888. Mack, W. B.: Intracellular bodies associated with equine anemia. Proc. Amer. Vet. Med. Assoc. 1911 (p. 378) Lansing, Michigan, 1911

889. Manninger, R.: Fertözési kisérletek a lovak fertözö kevésvérüségének ragályanyagával. (Experimental infection of horses with the virus of equine infectious anemia.) (*In Hungarian*) Állatorv. Lapok 1938, **61.** 341 (abstr.: V.B. **10.** 173)

890. Mantovani, G.: Contributo alla conoscenza del reperto anatomoistopatologico nella anemia infettiva del cavallo. Progresso Vet. (Torino) 1948, (No. 6) 91

891. Marbach, H.: Rectale Infektion des Kaninchens mit dem Virus der infektiösen Anämie der Pferde. Diss. Hannover, 1924 (abstr.: Tier. Rund. **32.** 413)

892. Marcato, A.: Le lesioni anatomoistopatologiche dell'anemia infettiva degli asini in Eritrea. Azione Vet. 1937, **6.** 144; Studio anatomoistopatologico su di un focolaio di anemia infettiva dell'asino in Eritrea. Nuova Vet. 1938, **16.** 227

893. Margalowski, G.: Beiträge zur Prophylaxe und Therapie der infektiösen Anämie des Pferdes. Diss. Hannover, 1924 (abstr.: Jber. **44.** 92)

894. Martin, A. D.: Equine infectious anemia. Vet. Bull. of U. S. Army 1933, **27.** 246

895. Mayer, A.: Ueber die Resistenz der Erythrozyten unter Berücksichtigung der Zahl der Leukozyten bei verschiedenen Krankheiten der Pferde. Monat. Tierheilk. 1913, **24.** 554

896. McGilvray, C. D.: Rarer forms of fever in horses. Report, Ann. Meeting Veterinary Assoc. Manitoba (p. 23) Winnipeg, Canada, 1910

897. Meier, H.: Gibt es eine ansteckende Virusanämie der Pferde in der Schweiz? Schweiz. Z. Path. 1945, **8.** 1

898. Mench, K.: Lymphadenose bei einem Pferde. (Ein Beitrag zur Differentialdiagnose bei ansteckender Blutarmut.) Berl. Tier. Woch. 1935, **51.** 467

899. Mench, K.: Maligne Endotheliome in der Milz eines Pferdes. (Ein Beitrag zur Differentialdiagnose bei ansteckender Blutarmut der Einhufer) Berl. Tier. Woch. 1936, **52.** 4

900. Mench, K.: Ueber ansteckende Blutarmut. Berl. Tier. Woch. 1936, **52.** 261

901. Merk, M.: Untersuchungen über fortschreitende, bösartige Blutarmut des Pferdes, unter besonderer Berücksichtigung der Erkrankung in der Ostschweiz. Schweiz. Arch. Tierh. 1923, **65.** 469

902. Metz: Zur perniziösen Anämie der Pferde. Z. Vet.kunde 1916, **28.** 381

903. Metzger: Die perniciöse Anämie des Pferdes. Mitt Ver. Bad. Tierärzte 1912, **12.** 165

904. Meyer, B.: Untersuchungen über das Vorkommen der ansteckenden Blutarmut bei Schlachtpferden aus dem Saarland. Diss. Hannover, 1939 (abstr.: D.T.W. **47.** 485)

905. Meyer, E.: Die infektiöse Anämie auf der Herrschaft Heinrichau. Ein Beitrag zur Epidemiologie und Klinik der Seuche. Diss. Hannover, 1924 (abstr.: D.T.W. **32.** 512)

906. Meyer, G.: Der Siderozytengehalt der Leber bei Anämiepferden. Diss. Hannover, 1924 (abstr.: D.T.W. **32.** 566)

907. Meyer, H.: Uebertragungsversuche der infektiösen Anämie der Pferde auf Hunde. Diss. Hannover, 1925 (abstr.: D.T.W. **34.** 809)

908. Meyer, H.: Untersuchungen über den diagnostischen Wert der Sublimatprobe nach Horgan, Bennett und Kenny bei der infektiösen Anämie der Pferde. Diss. Hannover, 1931

909. Meyer, H.: Haben sich die vom Oberkommando des Heeres am 21.12.1936 zur Bekämpfung der ansteckenden Blutarmut der Pferde erlassenen Bestimmungen als ausreichend zur Tilgung der Seuche innerhalb der Wehrmacht erwiesen? Diss. Berlin, 1938 (abstr.: D.T.W. **47.** 561)

910. Miégeville, M.: Contribution à l'étude de l'anémie infectieuse des équidés au Maroc. Rev. Vét. Toulouse 1927, **79.** 239

911. Miura, S., Kutii, T., Shionoya, K., and Ueda, S.: Experimental studies on the simple inactivation of infectious anemia virus present in the horse serum. Jap. J. Vet. Sci. 1947, **9.** 87, 113

912. Miyagawa, F., und Nakamura, N.: Ueber die Verwendbarkeit der Senkungsgeschwindigkeit für die Diagnose der ansteckenden Blutarmut beim Pferde. (*In Japanese*) Mitt. Regierungsinst. Tierseuch. Japan 1930, **13.** 77 (abstr.: Jber. **50.** 1059)

913. Mócsy, J.: Adatok a lovak fertözö anaemiája ragályanyagának ismeretéhez. (About the nature of the virus of equine infectious anemia.) (*In Hungarian*) Állatorv. Lapok 1937, **60.** 406 (abstr.: D.T.W. **46.** 153)

914. Mohler, J. R.: Infectious anemia or swamp fever of horses. Circular No. 138, Bureau of Animal Industry, U. S. Dept. Agric. Washington, 1909

915. Möhling, H.: Der Einfluss der Trabprobe auf Herz und Puls bei gesunden und kranken Pferden mit besonderer Berücksichtigung der infektiösen Anämie. Diss. Hannover, 1933 (abstr.: Jber. **57.** 90)

916. Mönkemeier, A.: Weitere vergleichende Untersuchungen über die Vereinfachung des Kaninchenversuches für die Diagnose der ansteckenden Blutarmut des Pferdes. Diss. Hannover, 1937 (abstr.: Jber. **63.** 470)

917. Moretti, B.: Klinisches Bild der infektiösen Anämie in einem Fall von Tuberkulose des Pferdes. Wien. Tier. Monat. 1941, **28.** 183

918. Moretti, B.: Osservazioni cliniche sull'anemia infettiva del cavallo. Nuova Vet. 1941, **20.** 51

919. Morot-Sir et Rossi: Typho-anémie infectieuse du cheval et traitement par le Stovarsol sodique. Bull. Soc. Sci. Vét. Lyon 1932, **35.** 119

920. Mossdorf, H.: Beiträge zur Biologie des Virus der infektiösen Anämie des Pferdes. Diss. Hannover, 1923 (abstr.: Jber. **43.** 30)

921. Moszczenski, Z.: Zur Frage der Spezifität der histopathologischen Veränderungen der Leber bei infektiöser Anämie. Diss. Zürich, 1943

922. Mrowka, F.: Die normale Milz des Pferdes und ihre pathologischen Veränderungen bei chronischer infektiöser Anämie. Z.Vet.kunde 1919, **31**. 49

923. Mrowka, F.: Ein weiterer Beitrag zur Pathogenese der infektiösen Anämie des Pferdes. V. Mitteilung. Arch. Tierheilk. 1937, **71**. 364

924. Mukhachev, A. V., and Yakimov, N. N.: Control of equine infectious anemia according to the method described by Boshyan. (*In Russian*) Veterinariya 1951, **28**. (No. 8) 36 (abstr.: V.B. **23**. 18)

925. Muller, E.: A propos de quelques cas de typho-anémie observée dans une clientele du département de la Moselle. Thèse, Paris, 1930 (abstr.: Jber. **50**. 1059)

926. Müller, W.: Kriegsveterinärbericht des deutschen Heeres 1914-1918. Das Pferd im Kriege. Berl. Tier. Woch. 1930, **46**. 983

927. Muratov, S. I.: Differential diagnosis of equine infectious anemia and piroplasmosis. (*In Russian*) Veterinariya 1944, **21**. (No. 11-12) 32 (abstr.: V.B. **17**. 535)

928. Müssemeier: Die Anämie der Pferde und ihre Verbreitung in Preussen. Mitt. Deut. Landw. Ges. 1922, **37**. 262

929. Mutelet, E.: Etiologie de l'anémie essentielle du cheval. Bull. Soc. Centr. Méd. Vét. 1896, **14**. 523

930. Nagao, M.: Die statistischen Beobachtungen über die Inkubationsstadien und den Verlauf bei der infektiösen Blutarmut der Pferde. (*In Japanese*) J. Jap. Soc. Vet. Sci. 1923, **2**. 101 (abstr.: Jber. **43**. 82)

931. Nakamura, N.: Equine infectious anemia. (*In Japanese*) J. Cent. Soc. Vet. Med. Tokyo 1938, **50**. Suppl. p. 75

932. Nakamura, N., Ishii, S., and Watanabe, S.: The virus of equine infectious anemia. I. Distribution in the organs of afebrile patients. J. Jap. Soc. Vet. Sci. 1938, **17**. (No. 3) 50

933. Nakamura, N., Ishii, S., and Watanabe, S.: Histopathology of equine infectious anemia. I. Brain and spinal cord. 2. Testis. J. Jap. Soc. Vet. Sci. 1938, **17**. (No. 3) 64

934. Nakamura, N., Matsuba, S., Kawamura, Y., und Miyagawa, F.: Ueber die Oppermannsche Reaktion für die Diagnose der infektiösen Anämie des Pferdes. (*In Japanese*) Mitt. Regierungsinst. Tierseuch. Japan 1930, **13**. 125 (abstr.: Jber. **50**. 1060)

935. Nakamura, N., und Miyagawa, F.: Ueber die Resistenz der roten Blutkörperchen bei der ansteckenden Anämie der Pferde. (*In Japanese*) Mitt. Regierungsinst. Tierseuch. Japan 1930, **13**. 99 (abstr.: Jber. **50**. 1059)

936. Nakamura, N., Miyagawa, F., und Watanabe, S.: Ueber den hemmenden Einfluss des anämischen Pferdeserums auf die Rinderhämolysinwirkung. (*In Japanese*) Mitt. Regierungsinst. Tierseuch. Japan 1930, **13**. 147 (abstr.: Jber. **50**. 1059)

937. Namikawa, S., Nakayama, T., Suto, H., and Kasai, K.: Experimental studies on equine paratyphoid due to *Salmonella abortivo-equina*. II. On the influence of association with infectious anemia upon the Salmonella infection. Jap. J. Vet. Sci. 1943, **5**. 371 (abstr.: Biol. Abstr. **25**. (No. 8) 27)

938. Natscheff, B.: Klinische Untersuchungen über die Gastrophiliase der Pferde. Tierärzt. Rund. **1938**. 85

939. Nemec, W.: Untersuchungen über das Vorkommen der infektiösen Anämie in der Ostmark mit einem vergleichenden histologischen Beitrag zur Diagnose. Berl.-Münch. Tier. Woch. **1939**. 689

940. Neser, C. P.: The blood of equines. 9th and 10th Report, Director Vet. Research, Dept. Agric. South Africa (p. 481) Pretoria, 1924

941. Neumann-Kleinpaul, K.: Anämie beim Pferde. Tierärzt. Rund. 1934, **40**. 862

942. Neumann-Kleinpaul, K., und Weyers, H.: Ueber die Erythrocytensenkung als diagnostisches und prognostisches Hilfsmittel bei verschiedenen inneren Erkrankungen des Pferdes. Arch. Tierheilk. 1937, **71**. 91

943. Neuwerth, K.: Infektionsversuche beim Meerschweinchen mit Virus der infektiösen Anämie der Pferde. Deut. Tier. Woch. 1925, **33**. 285

944. (New England): "Swamp fever" epizootic. Infectious anemia outbreak perils thoroughbred industry. (Editorials) J. Amer. Vet. Med. Ass. 1947, **111.** 303, 366

945. Nichols, R. E.: A study of the phenomenon of erythrocyte sedimentation. I-IV. J. Lab. Clin. Med. 1942, **27.** 1317, 1410, 1569; 1942, **28.** 75.

946. Nickel, C. C.: Infectious anemia. North Amer. Vet. 1930, **11.** (No. 7) 23

947. Nicol: Ein Fall von infektiöser Anämie bei einem Pferde. Deut. Tier. Woch. 1918, **26.** 49

948. Niemeyer, W.: Vermag das Präparat "Haemosal" den erythropoetischen Apparat bei mit infektiöser Anämie behafteten Pferden zu beeinflussen? Diss. Hannover, 1931 (abstr.: Jber. **51.** 1054)

949. Niendick, F.: Beiträge zur Diagnose der infektiösen Anämie der Pferde mit Hilfe des Tauben- und Hühnerversuches. Diss. Hannover, 1931 (abstr.: Jber. **51.** 1054)

950. Nobis, J.: Einleitende Untersuchungen über den Wert des vereinfachten Kaninchenimpfversuchs für die Differentialdiagnose der ansteckenden Blutarmut der Pferde. Diss. Hannover, 1937 (abstr.: Jber. **63.** 384)

951. Nörr, J.: Pulsbefunde bei infektiöser Anämie und symptomatischer Anämie der Pferde. Z. Infekt. Haustiere 1925, **28.** 1

952. Norton, O. M.: A practitioner's view of swamp fever. Amer. J. Vet. Med. 1911, **6.** 672

953. Obladen: Ueber einige Fälle von perniziöser Anämie. Deut. Tier. Woch. 1917, **25.** 91

954. Oellerich: Epidemiologisches über die ansteckende Blutarmut. Berl. Tier. Woch. 1935, **51.** 712

955. Oellerich: Ansteckende Blutarmut der Pferde. Deut. Tier. Woch. 1937, **45.** 23

956. (Office International des Epizooties, Paris): Décret ajoutant l'anémie infectieuse des équidés à la liste des maladies réputées légalement contagieuses. Bull. Off. Intl. Epizoot. 1936, **13.** 109

957. Okamura, H.: Biochemical studies of infectious anemia in horses. VIII. Residual nitrogen of blood in anemic horses. (*In Japanese*) J. Cent. Soc. Vet. Med. Tokyo 1937, **50.** 811

958. Okuntsov, I. V.: Differential diagnosis of infectious anemia, nuttalliosis and piroplasmosis in the horse. (*In Russian*) Sovyet Vet. 1939, **16.** (No. 10-11) 46 (abstr.: V.B. **12.** 347)

959. Oltmanns, H.: Untersuchungen über die Konservierung des Virus der infektiösen Anämie des Pferdes im Körper kleiner Versuchstiere. Diss. Hannover, 1923 (abstr.: Jber. **43.** 78)

960. Oppermann: Ziele und Wege der neueren Forschungsarbeiten über die infektiöse Anämie des Pferdes. Arch. Tierheilk. 1924, **51.** 260

961. Oppermann: Reflexionen über den Pferdeinfektionsversuch zur Diagnose der infektiösen Anämie. Deut. Tier. Woch. 1929, **37.** 115

962. Oppermann: Antikritisches zum Thema: Reflexionen über den Pferdeinfektionsversuch zur Diagnose der infektiösen Anämie. Deut. Tier. Woch. 1929, **37.** 343

963. Oppermann, T.: Die diagnostische Auswertung der Sublimatprobe (nach Bennett, Horgan, Kenny bzw. Fulton) bei der ansteckenden Blutarmut der Pferde. Arch. Tierheilk. 1933, **66.** 485

964. Oppermann, T.: Epikritische Betrachtungen über die klinische Diagnose der ansteckenden Blutarmut der Pferde. Deut. Tier. Woch. 1933, **41.** 353

965. Oppermann, T.: Untersuchungen über die ansteckende Blutarmut der Pferde. Deut. Tier. Woch. 1934, **42.** 495

966. Oppermann, T.: Anämische Blutbefunde bei sporadischen Krankheiten der Pferde. Deut. Tier. Woch. 1934, 42. 595

967. Oppermann, T.: Grundsätzliches zur Beurteilung des Kanincheninfektionsversuches und der Sublimatprobe bei der Diagnose der ansteckenden Blutarmut der Pferde. Arch. Tierheilk. 1935, **70.** 52

968. Oppermann, T.: Schwierigkeit bei der Diagnose der ansteckenden Blutarmut der Pferde. Deut. Tier. Woch. 1936, **44.** 169

969. Oppermann, T.: Diagnostische, therapeutische und forensische Gesichtspunkte bei heimischen Viruskrankheiten der Pferde. Deut. Tier. Woch. 1939, **47.** 369

970. Oppermann, T.: Ein Beitrag zur Differentialdiagnose der ansteckenden Blutarmut der Einhufer. Deut. Tier. Woch. 1939, **47.** 418

971. Oppermann, T.: Der Wert des Tierversuches für die Diagnose der ansteckenden Blutarmut der Einhufer. Deut. Tier. Woch. 1943, **51.** 21

972. Oppermann und Lauterbach: Die Diagnose der infektiösen Anämie des Pferdes mit Hilfe des Hühnerversuches. Deut. Tier. Woch. 1928, **36.** Festschrift der Tierärztlichen Hochschule Hannover, p. 61

973. Oppermann, T., und Oppermann, M.: Ueber die Symptomatologie der chronischen und latenten Form der ansteckenden Blutarmut der Einhufer. Deut. Tier. Woch. 1943, **51.** 130

974. Orlov, F. M.: Susceptibility of geese and ducks to the virus of equine infectious anemia. (*In Russian*) Sovyet Vet. 1940, **17.** (No. 6) 20 (abstr.: V.B. **13.** 16)

975. Otterich, E.: Ein interessanter Fall von infektiöser Anämie. Münch. Tier. Woch. 1922, **73.** 601

976. Pallaske, G.: Beitrag zur Diagnostik der infektiösen Anämie der Pferde mittels des Kaninchenübertragungsversuches. Diss. Leipzig, 1924 (abstr.: Jber. **44.** 94)

977. Pallaske, G.: Untersuchungen über das Vorkommen von Veränderungen der ansteckenden Blutarmut an Organen von Schlachtpferden der Grenz- und Neumark. (Beitrag zur Frage der Verbreitung der ansteckenden Blutarmut in Deutschland.) Z. Infekt. Haustiere 1940, **56.** 25

978. Palló, P.: Zur Diagnose der infektiösen Anämie der Pferde durch den Meerschweincheninfektionsversuch. Diss. Wien, 1926 (abstr.: Wien. Tier. Monat. **14.** 106)

979. Panisset, L.: La typho-anémie infectieuse du cheval. Rev. Zootechn. 1931, **10.** (No. 8) 73

980. Panisset, L.: Traité des Maladies Infectieuses des Animaux Domestiques (tome **1.** p. 181). Paris, 1938

981. Panisset, L., et Lamarre: Etude clinique, hématologique et anatomo-pathologique d'un cas de typho-anémie infectieuse du cheval. Cahiers Méd. Vét. 1932, **2.** 201

982. Panisset, L., et Pflieger, C.: Le rythme quotidien de la température dans l'anémie infectieuse du cheval. Bull. Acad. Vét. France 1936, **9.** 299

983. Panisset, M.: Historique et répartition géographique de l'anémie infectieuse des équidés au Canada. Cahiers Méd. Vét. 1937, **7.** 136

984. Parnes, J.: Beitrag zur Vielgestaltigkeit des klinischen Bildes der infektiösen Anämie der Pferde. Tierärzt. Rund. 1938, **44.** 473

985. Patriat, Rossi, et Vitu: Observations cliniques, hématologiques et anatomo-pathologiques de quelques cas de typho-anémie infectieuse du cheval. Bull. Soc. Sci. Vét. Lyon 1933, **36.** 250

986. Paul, J. R.: Infectious mononucleosis. Bull. New York Acad. Med. 1939, **15.** 43

987. Paulsen, J.: Untersuchungen über die prophylaktische Wirkung von "Bayer 205" bei der infektiösen Anämie der Pferde. Diss. Hannover, 1923 (abstr.: Jber. **43.** 81)

988. Payard, H.: Lésions oculaires sur un poulain atteint de typho-anémie. Rev. Path. Comp. 1938, **38.** 469

989. Payard, L. A.: Essai sur la typho-anémie infectieuse du cheval, dans la région de la Marne limitrophe de la Meuse. Diss. Alfort, 1926 (abstr.: Jber. **46.** 1064)

990. Penning, C. A.: Anaemia perniciosa infectiosa oder Surra bei Pferden in Niederländisch-Indien. (*In Dutch*) Veeartsenijkund. Blad. Nederl.-Indie 1899, **12.** 123 (abstr.: Jber. **21.** 88)

991. Penning, C. A.: Weitere Beobachtungen von Surra in Niederländisch-Indien. (*In Dutch*) Veeartsenijkund. Blad. Nederl.-Indie 1900, **13.** 25 (abstr.: Jber. **21.** 88)

992. Peters, A. T.: Malarial fever in horses. Press Bull. No. 22, Nebraska Agric. Exper. Station, Univ. Nebraska. Lincoln, 1906

993. Peters, J. T.: L'anémie infectieuse du cheval chez l'homme. Presse Méd. 1924, **32.** 105

994. Peters, J. T.: Ueber die Anaemia infectiosa chronica. Wien. Klin. Woch. 1928, **41.** 1741

995. Peters, T.: Weitere Beiträge zur Diagnose der ansteckenden Blutarmut der Pferde mit Hilfe des Kaninchenversuches. Diss. Hannover, 1937 (abstr.: Jber. **62.** 381)

996. Peters, W., und Bernard, M.: Das Meerschweinchen als Versuchstier für die Erkennung der ansteckenden Blutarmut. Arch. Tierheilk. 1926, **54.** 111

997. Petropavlovskii, V. P., Morev, V. I., and Semaev, V. A.: Electrolytic resistance of erythrocytes in equine infectious anemia. (*In Russian*) Trud. XV Plen. Vet. Sekt. Akad. Sel'khoz. Nauk, Moscow 1939 (Diseases of Horses) p. 17 (abstr.: V.B. **15.** 323)

998. Pfandler, L.: Untersuchungen mit der Sublimat-Serumprobe. Diss. Wien, 1936 (abstr.: Wien. Tier. Monat. **23.** 715)

999. Pfeil, C.: Beiträge zur Therapie der infektiösen Anämie des Pferdes. Diss. Hannover, 1925 (abstr.: Jber. **45.** 78)

1000. Pfeiler: Ansteckende Blutarmut der Pferde. Mitt. Deut. Landw. Ges. 1923, **38.** 391

1001. Pflieger, et Carpentier: Une épizootie d'anémie infectieuse sur les chevaux de la place de Belfort. Rev. Vét. Milit. 1936, **20.** 263

1002. Pieritz, B.: Elektive, durch das Virus der infektiösen Pferdeanamie bedingte Reizvorgänge im retikulozytären Blutbilde des Kaninchens. Diss. Hannover, 1931 (abstr.: Jber. **51.** 1054)

1003. Piérot, M.: Le rôle de l'eau dans la typho-anémie. Rev. Gén. Méd. Vét. 1935, **44.** 193

1004. Piérot, M.: Quelques remarques sur la typho-anémie. Ses rapports avec l'anémie infectieuse. Rev. Gén. Méd. Vét. 1936, **45.** 141

1005. Piérot, M.: Le bacille coli et la typho-anémie. Rev. Path. Comp. 1937, **37.** 345

1006. Piérot, M.: Si l'anémie infectieuse est une polynucléose, la typho-anémie est une lymphocytose. Rev. Path. Comp. 1937, **37.** 591

1007. Piérot: Du rôle de la rate dans la typho-anémie. Rev. Path. Comp. 1939, **39.** 173

1008. Pinus, A. A.: Die Punktion der Niere als Methode zum Studium der Pathogenese der infektiösen Anämie der Pferde. (*In Russian*) Sovyet Vet. 1938, **15.** (No. 1) 23 (abstr.: B.M.T.W. **1939,** 235)

1009. Pirog, P. P., and Vorontsov, S. M.: The value of pathological and histological diagnosis in equine infectious anemia. (*In Russian*) Trud. XV Plen Vet. Sekt. Akad. Sel'khoz. Nauk, Moscow 1939 (Diseases of Horses) p. 23, 1941 (abstr.: V.B. **15.** 78)

1010. v. Pirquet, C., und Schick, B.: Ueberempfindlichkeit und beschleunigte Reaktion. Münch. Med. Woch. 1906, **53.** 66

1011. Plote, H.: Beeinflussung des histologischen Blutbildes des Kaninchens durch Serum von anämiekranken Pferden. Diss. Hannover, 1924 (abstr.: Jber. **44.** 94)

1012. Pohle, J.: Beitrag zur Therapie der chronischen Form der infektiösen Anämie der Pferde. Diss. Hannover, 1932 (abstr.: D.T.W. **42.** 280)

1013. Polac, G.: Untersuchungen über die Beeinflussung des klinischen Befundes sowie des Blutbildes bei an ansteckender Blutarmut erkrankten Pferden durch Plastoserum-Präparate. Diss. Hannover 1936 (abstr.: D.T.W. **45.** 727)

1014. Preller, W.: Die sanitätspolizeiliche Beurteilung der infektiösen Anämie. Z. Fleisch Milchhyg. 1925, **35.** 196

1015. Presser, H.: Der Wert des Kaninchenimpfversuches für die Epidemiologie der ansteckenden Blutarmut der Pferde. Diss. Hannover, 1937 (abstr.: Jber. **62.** 382)

1016. Priebe, K.: Studien über die Beeinflussung des histologischen Blutbildes des Kaninchens durch wiederholte Injektion von Serum infektiös-anämiekranker Pferde. Diss. Hannover, 1925 (abstr.: Jber. **45.** 78)

1017. Protasov, A. I.: Differential diagnosis of equine infectious anemia and purulent hepatitis. (*In Russian*) Sovyet Vet. 1939, **16.** (No. 2) 19 (abstr.: Jber. **66.** 188)

1018. (Prussia): Ansteckende Anämie. Veröff. Jber. Beamt. Tierärzt. Preuss. für 1904 (II Teil, S. 37)

1019. (Prussia): Infektiöse Anämie der Pferde. Veröff. Jber. Beamt. Tierärzt. Preuss. für 1906 (II. Teil, S. 26)

1020. (Prussia): Die ansteckende Blutarmut der Pferde. Veröff. Jber. Beamt. Tierärzt. Preuss. für 1919 (II Teil, S. 2)

1021. (Prussia): Ansteckende Blutarmut. Deut. Tier. Woch. 1924, **32.** 746

1022. (Prussia): Ansteckende Blutarmut. Minist.bl. Preuss. Verw. Landw. 1926, **22.** (No. 2) 15

1023. (Prussia): Neue Bestimmungen betr. ansteckende Blutarmut in Preussen. Berl. Tier. Woch. 1934, **50.** 490

1024. (Prussia): Circulaire du Ministre de l'Agriculture concernant l'anémie contagieuse des équidés. Bull. Off. Intl. Epizoot. 1935, **11.** 353

1025. (Prussia): Blutuntersuchungen bei ansteckender Blutarmut der Einhufer. Deut. Tier. Woch. 1937, **45.** 383

1026. Quabeck, L.: Ueber das Vorkommen pathologisch-histologischer Veränderungen der infektiösen Anämie in der Leber von Schlachtpferden aus den anämiefreien Regierungsbezirken Köln und Aachen. Diss. Hanover, 1939 (abstr.: D.T.W. **47.** 482)

1027. Quentin: Recherches cliniques sur la typho-anémie infectieuse des équidés. Essais de "vaccination". Rev. Gén. Méd. Vét. 1933, **42.** 321

1028. Quentin, M.: Anémie infectieuse des équidés. Report, 14th International Veterinary Congress in London, 1949 (vol. **2.** p. 329) London, 1952

1029. Radomski, W.: Infectious anemia of horses in Czechoslovakia. (*In Polish*) Medycyna Wet. (Warsaw) 1951, **7.** 115

1030. Rasch: Beobachtungen bei der Feststellung der infektiösen Anämie der Einhufer. (Vortrag) Deut. Tier. Woch. 1937, **45.** 359; Tierärzt. Rund. 1937, **43.** 414

1031. Rastegaeva, A. M., Sirotkin, V. A., and Artemova, A. I.: The diagnosis of equine infectious anemia in artificially infected laboratory animals. (*In Russian*) Sovyet Vet. 1939, **16.** (No. 7) 31 (abstr.: V.B. **12.** 445)

1031a. Recherches sur l'anémie infectieuse expérimentale du cheval. (*Anonymous author.*) Bull. Acad. Vét. France 1936, **9.** 280

1032. Reinhardt, R.: Klinische und pathologisch-anatomische Beobachtungen bei der infektiösen Anämie der Pferde. Monat. Tierheilk. 1919, **29.** 526

1033. Reinhardt, R.: Infektiöse Anämie und infektiöse Bronchopneumonie. Berl. Tier. Woch. 1920, **36.** 174

1034. Reppin: Beobachtungen bei der Feststellung der infektiösen Anämie der Einhufer. (Vortrag) Deut. Tier. Woch. 1937, **45.** 360

1035. Richter, O.: Untersuchungen über die Auswertung der Erythrocyten von Kaninchen bei der serologischen Diagnose der infektiösen Anämie des Pferdes. Diss Hannover, 1924 (abstr.: Jber. **46.** 1063)

1036. Richters: Vergleichende Untersuchungen chemischer Desinfektionsmittel in ihrer Bedeutung für Rotz, Druse, Milzbrand und ansteckende Blutarmut der Pferde. Z. Vet.kunde 1927, **39.** 401

1037. Richters: Die Prüfung der Impfpferde im Heeresveterinäruntersuchungsamt auf das Freisein vom Virus der ansteckenden Blutarmut. Deut. Tier. Woch. 1929, **37.** 312

1038. Ricketts, W., and Sterling, K.: Comparative studies of "liver tests" and electrophoretic analyses of serum proteins in portal and biliary cirrhosis. Amer. J. Med. Sci. 1951, **221.** 38

1039. Rieken, F.: Beeinflussung des retikulocytären Blutbildes sensibler Kaninchen durch das Virus der infektiösen Anämie der Pferde. Diss. Hannover, 1932 (abstr.: D.T.W. 42. 251)

1040. Ries, J. N.: Sur le traitement et la pathogénie de l'anémie infectieuse et pernicieuse du cheval. Rec. Méd. Vét. 1916, **93**. 14

1041. Rietbrock, J.: Die "Sublimatprobe" im Dienste der Diagnostik der infektiösen Anämie des Pferdes. Diss. Leipzig, 1935 (abstr.: Jber. **58**. 198)

1042. Rievel, H.: Die Diagnose der infektiösen Anämie der Pferde mit Hilfe des Meerschweincheninfektions-Versuches unter Vermeidung der Erythrozyten-Zählung. Diss. Hannover, 1931

1043. Robert, J.: De l'anémie infectieuse du cheval dans la région de Montiers-sur-Saulx. Des diverses modalités cliniques. Appréciation de divers traitements. Thèse, Lyon, 1929 (abstr.: Jber. **49**. 975)

1044. Robin, V.: Le diagnostic de l'anémie infectieuse du cheval. Rev. Gén. Méd. Vét. 1933, **42**. 14

1045. Rodionov, I. M.: Dipterous insects as carriers of equine infectious anemia. (*In Russian*) Sovyet Vet. 1936, **13**. (No. 12) 11 (abstr.: V.B. **7**. 598)

1046. Rodionov, I. M.: Duration of preservation of the virus of infectious anemia in hay. (*In Russian*) Veterinariya 1947, **24**. (No. 6) 29

1047. Rodionov, I. M., and Oleynik, N. K.: Viability of the equine infectious anemia virus in water. (*In Russian*) Veterinariya 1946, **23**. (No. 10-11) 11 (abstr.: V.B. **20**. 81)

1048. Röhrer, H., und Möhlmann, H.: Experimenteller Beitrag zur Frage der natürlichen Ansteckung bei infektiöser Anämie der Pferde. Monat. Vet.-Med. 1950, **5**. 179

1049. Röhrs, A.: Beiträge zur Abtötung des Virus der infektiösen Anämie der Pferde im Serum. Diss. Hannover, 1924 (abstr.: Jber. **44**. 96)

1050. Romanov, N. A.: Experimental equine infectious anemia in a pig. (*In Russian*) Sovyet Vet. 1936, **13**. (No. 9) 12

1051. Romijn: The red blood picture of the horse. Tijdschr. Diergeneesk. 1948, **73**. 333

1052. Rossi, P.: Diagnostic de la typho-anémie infectieuse du cheval. Rev. Vét. Toulouse 1932, **84**. 545

1053. Rossi, P.: Sédimentation sanguine et réaction de Fulton dans la typho-anémie infectieuse du cheval. Bull. Soc. Sci. Vet. Lyon 1933, **36**. 265

1054. Rossi, P., et Saunie, L.: Sur le diagnostic de la typho-anémie infectieuse du cheval au moyen des examens de laboratoire. Rev. Vét. Toulouse 1934, **86**. 134

1055. Rottmann, W.: Einleitende Untersuchungen über die Diagnose der ansteckenden Blutarmut der Pferde mit Hilfe des vereinfachten Meerschweinchenimpfversuches. Diss. Hannover, 1937 (abstr.: Jber. **63**. 166)

1056. Rougieux: Mémoire sur la fièvre typhoide qui règne dans le département de la Meurthe. Rec. Méd. Vét. 1858, **35**. 280; 1859, **36**. 312 (Discussion pp. 319, 389, 435, 460)

1057. Rozhnov, D. I., and Potapov, G. G.: Differential diagnosis of broncho-pneumonia in horses and equine infectious anemia complicated by broncho-pneumonia. (*In Russian*) Sovyet Vet. 1940, **17**. (No. 6) 1 (abstr.: V.B. **12**. 490)

1058. Rózsa, P.: A lovak fertözö kevésvérüségének kezelése vérátömlesztéssel. (Treatment of equine infectious anemia by blood transfusion.) (*In Hungarian*) Állattani Közlem. **1925**, (No. 9-10) 26 (abstr.: Jber. **45**. 79)

1059. Ruddat, E.: Beiträge zur Epidemiologie der ansteckenden Blutarmut der Pferde im Saargebiet. Diss. Hannover, 1936 (abstr.: Jber. **61**. 425)

1060. Rust, W.: Epidemiologie der ansteckenden Blutarmut der Pferde im Regierungsbezirk Breslau. Diss. Hannover, 1923 (abstr.: B.T.W. **40**. 18)

1061. Rust, W.: Die Notwendigkeit der Einführung der Anzeigepflicht bei der ansteckenden Blutarmut. Deut. Tier. Woch. 1937, **45**. 38

1062. Rüther: Die Beziehungen der perniziösen Anämie zur infektiösen Bronchopneumonie. Tierärzt. Rund. 1917, **23**. 141

1063. Rüther: Chemotherapeutische Bekämpfung der perniziösen Anämie. Tierärzt. Rund. 1917, **23**. 245

1064. Rüther: Weitere Beiträge zur Erforschung der perniziösen Anämie. Tierärzt. Rund. 1917, **23**. 351

1065. Rutherford, J. G.: Equine surra. Vet. Rec. 1888, **1**. cited by Stein, 1941

1066. Rutherford, J. G.: Swamp fever. Report, Minister of Agric. Canada for 1902 (p. 85) Ottawa, 1903

1067. Rutherford, J. G.: Swamp fever. Report Vet. Director, Dept. Agric. Canada 1905 (p. 54); 1911 (p. 40). Ottawa, 1906, and 1911

1068. Ruwisch, J.: Beiträge zur Diagnostik der infektiösen Anämie der Pferde. Diss. Hannover, 1922 (abstr.: Jber. **41-42**. 147)

1069. Salow, H.: Ergebnisse verschiedener Untersuchungsmehoden in einem Bestand mit ansteckender Blutarmut. Monat. Vet.-Med. 1951, **6**. 109

1070. Sarata, U.: Studies in the biochemistry of copper. 38. Copper content of bone marrow in the horse in normal and anemic condition. (*In Japanese*) Jap. J. Med. Sci. 1938, **4**. 207 (abstr.: V.B. **13**. 333)

1071. Sarata, U., et al: Biochemical studies of equine infectious anaemia in the horse. Series I-VI. (*In Japanese*) J. Cent. Soc. Vet. Med. Tokyo 1935, **48**. 989, 1003, 1011, 1017, 1021, 1027

1072. Sauvage, L.: Contribution à l'étude de l'anémie infectieuse du cheval. Thèse, Lyon, 1928 (abstr.: D.T.W. **41**. 72)

1073. Scarborough, R. A.: The blood picture of normal laboratory animals. Yale J. Biol. Med. 1930, **3**. 64 (rabbit), 267 (mouse), 431 (horse)

1074. Schaaf, J.: Beitrag zur Kenntnis des Blutbildes von gesunden und kranken, namentlich an Anämie leidenden Pferden. Arch. Tierheilk. 1924, **51**. 512

1075. Schantz, F.: Das Blutbild des gesunden Schafes. Uebertragungsversuche mit infektiöser Anaemie bei Schafen. Monat. Tierheilk. 1920, **31**. 130

1076. Scharpwinkel, W.: Histologische Untersuchungen der Leber, Milz und Nieren von Schlachtpferden, ein Beitrag zur Epidemiologie der infektiösen Anämie. Diss. Hannover, 1927 (abstr.: Jber. **47**. 966)

1077. Schatzmann, H.: Ueber die Sublimatprobe und ihre Verwendung in der Diagnostik der infektiösen Anämie der Pferde. Diss. Bern, 1943

1078. Schebitz: Beobachtungen über infektiöse Anämie. Berl. Tier. Woch. 1918, **34**. 82

1079. Scheiber: Beitrag zur Kenntnis der infektiösen Anämie. Berl. Tier. Woch. 1918, **34**. 271

1080. Scheid, H.: Eigene Beobachtungen über das erste Auftreten der infektiösen Anämie in der Rheinprovinz. Diss. Hannover, 1922 (abstr.: Jber. **41-42**. 146)

1081. Schermer, S.: Ueber das Vorkommen von Blutgruppen bei unseren Haustieren. Deut. Tier. Woch. 1928, **36**. 797

1082. Schermer, S., und Hofferber, O.: Individualitätsreaktionen (Isohämagglutination, Isolysis, Heteroagglutination und Heterolysis) des normalen Pferdeblutes. Arch. Tierheilk. 1928, **57**. 77

1083. Schern, K.: Die japanische Anämieforschung und ihre Bestätigung durch Habersang, Lührs im Lichte des veterinären Auslandsdienstes. Berl. Tier. Woch. 1920, **36**. 226

1084. Schlathölter, P.: Infektiöse Anämie der Pferde. Veröff. Jber. Beamt. Tierärzt. Preuss. 1909 (II Teil, S. 27)

1085. Schlathölter, P.: Ueber die perniziöse Anämie der Pferde. Diss. Bern, 1910 (abstr.: Zbl. Bakt. I. Ref. **49**. 133)

1086. Schlegel, M.: Die infektiöse Anämie des Pferdes mit besonderer Berücksichtigung der neuzeitlichen Forschungsergebnisse. Mitt. Ver. Bad. Tierärzte 1930, **30**. 17

1087. Schmid, G.: Einige Versuche zur Therapie der infektiösen Anämie der Einhufer. Festschrift Prof. O. Bürgi, 1943 (abstr.: Schweiz. Arch. Tierh. **87**. 108)

1088. Schmidt, F. W.: Postmortale Schnelldiagnose der infektiösen Anämie der Pferde. Münch. Tier. Woch. 1935, **86**. 385

1089. Schmidt, J.: Die infektiöse Anämie des Pferdes und ihre Beziehungen zur praktischen Veterinärpolizei. Berl. Tier. Woch. 1928, **44**. 901

1090. Schmitt, F.: Vergleichende Untersuchungen über den Wert der Sublimatprobe (nach Horgan, Bennett und Kenny bzw. Fulton) und der Refraktometrie für die Diagnose der infektiösen Anämie der Pferde. Diss. Hannover, 1932

1091. Schnibbe, D.: Untersuchungen über die infektiöse Anämie des Pferdes. Diss. Hannover, 1923 (abstr.: Jber. **43**. 80)

1092. Schoening, H. W.: Conglutination test for the diagnosis of glanders. J. Agricult. Res. 1917, **11**. 65

1093. Schofield, F. W.: An unusual outbreak of swamp fever. Report, Ontario Veterinary College, 1942 (p. 29) Toronto, Canada, 1943

1094. Schöllner, F.: Ueber Amyloid bei Tuberkulose und infektiöser Anämie des Pferdes. Diss. Hannover, 1934 (abstr.: Jber. **55**. 154)

1095. Schopen, J. G.: Einige Versuche zur Vereinfachung der Diagnose der infektiösen Anämie des Pferdes mit Hilfe des Kaninchenversuches. Diss. Hannover, 1933 (abstr.: M.T.W. **85**. 601)

1096. Schotte, A.: Die ansteckende Blutarmut der Einhufer. Berl. Tier. Woch. 1928, **44**. 335

1097. Schrader, J.: Verteilung des mikrochemisch nachweisbaren Hämosiderins und des Fettes in der Leber des Pferdes. Diss. Hannover, 1938 (abstr.: Jber. **64**. 331)

1098. Schramm, W.: Versuche an Kaninchen über die Beeinflussung des Virus der ansteckenden Blutarmut des Pferdes durch das Wismutpräparat "Milanol". Diss. Hannover, 1939 (abstr.: D.T.W. **47**. 484)

1099. Schröder, K.: Beiträge zur Eigenblutbehandlung der infektiösen Anämie der Pferde. Diss. Hannover, 1927 (abstr.: Jber. **47**. 967)

1100. Schroeder, E. C.: Diseases of horses in the West. Ann. Reports, Bureau of Animal Industry, U. S. Dept. Agric. for 1891-1892 (pp. 104, 371). Washington

1101. Schuchmann, C., und Karmann, P.: Die Diagnose der infektiösen Anämie der Pferde durch den Kaninchenversuch nach Oppermann. Berl. Tier. Woch. 1924, **40**. 497

1102. Schuler, et Velu, H.: L'anémie infectieuse des équidés au Maroc en 1932. Bull. Soc. Path. Exot. 1933, **26**. 726

1103. Schultz, O.: Ein Beitrag zur alimentären Anämie. Berl. Tier. Woch. 1929, **45**. 177

1104. Schultze, O.: Therapeutische Versuche bei der infektiösen Anämie des Pferdes. Diss. Hannover, 1923 (abstr.: Jber. **43**. 79)

1105. Schultze: Die ansteckende Blutarmut der Einhufer. Berl. Tier. Woch. 1928, **44**. 335

1106. Schulze-Bertelsbeck, A.: Beiträge zur Diagnostik der infektiösen Anämie des Pferdes. Diss. Hannover, 1922 (abstr.: Jber. **41-42**. 148)

1107. Schulze-Gahmen, J.: Infektionsversuche am Meerschweinchen mit dem Virus der infektiösen Anämie des Pferdes. Deut. Tier. Woch. 1925, **33**. 850

1108. Schümann, D.: Therapeutische Versuche bei der Anämie der Pferde. Diss. Hannover, 1923 (abstr.: Jber. **52**. 81)

1109. Schwärzel: Behandlungsversuche mit "Bayer 205" bei der anstecekenden Blutarmut der Pferde. Monat. Tierheilk. 1921, **32**. 339

1110. Schwarzmaier, E.: Epidemiologie der ansteckenden Blutarmut in Hessen. Tierärzt. Rund. 1938, **44**. 729

1111. Schweizer, R.: Kritische Ueberprüfung des vereinfachten Kaninchenimpfversuches nach Oppermann zur Sicherung der Verdachtsdiagnose "Anaemia infectiosa equorum". Diss. Bern, 1945

1112. Schweizer, R.: L'anémie infectieuse dans le Canton de Vaud. (Observations des années 1947-1950.) Schweiz. Arch. Tierh. 1951, **93.** 540

1113. Scott, J. W.: Some experiments on the transmission of swamp fever by insects. Anat. Rec. 1917, **11.** 540

1114. Scott, J. W.: Further experiments on the transmission of swamp fever. Anat. Rec. 1918, **14.** 98

1115. Seibel, L.: Zur Epidemiologie und Bekämpfung der ansteckenden Blutarmut des Pferdes. Tierärzt. Umschau 1950, **5.** 278

1116. Seifried, O.: Die Veränderungen des Zentralnervensystems bei der infektiösen Anämie und ihre Abgrenzung von den übrigen Viruserkrankungen des Zentralnervensystems bei Pferden. Proc. Third International Congress for Microbiology in New York, 1939 (p. 300) New York, 1940

1117. Seifried, O., und Krembs, J.: Die Veränderungen des Zentralnervensystems bei der infektiösen Anämie der Pferde. Z. Infekt. Haustiere 1940, **56.** 157

1118. Semenov, M. A., and Kozlova, E. S.: Effect of temperature on the virus of equine infectious anemia in sera preserved with Chinosol. (*In Russian*) Trud. Vsesoyuz. Inst. Eksp. Vet. 1940, **15.** 23 (abstr.: V.B. **16.** 146)

1119. Semenov, M. A., and Kozlova, E. S.: Action of disinfectants on the virus of equine infectious anemia. (*In Russian*) Trud. Vsesoyuz. Inst. Eksp. Vet. 1940, **15.** 24 (abstr.: V.B. **16.** 146)

1120. Semenov, M. A., and Oldenborger, N. A.: Action of phenol on the virus of equine infectious anemia. (*In Russian*) Trud. Vsesoyuz. Inst. Eksp. Vet. 1936, **12.** 50 (abstr.: V.B. **8.** 27)

1121. Semenov, M. A., and Oldenborger, N. A.: Possible spontaneous infection of pigs by equine infectious anemia. (*In Russian*) Trud. Vsesoyuz. Inst. Eksp. Vet. 1936, **12.** 60 (abstr.: V.B. **8.** 27)

1122. Semmler: Ueber Versuche mit dem provokatorischen Aderlass. Z. Vet.kunde 1922, **34.** 272

1123. Serra, A.: L'anemia infettiva degli equini. Norme per la diagnosi e la profilassi. Bull. Istit. Zooprofilatt. Sperim. Torino. Novara, 1941 (abstr.: Jber. **70.** 257)

1124. Seyderhelm, K. R., und Seyderhelm, R.: Wesen, Ursache und Therapie der perniziösen Anämie der Pferde. Arch. Tierheilk. 1915, **41.** 50

1125. Seyderhelm, K. R., und Seyderhelm, R.: Zur Frage der perniziösen Anämie der Pferde. Z. Vet.kunde 1918, **30.** 289

1126. Seyderhelm, R.: Ueber die Eigenschaften und Wirkungen des Oestrins und seine Beziehung zur perniziösen Anämie der Pferde. Arch. Exp. Path. Pharm. 1918, **82.** 253

1127. Sickendiek, A.: Kutane Infektionsversuche mit dem Virus der ansteckenden Blutarmut der Pferde an sensibilisierten Kaninchen. Diss. Hannover, 1939 (abstr.: D.T.W. **47.** 546)

1128. Siegel, O.: Beitrag zur infektiösen Anämie der Pferde. Münch. Tier. Woch. 1918, **69.** 612; Z. Vet.kunde 1918, **30.** 358

1129. Simon, P.: Die Spezifität des Noltzeschen Sedimentierungsverfahrens zur Diagnose der ansteckenden Blutarmut und seine Verwendbarkeit mit konserviertem Blute. Diss. Hannover, 1922 (abstr.: Jber. **43.** 79)

1130. Sindram, W.: Untersuchungen über den Glykogengehalt verschiedener Organe von gesunden und anämiekranken Pferden. Diss. Hannover, 1933 (abstr.: Jber. **54.** 64)

1131. Sinev, A. V.: Refractometry of the blood serum in equine infectious anemia. (*In Russian*) Sborn. Rab. Leningr. Vet. Inst. **1937.** 87

1132. Singelmann, K.: Infektionsversuche am Kaninchen mit Blut, Serum, und Erythrozyten von infektiös-anämisch kranken Pferden. Diss. Hannover, 1925 (abstr.: Jber. **45.** 78)

1133. Slagsvold, L.: Epizootic anemia of horses. (*In Norwegian*) 2. Nord. Vet. Mötet 1921 (p. 325) Stockholm, 1922

1134. Sobra, K.: Diagnosis of equine pernicious anemia by the blood picture. (*In Czech*) Klin. Spisy Skoly Zverol. Brno 1933, **10.** 79 (abstr.: V.B. **4.** 654)

1135. Sobra, K.: Reaction of horses with infectious anemia to subcutaneous injection of tuberculin. (*In Czech*) Zverol. Rozpr. 1933, **7**. 239, 257 (abstr.: V.B. **5**. 346)

1136. Sobra, K.: The blood picture in equine infectious anemia. (*In Czech*) Voj. Zdravotn. Listy Praha 1935, **11**. 32 (abstr.: V.B. **7**. 330)

1137. Sohns, J. C. F., and Soetedjo, R.: Infectious anemia of horses. (*In Dutch*) Veeartsenijkund. Blad. Nederl.-Ind. 1917, **29**. 141

1138. Sokola, D.: Clinical and pathological findings in horses suffering from infectious anemia. (*In Serbian*) Jugoslov. Vet. Glasnik 1935, **15**. 211 (abstr.: V.B. **7**. 175)

1139. Sokola, D.: Einige Beobachtungen in Verbindung mit Fieberanfällen, bei an infektiöser Anämie latent kranken Pferden. (*In Serbian*) Jugoslov. Vet. Glasnik 1940, **20**. 240 (abstr.: Jber. **68**. 438)

1140. Söntgen, K.: Die diagnostische Bedeutung der amtlichen Blutuntersuchung bei der ansteckenden Blutarmut der Einhufer. Berl.-Münch. Tier. Woch. **1940**. 193

1141. Standfuss, R.: Zur Erkennung der ansteckenden Blutarmut des Pferdes durch den Kaninchenversuch. Berl. Tier. Woch. 1923, **39**. 451

1142. Standfuss, R.: Ansteckungsmöglichkeiten und Weidefrage bei der ansteckenden Blutarmut der Pferde. Landwirt. Z. 1926, **46**. 345

1143. Standfuss, R., und Peters, W.: Versuche über die Widerstandfähigkeit des Erregers der ansteckenden Blutarmut der Pferde gegenüber Witterungseinflüssen, Fäulnis und Eintrocknung mit besonderer Berücksichtigung der Weide. Berl. Tier. Woch. 1925, **41**. 517

1144. Standfuss, R., Schultz, E., Schnauder, F., Peters, W., und Frenzel, W.: Untersuchungen über die ansteckende Blutarmut der Pferde. Arch. Tierheilk. 1924, **51**. 154

1145. Steck, W.: Studien über die infektiöse Anämie der Pferde. II. Thermolabilität des Serums. Schweiz. Arch. Tierh. 1939, **81**. 531

1146. Steck, W.: Die gleichzeitige Bestimmung des Blutkörperchensedimentes und der Sedimentierungsgeschwindigkeit beim Pferd. Schweiz. Arch. Tierh. 1941, **83**. 281

1147. Steck, W.: Probleme und Untersuchungen um die infektiöse Anämie der Pferde. Mitt. Naturforsch. Ges. Bern 1945, **3**. 41

1148. Steck, W.: Studien über die infektiöse Anämie der Pferde. IV. Weitere Beobachtungen über Zungenpunktblutungen und Ausbreitung der Infektion. Schweiz. Arch. Tierh. 1946, **88**. 389

1149. Steck, W.: Nouvelles recherches sur l'épizootologie de l'anémie infectieuse des chevaux. Bull. Acad. Suisse Sci. Med. 1946, **1**. 454

1150. Steck, W.: Studien über die infektiöse Anämie der Pferde. V. Verlauf der Einzelerkrankung und der Enzootie. Schweiz. Arch. Tierh. 1947, **89**. 49

1151. Steck, W.: Infektiöse Anämie der Pferde. Schweiz. Arch. Tierh. 1949, **91**. 346

1152. Steck, W.: Studien über die infektiöse Anämie (Valléesche Krankheit) der Pferde. VII. Die Beurteilung des Zungenbefundes unter Berücksichtigung der epizootologischen Verhältnisse. Schweiz. Arch. Tierh. 1951, **93**. 665

1153. Stein, C. D.: Infectious anemia or swamp fever in horses. A review of the Bureau of Animal Industry's investigations. J. Amer. Vet. Med. Ass. 1935, **87**. 312

1154. Stein, C. D., Osteen, O. L., and Mott, L. O.: A resumé of studies and observations on infectious anemia, or swamp fever of horses, carried on by the Bureau of Animal Industry from 1935-1940. Path. Div., Bureau of Animal Industry, U. S. Dept. Agric. Washington, 1941 (Mimeographed)

1155. Stenius, P. I.: Diagnosis of equine infectious anemia. (*In Finnish*) Suom. Eläinlääkril. 1934, **40**. 154, 182

1156. Steudel, R. W.: Kolik und infektiöse Anämie. Diss. Hannover, 1931 (abstr.: Jber. **51**. 1053)

1157. Stilling, J.: Beiträge zur Diagnose der ansteckenden Blutarmut der Einhufer mit Hilfe des vereinfachten Kaninchenversuchs. Diss. Hannover 1939 (abstr.: Jber. **67**. 204)

1158. Stolle, O.: Beiträge zur Diagnose der infektiösen Anämie der Pferde. Diss. Hannover, 1922 (abstr.: Jber. **41-42.** 149)

1159. Stroh, G.: Ueber eine in Südbayern stationäre chronische progressive Anämie bei Pferden und deren vermutlichen Zusammenhang mit der Schweinsberger Krankheit. Münch. Tier. Woch. 1917, **68.** 855

1160. Stroh, G., und Ziegler, M.: Die "Schweinsberger Krankheit" in Südbayern. Z. Infekt. Haustiere 1924, **27.** 47, 141

1161. Stubbs, E. L., and Live, I.: Studies on the allergic and antigenic activity of sonic filtrate of *Brucella abortus*. Amer. J. Vet. Res. 1942, **3.** 146

1162. Suchin, M. J.: Secondary infections in infectious anemia of horses. (*In Russian*) Sovyet Vet. 1938, **15.** (No. 12) 13 (abstr.: Jber. **66.** 601)

1163. Sugano, S., Kobayashi, T., and Yamagiwa, S.: Pathological studies on the bacterial infections associated with infectious anemia. I. The significance of the mixed infection with *Shigella equirulis* in infectious anemia. (*In Japanese*) Jap. J. Vet. Sci. 1949, **11.** 127

1164. Sundberg, R.: Therapeutic attempts in pernicious anemia of horses. (*In Swedish*) Svensk. VetTidskr. 1936, **41.** 17

1165. Suto, H., Kutii, T., Shoho, C., and Kasai, K.: Experimental studies on the superinfection of *Salmonella abortivo-equina* in horses infected with infectious anemia. II. Jap. J. Vet. Sci. 1948, **10.** 19

1166. (Switzerland): Bundesratsbeschluss über vorläufige Massnahmen zur Bekämpfung der ansteckenden Blutarmut der Einhufer. Schweiz. Arch. Tierh. 1943, **85.** 22

1167. Szekeres, V.: Vizsgálatok a lovak fertözö kevésvérüségéröl. (Untersuchungen über die ansteckende Blutarmut der Pferde.) (*In Hungarian*) Diss. Budapest, 1923 (abstr.: B.T.W. **39.** 339)

1168. Taubitz, W.: Untersuchung des Zirkulationsapparates bei gesunden und anämie-kranken Pferden. Diss. Berlin, 1924 (abstr.: Jber. **44.** 95)

1169. Taylor, H.: A case of malarial fever. Vet. Journ. 1899, **49.** 1

1170. Tevosov, A. M.: The susceptibility of mules and asses to equine infectious anemia. (*In Russian*) Trud. XV Plen. Vet. Sekt. Akad. Sel'khoz. Nauk, Moscow 1939 (Diseases of horses) p. 36 (abstr.: V.B. **15.** 323)

1171. Thatcher, R. W.: Pernicious anemia in horses. Ann. Report, Washington State Agric. Exper. Station 1910 (p. 13) Pullman, 1910

1172. Theiler, A.: Ann. Report, Director Vet. Research, Dept. Agric. Union of South Africa, 1915-1916 (p. 45). Pretoria, 1916

1173. Thierry, E.: Note sur l'anémie infectieuse du cheval. J. Agric. Prat. 1904, **8.** 243; 1905, **9.** 149

1174. Thiéry, J. P., et Lucas, A.: Sur l'anémie infectieuse des équidés. Rev. Path. Comp. 1950, **50.** 717

1175. Thomssen, H.: Vergleichende Untersuchungen über die Diagnose der infektiösen Anämie mittels des Kaninchenversuches nach Oppermann. Diss. Leipzig, 1924 (abstr.: D.T.W. **34.** 176)

1176. Thorshaug, N.: Verbreitung und Bekämpfung der infektiösen Anämie beim Pferde in Norwegen. Münch. Tier. Woch. 1936, **87,** 349, 365

1177. Titze, C.: Auf die Entgegnung von Reinhardt und Wirth: Infektiöse Anämie und infektiöse Bronchopneumonie. Berl. Tier. Woch. 1920, **36.** 175

1178. Todoroff, A.: Die infektiöse Anämie des Pferdes und die Rolle des Kaninchens bei der Feststellung ihrer Diagnose. (*In Russian*) Veterin. Sbirska. 1926, (No. 1-2) 1 (abstr.: Jber. **46.** 1062)

1179. Topolnik, E.: Effect of phenyl hydrazine administration on the diagnosis of equine infectious anemia in experimentally infected rabbits. (*In Croatian*) Vet. Arhiv. Zagreb 1943, (No. 7) 249 (abstr.: V.B. **16.** 348)

1180. Torrance, F. W.: Swamp fever in the horse. Report on Health of Animals by Dept. Agric. Canada for 1903 (p. 85); same for 1904 (p. 112). Ottawa, 1904, and 1905

1181. Torrance, F. W.: Report of swamp fever investigations. Report, Vet. Director, Dept. Agric. Canada 1905 (p. 125) Ottawa, 1906; same for 1908 (p. 71) Ottawa, 1909

1182. Troitskii, I. A., and Klimov, N. M.: The part played by the gastrointestinal tract in the spread of equine infectious anemia. (*In Russian*) Sovyet Vet. 1940, **17.** (No. 6) 15 (abstr.: V.B. **12.** 532)

1183. Tsuwerkalow, D. A.: Urine as an antigen for the diagnosis of equine infectious anemia. (*In Russian*) Sovyet Vet. 1936, **13.** (No. 1) 37 (abstr.: V.B. **6.** 864)

1184. Tunkunas, P.: Die Aetiologie der infektiösen Anämie des Pferdes. Kritische Darstellung bisheriger Forschungsergebnisse unter besonderer Berücksichtigung ausländischen Schrifttums. Diss. Giessen, 1950

1185. Udall, D. H., and Fitch, C. P.: Preliminary report on the recognition of swamp fever or infectious anemia in New York state. Cornell Vet. 1915, **5.** 69

1186. Umezu, M., Nobuto, K., Asami, N., Haga, T., Kamoto, K., and Tuda, T.: Judgment on the laboring ability of the horse infected with chronic infectious anemia. Tohoku J. Agric. Res. 1950, **1.** 43 (abstr.: Biol. Abstr. **26.** 175)

1187. (United States): Infectious anemia or swamp fever of horses. Circular No. 138, Bureau of Animal Industry, Dept. of Agricult. Washington, 1909

1188. (United States, Department of Agriculture): Keeping Livestock Healthy. Yearbook of Agriculture, 1942 (p. 392) Washington, 1942

1189. Vaessen, C.: Ueber die Beeinflussung der retikulozytären Blutbildes des Meerschweinchens durch das Virus der infektiösen Anämie der Pferde. Diss. Hannover, 1932 (abstr.: Biol. Abstr. **10.** 682)

1190. Van Es, L.: Swamp fever. Dakota Farmer 1910, **30.** (No. 18-19)

1191. Vellguth, K.: Einige Untersuchungen über die latente Form der infektiösen Anämie des Pferdes. Diss. Hannover, 1923 (abstr.: Jber. **43.** 144)

1192. Velu, H.: L'anémie infectieuse des équidés au Maroc en 1932. Rev. Vét. Milit. 1933, **17.** 199

1193. Velu, H., et Barotte, J.: Anémie infectieuse les équidés. Etude générale. Etude spéciale de l'infection au Maroc. Rev. Vét. Milit. 1923, **7.** 349; 1924, **8.** 438

1194. Velu, H., David, M. L., Faure, L., et Carpentier, C. J.: Essais de diagnostic de l'anémie infectieuse des équidés par réactivation. Bull. Soc. Path. Exot. 1934, **27.** 306

1195. Velu, H., et Faure, L.: Essai de diagnostic de l'anémie infectieuse du cheval par la méthode de W. Sarnowiec. Compt. Rend. Soc. Biol. 1934, **115.** 713

1196. Velu, H., Zottner, G., et Weyland, H.: Anémie et paraplégie infectieuses au Maroc: Diagnostic différential. Bull. Acad. Vét. France 1935, **8.** 132

1197. Verge, J.: Les maladies communes à l'homme et aux animaux. VI. L'anémie infectieuse des équidés ou maladie de Vallée. Rev. Gén. Méd. Vét. 1933, **42.** 729

1198. Vianello, G.: L'anemia infettiva del cavallo in Lombardia. Clinica Vet. 1940, **63.** 60

1199. Vogelsang, E. G., y Gallo, P.: Ensayos de infección en la anemia infecciosa de los equinos. Rev. Med. Vet. Caracas 1942, **4.** 59

1200. Voss, H.: Beiträge zur Diagnostik der infektiösen Anämie der Pferde. Diss. Hannover, 1922 (abstr.: Jber. **41-42.** 148)

1201. Vrede, K.: Passageversuche mit dem Virus der ansteckenden Blutarmut der Pferde an sensibilisierten Kaninchen. Diss. Hannover, 1937 (abstr.: Jber. **63.** 569)

1202. Wagner, C.: Die infektiöse Anämie der Pferde im staatlich-preussischen Halbblutgestüt Repitz. Diss. Hannover, 1923 (abstr.: B.T.W. **40.** 18)

1203. Wall, S.: Die Veränderungen an der Leber und an den Nieren bei der infektiösen Anämie des Pferdes. Tierärzt. Mitt. 1938, **19.** 23

1204. Walther, C.: Die Bewertung der Erythrozytenkurve des Kaninchens und Schweines im Hinblick auf Infektionsversuche mit dem Virus der infektiösen Anämie des Pferdes. Diss. Hannover, 1923 (abstr.: Jber. **43.** 145)

1205. Warringsholz: Infektiöse Anämie. Sammelreferat und Beobachtungen beim Seuchengange in Norderdithmarschen. Berl. Tier. Woch. 1924, **40.** 75

1206. Wehrle, E.: La prophylaxie actuelle; succès et insuccès. Bull. Off. Intl. Epizoot. 1933, **7**. 29, Discussion pp. 52, 314

1207. Weidlich, N.: Beitrag zur histologischen Diagnose der ansteckenden Blutarmut der Pferde. Berl.-Münch. Tier. Woch. **1942**. 85

1208. Weinberg: Action de l'extrait de sclérostomes sur le sang de cheval. Ann. Inst. Pasteur 1907, **21**. 798

1209. Weissgräber, und Notz: Perniciöse Anämie. Woch. Tierheilk. Viehzucht. 1891, **35**. 40

1210. Westerbuhr, H.: Beiträge zur Diagnose der latenten Form der infektiösen Anämie des Pferdes. Diss. Hannover, 1924 (abstr.: Jber. **44**. 95)

1211. Whitehouse, A. W.: Notes on swamp fever or infectious anemia of horses. Ranchman's Reminder (Laramie, Wyoming) 1909, **6**. 3

1212. Wilhelmi, J.: Die Ueberträgerfrage bei der infektiösen Anämie der Pferde. Berl. Tier. Woch. 1922, **38**. 277

1213. Wilking, R.: Uebertragungsversuche der infektiösen Anämie des Pferdes auf Tauben. Deut. Tier. Woch. 1925, **33**. 703

1214. Wilmes, H.: Kann durch Verwendung des chirurgischen Nahtmaterials "Carnofil-Bost" die ansteckende Blutarmut der Pferde auf den Menschen übertragen werden? Berl. Tier. Woch. 1936, **52**. 249

1215. Wilmes, H.: Pathologisch-histologische Untersuchungen über das Vorkommen der ansteckenden Blutarmut bei Schlachtpferden des Regierungsbezirks Kassel. Z. Infekt. Haustiere 1937, **51**. 50

1216. Windmeier, G.: Beiträge zur Therapie der infektiösen Anämie des Pferdes. Diss. Hannover, 1923 (abstr.: Jber. **43**. 81)

1217. Wirth, D.: Infektiöse Bronchopneumonie, infektiöse Anämie. Berl. Tier. Woch. 1920, **36**. 173

1218. Wirth, D.: Die Methoden zur Diagnose der infektiösen Anämie des Pferdes. (Vortrag) Wien. Tier. Monat. 1924, **11**. 433

1219. Wirth, D.: Kommt die infektiöse Anämie derzeit in Oesterreich vor? Wien. Tier. Monat. 1933, **20**. 486

1220. Wirth, D.: Infektiöse Anämie, Beschälseucheverdacht. Wien. Tier. Monat. 1936, **23**. 104

1221. Wirth, D.: Die besondere Reaktionsweise der hämatopoetischen Organsysteme bei unseren Haussäugetierarten. Dreizehnter Internatl. Tierärztl. Kongress, Zürich-Interlaken, 1938 (Bd. **1**. S. 273). Bern, 1938

1222. Wirth, D., und Hnatek, R.: Hämolytische Anämien schwerster Art bei Pferden nach Anwendung von Immunserum. Wien. Tier. Monat. 1925, **12**. 273

1223. Wirth, D., Wagner, H., und Gerbin, S. C.: Zur Diagnose der infektiösen Anämie des Pferdes durch den Kaninchenimpfversuch nach Oppermann. Deutsch-Oester. Woch. Tierheilk. 1925, **7**. 135

1224. Wisniewski, T.: Histiocytic reaction in equine infectious anemia. (*In Polish*) Ann. Univ. M. Curie-Sklodowska (Lublin) 1950, **5**. 151 (abstr.: V.B. **21**. 740)

1225. Witt: Zur Bekämpfung der infektiösen Anämie der Pferde. Tierärzt. Rund. 1922, **28**. 823

1226. Witte, G.: Rektale Infektionsversuche an sensibilisierten Kaninchen mit dem Virus der ansteckenden Blutarmut der Einhufer. Diss. Hannover, 1939 (abstr.: Jber. **67**. 289)

1227. Wittfogel, H.: Die Leberpunktion im Dienst der Erkennung der ansteckenden Blutarmut der Einhufer. Berl.-Münch. Tier. Woch. **1939**. 261

1228. Wittmann, F.: Kontaktinfektion und Wismutbehandlung der ansteckenden Blutarmut der Pferde. Berl. Tier. Woch. 1925, **41**. 353

1229. Wright, L. H.: Further investigations of infectious equine anemia in Nevada. J. Agricult. Res. 1925, **30**. 683

1230. Wulff, H. J.: Untersuchungen über die Histologie des Blutbildes bei der latenten Form der infektiösen Anämie der Pferde. Diss. Hannover, 1931 (abstr.: Jber. **51**. 1053)

1231. Wunderly, C., und Leemann, W.: Ueber neue klinisch-chemische Untersuchungsergebnisse an Pferdeblut. Schweiz. Arch. Tierh. 1946, **88.** 181

1232. Wyssmann, E.: Zur perniziösen Anämie der Pferde. Schweiz. Arch. Tierh. 1915, **57.** 427

1233. Yamashita, J.: Transmission of equine infectious anemia by parasites. A review on the subject. (*In Japanese*) Rep. Bur. Anim. Industr. Tokyo 1942 (vol. **1.** p. 99) (abstr.: V.B. **22.** 466)

1234. Yampolskii, I.: Diagnostic value of histopathological lesions in infectious anemia. (*In Russian*) Sovyet Vet. 1940, **17.** (No. 8-9) 28 (abstr.: V.B. **13.** 124)

1235. Zakrzewski, A.: Ein Betrachtung über das Problem der infektiösen Anämie des Pferdes. (*In Polish*) Przegl. Wet. (Lwow) 1935, **48.** 36 (abstr.: Jber. **58.** 181)

1236. Zeiller: Ein Beitrag zur Beurteilung der ansteckenden Blutarmut. Z. Vet.kunde 1923, **35.** 161

1237. Zeller, Lührs, und Nöller: Diskussion über infektiöse Anämie. 88. Versammlung Deutscher Naturforscher und Aerzte in Innsbruck, 1924 (abstr.: Tier. Rund. **30.** 764)

1238. Zieger, W.: Ueber Erschöpfungskrankheiten der Pferde unter besonderer Berücksichtigung der infektiösen Anämie. Deut. Tier. Woch. 1948, **55.** 215

1239. Ziegler, M.: Weitere Untersuchungen über die stationäre chronische progressive Anämie des Pferdes in Südbayern (Augsburger Anämie). Münch. Tier. Woch. 1925, **76.** 41, 69

1240. Ziegler, M.: Die pathologisch-anatomische Diagnose der infektiösen Anämie des Pferdes. Seuchenbekämpfung 1925, **2.** 245

1241. Ziegler, M.: Zur Histologie der ansteckenden Blutarmut. Berl. Tier. Woch. 1925, **41.** 751

1242. Ziegler, M.: Die histologische Diagnose der ansteckenden Blutarmut. Deut. Tier. Woch. 1925, **33.** 253

1243. Ziegler, M., und Grosse, H.: Weitere Untersuchungen über die ansteckende Blutarmut des Pferdes (Mit besonderer Berücksichtigung des Kaninchenübertragungsversuches nach Oppermann). Z. Infekt. Haustiere 1925, **27.** 288

1244. Ziegler, M., und Wolf, E.: Histochemische Untersuchungen über das vorkommen eisenhaltigen Pigments (Hämosiderins) in der Milz und Leber der Haussäugetiere unter normalen und einigen pathologischen Verhältnissen. Virchow's Arch. Path. Anat. 1924, **249.** 374

1245. van Zijl, W. J.: Blood sedimentation rate in the horse. Tijdschr. Diergeneesk. 1948, **73.** 485

1246. Zweig, J.: Beitrag zur Histopathogenese der infektiösen Anämie, ihre Bedeutung bei der Sicherung der Diagnose. Zverol. Rozpr. 1933, **7.** 94, 118, 129, 139, 151 (abstr.: Jber. **58.** 182)

INDEX

Design by Guenther K. Wehrhan — Composition by University of Pennsylvania Printing & Duplicating Service and part of Chapter 7 & 8 and Chapter 9 by National Typesetting Corporation, Philadelphia, in Times-Roman and Bulmer Display Type — Printing by Alliance Printing Company, Philadelphia, on basis 60 white Multifect made by the Kimberley Clark Mill supplied by Whiting-Patterson Company, Philadelphia — Binding by John W. Clark's Sons, Inc., Philadelphia — Color Plate printed by Princeton Polychrome Press, Princeton, N. J., on Kromekote made by the Champion Paper & Fibre Company — Microphotos were made by Dr. John W. Mills and Dr. Steven C. Mohos — Line drawings by Guenther K. Wehrhan — All engravings by American Photoengraving Company, Philadelphia.